Beating Type 2 Diabetes

Michael Gleeson, PhD

BEATING
TYPE 2 DIABETES

A Healthy
Lifestyle
Guidebook

Natural and
Simple Methods to
Reverse Diabetes for Good

Meyer & Meyer Sport

British Library Cataloguing in Publication Data
A catalogue record for this book is available from the British Library

Beating Type 2 Diabetes
Maidenhead: Meyer & Meyer Sport (UK) Ltd., 2020
ISBN: 978-1-78255-199-7

Aachen, Auckland, Beirut, Dubai, Hägendorf, Hong Kong, Indianapolis, Cairo, Cape Town, Manila, Maidenhead, New Delhi, Singapore, Sydney, Tehran, Vienna

Member of the World Sport Publishers' Association (WSPA), www.w-s-p-a.org

Printed by: C-M Books, Ann Arbor, MI
ISBN: 978-1-78255-199-7
Email: info@m-m-sports.com
www.thesportspublisher.com

CONTENTS

Chapter 8   **What Can I Do to Beat Diabetes?**.. **144**

Chapter 1

What Is Type 2 Diabetes?

Objectives

After studying this chapter, you should:

- Understand the scope of this book.

- Know something about the author.

- Have a basic understanding of what diabetes is and the difference between type 1 and type 2 diabetes.

- Understand the role of insulin in the control of blood sugar.

- Know the basics of what goes wrong in type 2 diabetes.

- Appreciate the potential long-term health problems caused by being overweight and having type 2 diabetes.

- Know what having the "metabolic syndrome" means and its impact on cardiovascular disease risk.

- Appreciate that type 2 diabetes can be reversed and effectively cured.

INTRODUCTION

Firstly, I want to thank you for buying this book and congratulate you on your decision. The book contains everything that I think you should know about **type 2 diabetes** which includes not only explanations about the diagnosis of the condition, what causes it, how it is treated, managed, and monitored but also how you can reduce your risk of health consequences, and how – if you are determined enough – you can beat it. In this book I provide advice and recommendations about living with type 2 diabetes and how to get rid of it. I also explain the scientific reasons for the guidance that is given in a way that any reasonably intelligent person can understand.

In this book I use my extensive experience of working with elite athletes and games players to help people with both **prediabetes** (the prelude to type 2 diabetes, sometimes also referred to as borderline diabetes) and type 2 diabetes learn how to safely and effectively lose weight, get fitter, sleep better, avoid illness, and live healthily for longer. Much of my career has been spent researching the impact of food and exercise on health and performance in sport. I have conducted research projects on how athletes can stay healthy and in peak condition so that they can perform at their best, which includes training to maximize adaptation but avoid burnout, avoiding being underweight or overweight, improving the quality of sleep, promoting robust immunity, and eating the right foods at the right time to maximize performance. This means I have an excellent understanding of energy metabolism, nutrition, exercise, and fitness. What's more is that I have had type 2 diabetes myself and have successfully reversed it by applying the science that I have learned in my work with athletes. The advice I give in this book is all based on the latest scientific evidence, and my aim is to explain in clear and simple terms how this can be applied to help others get rid of their type 2 diabetes. I do not promote any fad diets or exercise regimens, just ones that have been proven to be safe and effective. From me you will learn the principles of healthy eating and what you can do to make your health optimal...that is as good as your health can possibly be.

Although this book is mainly for people who have been diagnosed with either prediabetes or type 2 diabetes it will also be a useful resource for their family members, friends, carers, or healthcare practitioners who want to be able to help them with their condition. If other members of your family have prediabetes, type 2 diabetes, or suspect that they may be at risk of the condition, pass this book on to them. If you are interested in how to actually avoid type 2 diabetes altogether, then you should read my previous book *Eat, Move, Sleep, Repeat*, published by Meyer and Meyer January 2020.

Type 2 diabetes is known as a metabolic disease. This is because it affects how your body deals with **glucose**, the primary source of **energy** that our **cells** rely on. This change in your body's handling of glucose results in the main dangers of type 2 diabetes: substantially higher risks of health complications that can include **coronary heart disease**, **stroke**, kidney disease, infections, ulcers, and blindness.

Please note that any word that appears in **bold** font in this book is defined in the glossary which you will find at the end of the book. I have tried to identify some of the key words or terms, as well as words that may be unfamiliar to some readers, and those that it is simply useful to know the exact meaning of.

One of the main problems with type 2 diabetes is that it creeps up on you, and there are probably many people out there that have the condition but aren't actually aware of it. In fact, we know for sure that there are millions of people who have high blood glucose levels but don't actually realize they have a developing metabolic problem because they have not had a blood test to diagnose it, and nor do they yet feel ill or abnormal in any way. This is because, especially in the early stages of the disease, the symptoms may be absent or not obvious with no overt signs of feeling unwell. But high blood **sugar** levels are the first real indication that something is wrong and always precede the onset of type 2 diabetes.

However, the lack of obvious symptoms is no reason to ignore high blood sugar levels. The big danger with type 2 diabetes is that it increases the risk of associated major health problems only a few years down the line. The biggest single risk factor for diabetes – by far – is being overweight. Therefore, it is important, particularly if you are overweight or have high blood pressure, to have regular health checks by your local medical practitioner, including an annual blood test which can reveal if you have prediabetes or type 2 diabetes. More detail about these conditions will follow shortly, but first let me tell you a little about myself and why I have written this book.

WHO AM I?

I am a recently retired university professor who has spent the last 40 years of my life teaching and researching in the field of exercise physiology, metabolism, immunology, and health with a particular interest in sport nutrition. So essentially much of my work has been spent examining the body's reactions to food and exercise. The last 20 years of my career were spent working at two of the top universities in the world for sport, exercise, and health science (Birmingham and Loughborough in the UK). I have coauthored several books on metabolism, immunology, and nutrition in sport and exercise, and have published over 200 research papers in scientific and medical literature journals; much of which has been focused on the well-being of athletes and the factors influencing their health and performance. After retiring and joining the ranks of the aging general public I turned my attention to the issue of living a healthy lifestyle (in part, to improve my own quality of life and longevity) and spent the first couple of years of my retirement putting together the material for my healthy lifestyle guidebook *Eat, Move, Sleep, Repeat*.

About 10 years ago I was diagnosed with high blood pressure (**hypertension**) and high serum **cholesterol**, both of which are major risk factors for coronary heart disease and stroke. This was not too surprising because despite working in a university sport, exercise, and health science department, my working days were mostly sedentary with much of my time spent sitting at a desk or standing to deliver a lecture. Also, my mother suffered from hypertension from her mid-50s, and some conditions like hypertension tend to run in families. Although both conditions can be managed to some degree by alterations to diet and lifestyle, some medication is required to get them back down into the normal "healthy" range. So since then I have had a daily tablet (what is known as an angiotensin converting enzyme or ACE inhibitor) to lower my blood pressure and a daily statin tablet to lower my cholesterol. These work relatively quickly for most people, and my values were back in the normal range within a few months.

However, five years ago, after another annual blood test I was told that I had developed type 2 diabetes and was advised to change my diet and do more exercise. I researched the literature on type 2 diabetes and realized that it is possible to cure the condition without the need for medication, and that is what set me on the road to writing this book. I also discovered for myself that losing some weight by being more active and eating a healthier diet does actually work. Five years ago my body weight (also known as **body mass**) was close to 80 kg with a **body mass index (BMI)** of 27.0 kg/m² (BMI is just your weight in kilograms divided by your height in meters, and then divided again by your height in meters; more on this in chapter 6). Within a few months I got my weight down to 70 kg and my BMI dropped to 23.7 kg/m²; my diabetes went into remission, and I intend to keep it that way.

I did not achieve this 10 kg weight loss by drastic dieting. My main dietary changes were to reduce my **fat** intake; eat fruit with yogurt rather than pies, sweets, or puddings for dessert; cut down on **alcohol** to just one glass of wine per day; and eat more low **energy density** vegetables, rice, and noodles in place of boiled potatoes, French fries, and bread. I enjoy both Mediterranean and Asian cuisine so fish, stir-fry, tagine, and curry are all on the menu at least once per week and some kind of salad features at least twice per week. I also now have a much more active lifestyle: I aim to walk at least six miles (10 km) on average per day. I play the occasional game of doubles tennis and do two or three 10- to 15-minute **resistance exercise** sessions (at home, not in the gym) each week. So, if you were wondering if it is actually possible to reverse and essentially get rid of type 2 diabetes after it has been diagnosed, the answer is yes. If it wasn't, I wouldn't have written this book!

THE MAIN PURPOSE OF THIS BOOK

I decided this book was needed while researching the literature on type 2 diabetes. I found many websites on the subject of diabetes, and some gave excellent advice about the condition and its management. But much of the advice about diabetes was concerned with its diagnosis and treatment and how to live with the condition. There was little information about how to get rid of it for good. I decided that many people with type 2 diabetes, prediabetes, or who are at risk of the condition would appreciate a single, reliable, evidence-based resource on the subject, Therefore, in this book I have tried to include everything that I think you should know about type 2 diabetes and how you can reverse it.

I begin by explaining exactly what type 2 diabetes is (and how it differs from type 1 diabetes), how the condition is diagnosed, how it is treated (with medication and encouraging changes to lifestyle behavior), and how the condition is monitored and managed. Then I explain what is known about the causes of type 2 diabetes, the main risk factors, and why it is linked so strongly to having an excess of **body fat** (i.e., being overweight or obese), how you can tell if (or by how much) you are overweight or overfat, what you can do to reduce your risk of serious health complications, and – if you are determined enough – how you can beat the condition.

I will take you through a novel and effective weight loss plan that uses sensible, varied, non-extreme dieting, combined with enjoyable and exhilarating (but not exhausting) exercise that should kick your diabetes into remission and improve many other aspects of your health in the process. The great thing about the diet part of my weight loss plan is that it does not require you to stick with the same boring diet week after week. I utilize a variety of different, but equally effective diets that are well suited to people with type 2 diabetes and that you can change on a weekly basis. And none of the exercises I recommend will leave you with aching muscles, or feeling sick, or tired. Finally, I have devoted a chapter to describing some meal ideas for the dieting part of the weight loss plan.

TYPE 1 AND TYPE 2 DIABETES: WHAT IS THE DIFFERENCE?

The full clinical name for diabetes is **Diabetes mellitus** which is derived from the Greek word diabetes meaning siphon – to pass through – and the Latin word mellitus meaning honeyed or sweet. This is because in diabetes, excess sugar is found in both the urine and the blood, making it taste sweet – if you were daft enough to drink it that is! Having said that, tasting urine to see if it was sweet was actually how diabetes was diagnosed in the old days. It wasn't until the 1800s that scientists developed chemical tests to detect the presence of sugar in the urine. There are two main forms of diabetes mellitus, and both result from a problem related to the hormone insulin.

Type 1 diabetes mellitus, also known as insulin-dependent diabetes mellitus is a **chronic disease** (one that persists over a long time, like arthritis, cancer, coronary heart disease, stroke, etc.) in which the pancreas (an accessory digestive organ located below the liver in the abdomen) produces little or no insulin. Type 1 diabetes usually results from a highly specific immune-mediated destruction of pancreatic islet β-cells – specialist cells that detect the level of blood glucose and secrete the hormone insulin when it rises above normal. This is commonly described as an autoimmune type of disease. Insulin stimulates the tissues to take up insulin from the blood such that the blood glucose concentration returns to its normal fasting level within a few hours following a meal. For type 1 diabetics, the absence of insulin production results in chronic elevated blood glucose concentration (known as hyperglycemia). The condition usually occurs in early childhood and can lead to many serious complications if not properly managed. The patient and their physician must work together to optimize glucose control involving both regular insulin injections and management of food intake. Around 5-10% of people who are diagnosed as diabetic have type 1 diabetes mellitus. Although much rarer (less than 1% of cases), type 1 diabetes can also be caused by a genetic defect in β-cell function that prevents normal levels of insulin production.

Another form of type 1 diabetes is the acquired type which develops when there is damage to the pancreas caused by infection or **inflammation** resulting in a condition called **pancreatitis**. In some cases, this can be caused by stones that are formed in the gall bladder coming down the shared pancreatic duct and getting trapped in the pancreas and later forming a cyst. This form of diabetes may resolve itself within a year or two as the inflammation disappears and the pancreas repairs itself. It depends on the extent of damage to the β-cells; if the damage is too extensive, the affected person may be stuck with diabetes for life just like other type 1 diabetics.

Type 2 diabetes mellitus, also known as **non-insulin-dependent diabetes mellitus**, usually comes on slowly, is relatively rare below the age of 40, and most often develops in people who are overweight and sedentary. The main problem in type 2 diabetes is that the body tissues (e.g., **adipose tissue**, liver, and skeletal muscle) become resistant to the action of insulin which normally stimulates these tissues to take up blood-borne glucose when the blood glucose level is elevated such as after a meal. The lack of tissue response to insulin – often referred to as **insulin resistance** – results in sustained hyperglycemia (higher than normal blood glucose concentration) with many serious complications including reduced life expectancy if it is not properly managed.

These consequences are described in detail later in this chapter. The main differences between type 1 and type 2 diabetes are illustrated in figure 1.1.

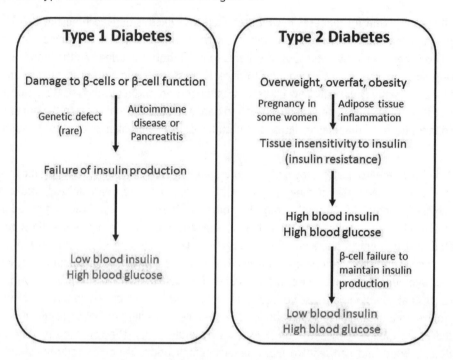

Figure 1.1 A simplified illustration of the main differences between type 1 diabetes and type 2 diabetes. A form of type 2 diabetes called gestational diabetes that develops during pregnancy in 6-8% of women is usually temporary but puts the mother at higher risk of type 2 diabetes later in life.

A temporary form of diabetes called **gestational diabetes** that has some similarities to type 2 diabetes can occur during pregnancy, particularly in overweight women. The hormones produced by the placenta during pregnancy (estrogen, **cortisol** and human placental lactogen) can block the actions of insulin putting the mother-to-be at an increased risk of insulin resistance, and some women are not able to produce enough insulin to overcome this resistance. This makes it difficult for the tissues to take up glucose from the blood, so the glucose remains in the blood and the levels rise, leading to gestational diabetes. The condition develops during the second and third trimester and currently affects 6-8% of pregnant women, though its prevalence is on the increase and is higher in 35- to 45-year-old women than in younger women. Some women diagnosed with gestational diabetes may already have had type 2 diabetes before they conceived. If they didn't have type 2 diabetes already, having gestational diabetes means that there is a higher chance of developing type 2 diabetes later in life. That's why mothers are usually offered a blood test for diabetes at their postnatal check, and annually from then on.

THE 21ST CENTURY DISEASE

Type 2 diabetes has exhibited increasing prevalence in the adult population since the late 1950s. In 1960 the percentage of the US population with diagnosed diabetes was close to 1.0%, by 1990 it had risen to 2.7%, in 2000 it was 4.7%, and in 2018 it stands at 9.0% (figure 1.2). It is projected to rise to close to 12% by 2030, and this does not include people (estimated to be approximately 3% of the population) who may have type 2 diabetes but have not yet had a confirmed diagnosis. Alarmingly, about 34% of the US population in 2018 were confirmed to have prediabetes, a condition that if not treated often leads to Type 2 diabetes within 5 years. So it is rapidly becoming the disease to beat in the 21st century.

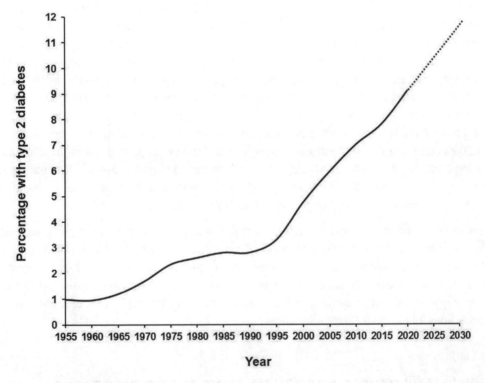

Figure 1.2 Percentage of the US population with diagnosed diabetes since 1958 (solid line) and the projected increase to 2030 (dashed line). From US Center for Disease Control Division of Diabetes Translation. Available at http://www.cdc.gov/diabetes/data.

In the past we have beaten other diseases. Before the 19th century the major diseases were infections caused by viruses (e.g., measles, mumps, polio, smallpox) or bacteria (e.g., bubonic plague, tuberculosis, typhoid, whooping cough). The introduction of vaccines in the 19th century and antibiotics in the 1940s has resulted in these diseases being eliminated or greatly reduced in incidence. Improved **nutrition**, better medications, and improved sanitation and hygiene practices have also contributed to the much lower prevalence of infectious diseases that we now take for granted. Lung cancer became a big problem in the 20th century due to the smoking of tobacco products and increasing air pollution, but in recent years the incidence of lung cancer has dropped as many people have quit smoking or switched to less harmful vaping. In the early 1980s we had the start of the Acquired Immunodeficiency Syndrome (AIDS) epidemic caused by the Human Immunodeficiency virus (HIV) which attacks and destroys crucial **white blood cell**s (called CD4+ T-helper **lymphocyte**s) and is transmitted through sexual contact or blood. These cells direct the body's immune responses to other viral and bacterial infections. The loss of these T cells leads to the point where opportunistic infections can become fatal; although, nowadays, while there is still no cure for HIV, there are very effective treatments that enable most people with the virus to live a long and healthy life.

Becoming much more prevalent now are other forms of what we could call "self-inflicted disease", namely obesity, type 2 diabetes and hypertension and the health complications that result from them including increasing fatality from cardiovascular disease and cancers. For these diseases of modern society that affect increasing numbers of people in developed countries, medication will almost certainly not be the answer. Although there may be some improvements to drug treatment to help the management of type 2 diabetes, it is very unlikely that a drug will be found to cure the condition. Changes to diet and lifestyle are the things that are needed. Simply put, weight loss is the key to curing type 2 diabetes, and avoiding excessive weight gain in the first place is the key to its prevention. This will require government investment in health and nutrition education, the introduction of taxes on high **calorie** and high sugar food products to discourage people from buying them, and healthcare programs to help people get rid of type 2 diabetes by dieting and/ or doing more exercise. Most importantly, it needs people to take these messages on board and make a conscious decision to change their unhealthy lifestyle.

Current projections of the incidence of type 2 diabetes suggest that the numbers of people with the condition and those that die prematurely from it (we're talking about living 5-10 years less than average here) will increase considerably more in the next 10-30 years unless something is done about it very soon. The good news for people with type 2 diabetes, and especially those who have only recently been diagnosed with the condition, is that you can get rid of it through your own actions. In this book I will explain how.

HOW MANY PEOPLE CURRENTLY HAVE TYPE 2 DIABETES?

Globally, the estimated diabetes prevalence for 2017 was 425 million and is expected to affect about 629 million people by 2045 if current trends continue. According to a 2017 report from the US Centers for Disease Control and Prevention (CDC) over 30 million Americans – almost 10% of the US population – have type 2 diabetes. Another 84 million have prediabetes, a condition that if not treated often leads to type 2 diabetes within five years. In the UK about 9% of adults (aged over 16) have diabetes. This means that, including the number of undiagnosed people who have the condition but don't yet realize they have it (estimated to be about one million), there are about five million people living with diabetes in the UK at present. Furthermore, an estimated 12.3 million people (that is almost 20% of the total population) in the UK are currently considered to be at increased risk of the disease. The situation is similar in many other developed countries including other parts of Europe, Canada, and Australasia. There are huge economic costs to society. In 2018 it was estimated that the cost of medications to treat type 2 diabetes alone for the National Health Service in the UK was over one billion pounds sterling.

The proportion of people who have diabetes increases with age: 9% of people aged 45 to 54 have diabetes, but for over 75s it is 24%. Diabetes at older ages has even bigger health implications as people are more likely to be suffering from other health problems, particularly cardiovascular diseases. Diabetes is more common in men (10% compared with 8% for women) and people from south Asian, Hispanic, and black ethnic groups are nearly twice as likely to have the disease compared with people from white, mixed, or other ethnic groups (15% compared with 9%).

INSULIN ACTION AND THE CONTROL OF BLOOD SUGAR

Let me explain a little more about what insulin is and what it actually does in a normal healthy person. Insulin is a small **protein** hormone consisting of 51 **amino acids** in the form of two linked chains (figure 1.3 and photo 1.1). Insulin is synthesized by specialized **endocrine** β-cells which are arranged in small clusters (called the islets of Langerhans) in the pancreas. The name insulin comes from the Latin insula for island. The main function of the pancreas is as a digestive accessory organ and it is located just behind and below the stomach. The pancreas produces pancreatic juice containing **enzymes** that break down protein, fat, and **carbohydrate** when the juice is secreted into the small intestine. The pancreas's β-cells can detect the concentration of glucose (blood sugar) in the circulation and increase their production and release of insulin when the blood glucose concentration rises above its normal fasting level of about 5 **millimoles** per liter (**mmol/L**) or 900 milligrams per liter (mg/L). Another hormone called **incretin** that is produced and released by cells in the small intestine after eating helps the body produce more insulin when it is needed and reduces the amount of glucose being produced by the liver when it is not needed. Insulin travels in the circulation to its target tissues which include adipose tissue, the liver, and skeletal muscle where it binds to specific **insulin receptors** located on the surface of the cells. The binding of insulin to its receptor activates **insulin receptor substrate 1** (IRS-1) which then initiates a cascade of reactions inside the cell that constitute a signaling pathway that brings about the actions of insulin in these target tissues as illustrated in figure 1.4. Insulin increases glucose uptake by causing glucose transporter proteins (e.g., **GLUT4** in muscle and adipose tissue; GLUT2 in the liver) which are located in vesicles (small bags of liquid encased within a lipid membrane) in the **cytoplasm** of the target cells to move to the cell membrane which then allows glucose transport from the blood into the target tissue cells. This causes the blood glucose concentration to fall back to its normal (pre-feeding or fasting) level and the stimulus for insulin secretion is no longer present. The insulin gets cleared from the circulation and when **plasma** insulin levels fall, the glucose transporters move back into the cytoplasm and tissue glucose uptake drops.

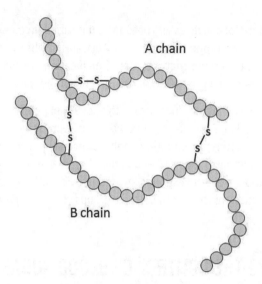

Figure 1.3 Diagrammatic illustration of the structure of the human insulin molecule. It consists of two linked chains of amino acids: an A chain containing 21 amino acids and a B chain containing 30 amino acids. The circles in the diagram represent individual amino acids which are linked together by **peptide** *bonds. The A and B chains of the insulin molecule are linked together by disulfide bonds formed between cysteine (a sulfur containing amino acid) residues in the two chains.*

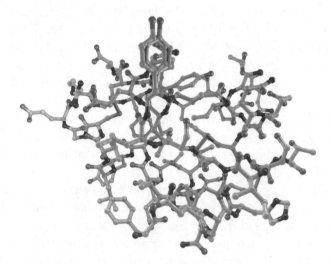

Photo 1.1 A three-dimensional picture of the human insulin molecule.

The main action of insulin is to promote the uptake of glucose (blood sugar) from the blood into the cells of its target tissues. When glucose is taken up into adipose tissue cells (**adipocytes**) it is converted into fat. Glucose taken up by skeletal muscle is converted to **glycogen** (a glucose polymer that acts as a store of carbohydrate for later use) or is used as a fuel for muscle contraction (i.e., exercise). Glucose that enters the liver is mostly converted to glycogen with excess amounts being converted to fat. This uptake of glucose by various tissues in response to insulin returns the blood glucose concentration back to its normal level. Other actions of insulin are to promote the storage of glucose into glycogen and increase amino acid uptake from the blood into skeletal muscle when the blood concentration of certain amino acids rises above normal such as after eating a meal containing protein (e.g., from meat, fish, eggs, milk, cheese, nuts, beans, or **legumes**). Insulin action also inhibits the breakdown of fat in adipose tissue.

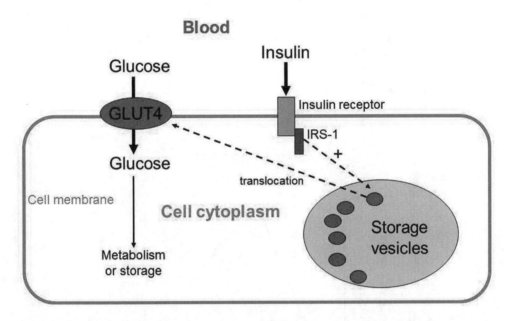

Figure 1.4 The mechanism of insulin action. See text for details. IRS-1: Insulin receptor substrate 1.

Insulin secretion is increased as soon as the blood glucose concentration starts to rise above about 5 mmol/L. The carbohydrate in our diet comes mostly from **starch**, a glucose polymer in plants that has a similar structure to glycogen, and is abundant in potatoes, rice, corn, and foods made from cereal grains such as bread, breakfast cereals, and pasta). The other major source of dietary carbohydrate is in the form of free sugars (e.g., **sucrose**, **lactose**, **maltose**, and **fructose**). Our digestive system breaks down the **starch** into glucose which is absorbed into the blood together with free glucose released from the enzymatic breakdown of sucrose (cane sugar which is formed of two sugars – glucose and fructose – linked together), lactose (milk sugar formed from glucose and galactose), and maltose (malt sugar formed from two linked glucose **molecules**). The glucose in the gut is then absorbed via the intestinal cells into the blood. Fructose is also absorbed separately and is converted into glucose by the liver. After eating a meal containing carbohydrate, the blood glucose concentration rises – usually to a peak of about 7-9 mmol/L – as its rise is countered by the action of insulin. Figure 1.5 illustrates the change in the blood glucose and insulin concentrations that occurs following a meal containing 75 grams (g) of glucose. As you can see, the blood glucose concentration remains elevated for several hours after a meal and the insulin concentration changes according to the level of blood glucose.

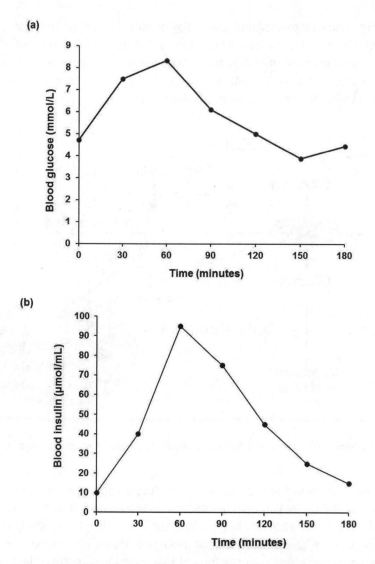

Figure 1.5 Changes in the blood concentration of (a) glucose and (b) insulin following a meal containing 75 g of glucose in a healthy adult.

Apart from the gut, the only other main source of glucose in the blood is the glucose that is released from the liver, an organ which can make glucose and stores it as a glucose polymer called glycogen. When you haven't eaten for quite some time (e.g., when you wake up in the morning after a night's sleep), your blood glucose levels will be lower than normal and the liver responds by breaking down stored glycogen into glucose and releasing it into the circulation to keep your blood glucose level within the normal range. This response occurs because when your blood glucose level drops below normal (e.g., due to a prolonged fast or performance of prolonged exercise without prior food intake) the drop in glucose availability is detected and your **neuroendocrine system** secretes several other hormones (**epinephrine** and cortisol from the adrenal glands and **glucagon** from the α-cells of the pancreas) that stimulate greater liver glucose production and glycogen breakdown. These hormones essentially prevent the blood glucose levels from falling too low (known as **hypoglycemia** or just "hypo" for short) which is important as the brain, nerve cells, and blood cells all rely on glucose as their main source of energy. Hypoglycemia (a blood glucose level below 3 mmol/L) causes symptoms of fatigue, dizziness, lack of coordination, impaired cognitive function, and fainting. If too prolonged, hypoglycemia can result in coma and death.

WHAT GOES WRONG IN TYPE 2 DIABETES?

In prediabetes and at least in the early stages of type 2 diabetes, normal (or above normal) amounts of insulin are still usually produced when the blood glucose concentration rises above the normal fasting level of 5 mmol/L. So the problem is not a lack of insulin production as in type 1 diabetes but is one of insulin resistance. In other words, the tissues are less sensitive (or more resistant) to insulin and do not respond in the usual way to increase their uptake of glucose from the blood (some uptake will occur but nowhere near as much as normal). Exactly why this happens is unknown, although genetics and environmental factors, such as excess weight and inactivity, seem to be contributing factors. What this means is that after a carbohydrate containing meal the blood glucose concentration will rise much higher than normal (e.g., to something like 11-50 mmol/L) and will only gradually return back towards normal over many hours as illustrated in figure 1.6. As most people eat three or four meals per day, in type 2 diabetics the blood glucose concentration remains chronically high. Even after a night's sleep with a 10-12 hour period of fasting it is usually still above 7 mmol/L. Type 2 diabetes usually begins with insulin resistance, a condition in which muscle, liver, and fat cells cannot take up glucose from the blood as normal, and at this stage it is referred to as prediabetes. As a result, your body needs more insulin to help glucose enter cells. At first, the pancreas makes and releases more insulin to keep up with the added demand. Over time, the β-cells of the pancreas become worn out and can't make enough insulin to meet the body's demands and blood glucose levels rise even more. When this occurs full-blown type 2 diabetes has developed, and medication will soon be needed to treat the condition and slow its progression.

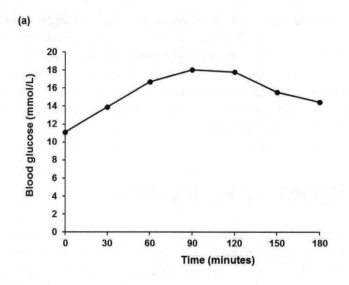

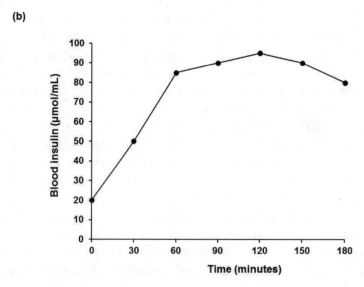

Figure 1.6 Changes in the blood concentration of (a) glucose and (b) insulin following a meal containing 75 g of glucose in an adult who is a type 2 diabetic.

WHAT ARE THE CONSEQUENCES OF TYPE 2 DIABETES?

If uncontrolled blood glucose stays much higher for longer after feeding and even in the fasting state, blood glucose concentrations can remain extremely high. Fat breakdown and mobilization is normally inhibited by insulin, and reduced insulin action therefore results in increased **fatty acid** concentrations in the blood. Some of these fatty acids are taken up by the liver and incorporated into **triglycerides** or converted into cholesterol and then released as **low-density lipoprotein**

(LDL) particles which contribute to the development of fatty deposits (called **plaques**) on the walls of blood vessels. This reduced insulin sensitivity (which is also called increased insulin resistance) has far-reaching consequences and may result in many serious clinical complications including hypertension, coronary heart disease, **atherosclerosis**, **peripheral vascular disease**, **cerebrovascular disease**, kidney disease, nerve damage, blindness, leg ulcers, more frequent infections, and poor wound healing (figure 1.7). Being a type 2 diabetic typically reduces life expectancy by 5-10 years. For further details of these complications see the sidebar.

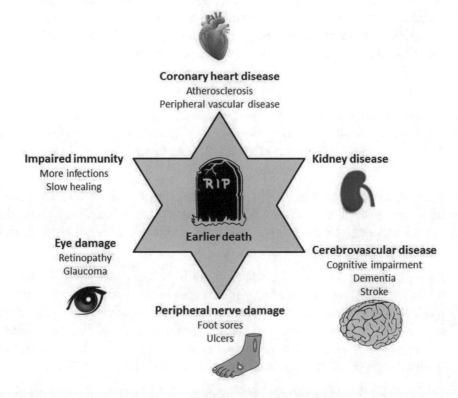

Figure 1.7. The serious and life-threatening health complications that come with type 2 diabetes.

The complications that can come with diabetes

Too much glucose in your blood and other body fluids, together with the associated changes in blood fats (higher cholesterol and triglyceride), can damage organs, blood vessels, and nerves which can lead to long-term health problems such as:

- Hypertension (high blood pressure) which increases the risk of stroke and coronary heart disease.

- Coronary heart disease which can lead to heart attacks that can be fatal. In diabetics the relative risk of a fatal heart attack is double that of the nondiabetic population.

(continued)

- Atherosclerosis (or **arteriosclerosis**), known as hardening or clogging up of the arteries is the build-up of cholesterol, fatty cells, and inflammatory deposits (called plaque) on the inner walls of the arteries that restrict blood flow to the heart and organs such as the brain and kidneys.

- Peripheral vascular disease is a type of atherosclerosis that can affect the arteries in the arms, legs, and feet. It is also known as peripheral arterial disease and lower extremity vascular disease. If the arteries become narrowed or blocked, blood cannot get through to supply oxygen to the tissues, causing the muscles of the lower extremities to cramp; when this occurs during walking it is called "intermittent **claudication**". In diabetics the relative risk of an obstruction (claudication) in a peripheral artery is eight-fold higher in women and four-fold higher in men than in nondiabetics.

- Cerebrovascular disease. This is when blood vessels in the brain that are damaged due to atherosclerosis cause cognitive impairment, dementia, and higher risk of stroke. About one third of people with type 2 diabetes suffer from cerebrovascular disease and the risk of stroke is 50% higher than in nondiabetics.

- Kidney disease which can lead to kidney failure with life-threatening **toxemia** (a build-up of toxins in the blood) and the need for a kidney transplant. In diabetics the relative risk of kidney disease is 3-fold and 2-fold higher in women and men, respectively than in nondiabetics.

- Diabetic retinopathy which is a condition in which the back of the interior of the eyes (called the **retina**) is damaged which leads to impaired vision and often results in total blindness. In diabetics the relative risk of blindness is five times that of the nondiabetic population. You can see a simulation on your phone or tablet of how this condition affects your vision as it develops over time if you download the Royal National Institute of Blind People (RNIB) app (it's called the RNIB Diabetic app) from the App Store.

- **Glaucoma** which is a common eye condition where the optic nerve, which connects the eye to the brain, becomes damaged. It's usually caused by fluid building up in the front part of the eye, which increases pressure inside the eye. Glaucoma can lead to loss of vision if it isn't diagnosed and treated early. In diabetics the relative risk of glaucoma is about 40% higher than that of the nondiabetic population.

- Nerve damage (known as neuropathy) which impairs sensation (loss of feelings of touch and pain) in the skin that increases the risk of complications such as increased risk of damage, infections, and slow healing of cuts, abrasions, and wounds. This is most noticeable for the hands and feet and can also affect the penis or vagina of sufferers.

- Leg and foot ulcers caused by poor circulation. These are slow to heal and prone to infection.

- Poor wound healing in general due to poor circulation and nerve damage.

- Foot problems because of poor or obstructed circulation and nerve damage which result in injuries, wounds, and ulcers that are prone to worsen and become infected. In extreme cases this can lead to the need for toe, foot, or even lower leg amputations. In diabetics the relative risk of a having a lower limb amputation is 13 times higher than in the nondiabetic population. Among 65- to 75-year-olds it is over 23 times higher.

- More frequent infections (e.g., the common cold) due to impaired immunity. Also, having the flu (influenza) is more dangerous for diabetics as there is a 25% higher risk of developing pneumonia which is the seventh leading cause of death in the US.

- Gingivitis (gum inflammation) caused by bacterial infection which can progress to periodontitis – a condition in which the tissues that surround and support the teeth become infected and inflamed – resulting in the breakdown of connective tissue, bone, and the base of the tooth, leading to tooth loss.

- Men who have diabetes are two to three times more likely to develop erectile dysfunction (the inability to get or maintain an erection firm enough for sex). Although diabetes and erectile dysfunction are two separate conditions, they tend to go hand-in-hand. Like the other vascular (blood vessel) problems that develop with type 2 diabetes, erectile dysfunction is caused by damage to nerves and blood vessels caused by poor long-term blood sugar control. Sexual dysfunction can also affect females with type 2 diabetes and studies have found that the prevalence in women is similar to that in men. Sexual dysfunction in women can affect sexual desire and arousal and can also lead to pain during sex. Vascular damage can limit blood supply to the vagina and clitoris which can cause problems with dryness and arousal. Neuropathy (nerve damage) can have a similar effect in that it can reduce sensitivity. Type 2 diabetes can also lead to lower than normal estrogen levels which can also affect lubrication of the vagina. However, it does not affect the ability of a woman to become pregnant.

WHAT IS THE METABOLIC SYNDROME?

Type 2 diabetes also forms part of the **metabolic syndrome**, a term that is used by scientists and clinicians to describe the common co-occurrence of several known cardiovascular disease risk factors that include elevated blood glucose levels and insulin resistance that are main features of type 2 diabetes. The metabolic syndrome is not actually a disease but a group of characteristics. These characteristics include:

- Obesity.

- Hypertension (high blood pressure).

- Elevated blood sugar levels.

- Insulin resistance.

- **Dyslipidemia**: A collective term for non-healthy levels of blood **lipids** (fats) including high levels of triglycerides (a storage form of fat), cholesterol, and LDL, and low levels of **high-density lipoproteins** (HDL).

Each of these characteristics is an individual risk factor for cardiovascular diseases including atherosclerosis, coronary heart disease, and stroke. Having just one of these characteristics doesn't mean you have metabolic syndrome; you need to have three or more of them. However, having any of them increases your relative risk (see the following sidebar about what relative risk means) of serious disease and the more you have increases your risk even further. The following factors increase your chances of having metabolic syndrome:

- Age: Your risk of metabolic syndrome increases with age.

- Race: In the US, Mexican Americans appear to be at the greatest risk of developing metabolic syndrome. In the UK it is the South Asians who are at highest risk for metabolic syndrome.

- Obesity: Carrying too much weight (fat) increases your risk of metabolic syndrome. People with central obesity – which is when you store fat around your middle (abdomen), rather than around the hips and thighs – and people with a BMI of 30 kg/m² or more are particularly at greater risk of metabolic syndrome.

- Type 2 diabetes: Your risk of metabolic syndrome increases the longer you remain diabetic.

- Gestational diabetes: You're more likely to develop metabolic syndrome if you have had diabetes during pregnancy (known as gestational diabetes). In 90% of women gestational diabetes will resolve after the baby is born but leaves the mother with an increased risk of developing both type 2 diabetes and metabolic syndrome.

- Other diseases: Your risk of metabolic syndrome is higher if you've ever had cardiovascular disease, nonalcoholic fatty liver disease, or polycystic ovary syndrome.

What does relative risk really mean?

In this book you will read about relative risks to health of certain characteristics such as being obese or over the age of 50 and certain lifestyle behaviors such as being sedentary, eating too much sugar, smoking, or drinking alcohol. It is important to realize that the comparisons of risk are made relative to the average person who, for example, does some exercise, consumes an average amount of sugar, does not smoke, or does not drink alcohol. It is not to say that the risk of health problems in these people with healthy habits is zero. Everyone has a certain degree of risk for a particular health problem like type 2 diabetes, coronary heart disease, or cancer but the risk of some diseases can be increased above average by unhealthy lifestyle behaviors such as consuming too much fat, sugar, or alcohol.

Sometimes the risk is not simply linearly related to the intake of "unhealthy" food items or the degree of other bad behaviors such as lack of exercise or smoking tobacco products.

Let's take alcohol as an example. A massive global study published in the Lancet in 2018 concluded that there is no safe level of drinking alcohol. In other words, even drinking one glass of wine or beer per day increases the risk of health problems such as cancer, injuries (e.g., accidents, burns, falls, violence, and road traffic incidents), and infectious diseases. But the increased risk to health of having just one alcoholic beverage per day is only 0.5% and this would probably not dissuade people from having a daily glass of wine with their meal. Specifically for the risk of developing type 2 diabetes, moderate alcohol consumption is actually beneficial. A **meta-analysis** (a pulling together of multiple studies in an effort to increase statistical power and help resolve uncertainty) of 20 studies concluded that moderate alcohol consumption was associated with a 30% reduced risk of developing type 2 diabetes in both men and women. Optimal alcohol consumption (compared with being teetotal) was 22 g/day for women and 24 g/day for men (20 g of alcohol is equivalent to one 175 mL glass of wine or a 330 mL bottle of beer). However, alcohol intake worsened the risk of type 2 diabetes when it exceeded 50 g/day for women and 60 g/day for men. Note that many food and health agencies report intakes as **units of alcohol**. One unit of alcohol is equivalent to 8 g or 10 mL of pure alcohol, so a 175 mL glass of wine or a 330 mL bottle of beer both contain just over two units of alcohol, and the maximum recommended intake for adult is 14 units per week.

So relative risk depends on the nature of the risk factor, its magnitude or dose, and on the specific outcome measure that is under examination. Studies that only concentrate on type 2 diabetes may be misleading with regard to the risks of other diseases such as coronary heart disease, cancer, or infectious illness so bear this in mind when you read about studies on characteristics or behaviors that influence the risk of developing type 2 diabetes. You also need to take into account the magnitude of any relative risk before making any decisions on changing your current lifestyle.

ARE TYPE 2 DIABETES AND THE METABOLIC SYNDROME REVERSIBLE?

The latest research indicates that type 2 diabetes can be reversed and gotten rid of by dieting that results in a sufficient loss of body weight and abdominal fat. Increased physical activity can also assist with weight loss and both acute and chronic exercise is known to improve insulin sensitivity. In other words, going for a run or a long walk will not only burn some fat but will also temporarily increase your insulin sensitivity and doing that sort of activity regularly will further improve your insulin sensitivity. Type 2 diabetes gets more difficult to reverse the longer you have it so it is best to act as soon as you are diagnosed with the condition. Now many people may think that because there are no immediate symptoms and there is some medication available to help control blood glucose, they should not bother to change their lifestyle. But that would not be my advice. A 2010 report by Diabetes UK claimed that type 2 diabetes reduces life expectancy by roughly 10 years, and a 2012 Canadian study found that women aged 55 years and over with diabetes lost on average 6 years of life while men lost 5 years. But that is not all. Because type 2 diabetes increases the risk of developing the host of clinical problems listed in the first sidebar, it is likely that the last 5-10 years of your life will be accompanied by illness, discomfort, and pain and that you will lose your independence, and possibly your sight and mobility. Those are things that any sane person should want to avoid.

A study in 2015 concluded that the risk of death associated with type 2 diabetes could be reduced by regular screening to identify the condition at an early stage, the use of new medications that enable better control of blood sugar levels, and improved awareness of the condition and its health risks by both medical practitioners and diabetic patients. The recent advancements in diabetes screening and treatment may mean that life expectancy increases for type 2 diabetics compared with 10 years ago. Even so, not having diabetes is far better than having it so the best policy is always going to be to try to reverse the condition when it is diagnosed and to try and prevent the condition recurring by making permanent changes to diet and lifestyle behaviors.

Some of the characteristics of the metabolic syndrome such as **obesity** and high blood sugar, triglyceride, cholesterol, and LDL levels can also be reversed by losing weight through dieting and doing more exercise. Hypertension can also be reduced to some degree by regular **aerobic exercise** and appropriate changes to the diet which include consuming leafy green vegetables (e.g., kale, spinach, and cabbage), beetroot, carrots, green beans, celery, and rhubarb. These vegetables – and in particular beetroot and rhubarb – contain abundant amounts of **nitrate** that in the body gets converted to nitric oxide which causes opening up of blood vessels (known as vasodilation) and a reduction in blood pressure. You can get a sufficient daily dose of nitrate (that's about 400 mg) in the form of commercially available concentrated beetroot drinks that are available in some supermarkets and health food shops. If you like sport you may see athletes and games players consuming beetroot juice in the hours before competing. However, they are not drinking it to lower their blood pressure. The nitrate in beetroot juice makes athletes more efficient in their use of oxygen and improves their endurance exercise performance.

Key Points

- Type 1 diabetes is a chronic condition in which the pancreas produces little or no insulin. The condition most commonly results from a highly specific immune-mediated destruction of pancreatic islet β-cells in early childhood.

- Type 2 diabetes usually develops from the age of 40 and usually in people who are overweight and sedentary. The body tissues become resistant to the action of insulin. Although the pancreas compensates by increasing its insulin production this is only maintained for maybe a few years and after that the β-cells start to fail and insulin secretion falls.

- Insulin is a hormone that normally stimulates the tissues to take up blood-borne glucose when the blood glucose level is elevated such as after a meal.

- The main consequences of both type 1 and type 2 diabetes are high levels of blood glucose and increased levels of blood fats including triglyceride, cholesterol, and LDL.

- Too much glucose and fat in the blood can damage organs, blood vessels, and nerves which can lead to long-term health problems such as hypertension, coronary heart disease, kidney disease, nerve damage, blindness, leg ulcers, more frequent infections, and poor wound healing.

- The metabolic syndrome is a term used to describe the common co-occurrence of several known cardiovascular disease risk factors that include elevated blood glucose levels and insulin resistance that are main features of type 2 diabetes. The metabolic syndrome is not actually a disease but a group of characteristics that include obesity, hypertension, elevated blood sugar levels, insulin resistance, and dyslipidemia.

- Type 2 diabetes can be reversed and be gotten rid of by losing weight through dieting and doing more exercise.

- Prevention is always better than cure, and, for the vast majority of people, type 2 diabetes can be prevented from occurring by eating a healthy diet, maintaining a normal body weight, and doing some form of regular exercise.

Chapter 2

How Do I Know If I Have Type 2 Diabetes, and How Will It Be Treated?

Objectives

After studying this chapter, you should:

* Know the most common symptoms of type 2 diabetes.

* Understand how type 2 diabetes is diagnosed and what the results of the blood tests mean.

* Know how type 2 diabetes is usually treated.

* Appreciate that the condition can get better, be kept stable, or get worse.

Type 2 diabetes usually develops in people aged over 40 years. It develops relatively slowly and has less obvious symptoms than type 1 diabetes, so it often goes unnoticed until its presence is confirmed by blood testing. Prediabetes is a "pre-diagnosis" of diabetes—you can think of it as a warning sign. It's when your blood glucose level (blood sugar level) is higher than normal, but it's not high enough to be considered diabetes. Appropriate changes to diet and exercise habits at this stage can prevent prediabetes from developing into type 2 diabetes.

SYMPTOMS OF TYPE 2 DIABETES

Some of the more common signs and symptoms of type 2 diabetes are illustrated in figure 2.1. These signs and symptoms of type 2 diabetes often develop slowly and usually don't make you feel ill. In fact, you can have prediabetes or type 2 diabetes for several years and not know it unless you happen to have a blood test. The things to look out for include:

* Increased thirst and frequent urination. High levels of sugar in your blood draws fluid from your tissues into the circulation. This makes you feel thirsty. As a result, you tend to drink more

which in turn makes you urinate more than usual. You might become aware of this if you start having to keep getting out of bed during the night to go to the toilet.

- Blurred vision. When your blood sugar levels are too high some fluid may be drawn out from the lenses of your eyes which can affect your ability to focus so that your vision becomes rather blurred.

- Increased hunger and **appetite**. As your tissues become more resistant to the actions of insulin (which normally helps to move glucose from the blood into the cells of your muscles, adipose tissue, liver, and other organs) your tissues become depleted of energy which can make you feel hungry and crave for sweet foods.

- Fatigue. If your cells are deprived of sugar, it can make you feel tired and irritable. Lower than normal glycogen in your muscles will impair your ability to sustain aerobic exercise.

- Weight changes. Some people may put on weight because their increased appetite means they eat more food. However, some people, even despite eating more than usual to relieve hunger, may lose weight. When blood glucose levels are high, significant amounts of glucose can be lost in the urine because there is just too much glucose for the kidneys to reabsorb. Essentially the diabetic is excreting calories in the form of glucose.

- Frequent infections like the common cold because type 2 diabetes impairs immunity.

- Slow-healing sores or ulcers because type 2 diabetes impairs wound repair and healing.

- Areas of darkened skin start to appear. Some people with type 2 diabetes develop patches of dark, velvety skin in the folds and creases of their bodies. This is usually most noticeable in the armpits, groin, and neck. This condition is called **acanthosis nigricans**, and it is thought to be caused by high levels of insulin in the blood which stimulate the growth of cells in the outer layer of the skin.

- When men aged 45 and under develop erectile dysfunction, it may be a sign that they have developed type 2 diabetes which is associated with impaired sensitivity and blood flow in the hands, feet, and genitals.

- A urine test may reveal the presence of glucose which should not be there in a normal healthy person.

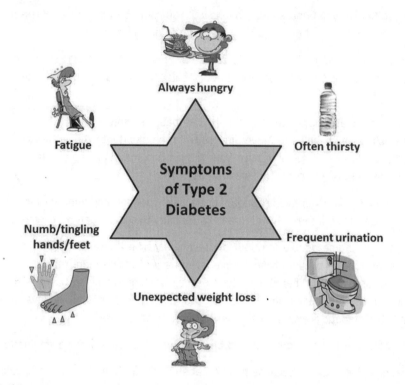

Figure 2.1 Six common symptoms of type 2 diabetes.

DIAGNOSIS OF TYPE 2 DIABETES

If you have several of the above symptoms you should visit your physician who may ask you for a urine sample to be tested for glucose. The presence of glucose in your urine is an indicator that you may be diabetic (see the sidebar for an explanation). Urine glucose measurements are less reliable than blood glucose measurements but can be used as an initial screening test which if positive indicates the need for a blood test to confirm the diagnosis.

Why does glucose appear in the urine of an untreated diabetic?

The kidneys filter the blood to produce urine and normally reabsorb all the glucose that is present to conserve it in the body. Therefore, in a normal, healthy person no glucose can be detected in the urine. However, the kidneys can only reabsorb a limited amount of glucose, and when the blood glucose level exceeds about 9-10 mmol/L (160-180 mg/dL), the kidneys become overwhelmed and begin to excrete glucose in the urine (this level is called the **renal threshold** for glucose; see figure 2.2). Chemical test strips can be dipped into a sample of urine to determine if glucose is present. Urine glucose measurements are less reliable than blood glucose measurements and are not used to diagnose diabetes or evaluate treatment for diabetes. They may be used for an initial screening test when you visit your physician as they give an immediate result which could indicate the need for a blood test.

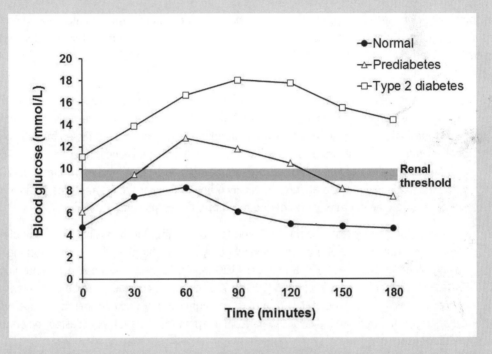

Figure 2.2: The results of an oral glucose tolerance test showing the blood glucose response to the ingestion of 75 g glucose in a normal person, a person with prediabetes, and a person with type 2 diabetes. The grey shaded bar indicates the normal renal threshold for glucose. Above this concentration some glucose will appear in the urine.

An increasing number of people are being diagnosed as suffering from type 2 diabetes by their medical practitioner. The diagnosis is usually made after a blood test reveals a **glycated hemoglobin** A1c concentration of 48 **mmol/mol** (or 6.5%) or higher (see table 2.1). **Hemoglobin** is the red pigment in your red blood cells (**erythrocytes**) that carries oxygen, and it is said to be glycated when some sugar (glucose) molecules become attached to it which happens when the blood sugar levels remain higher than normal for too long. As red blood cells have an average lifespan in the circulation of about four months, the level of glycated hemoglobin reflects the average blood glucose concentration over the previous two to three months. A high level indicates that the body tissues are becoming less responsive to the hormone insulin which normally stimulates glucose uptake from the blood by muscle, liver, and adipose tissue. If uncontrolled blood glucose stays much higher for longer after feeding, and even fasting, blood glucose concentrations can become extremely high (table 2.1). Your blood sample will be taken to the local hospital for analysis and the results are usually available within a few days. People with glycated hemoglobin (**HbA1c**) levels just below the threshold for diagnosis of type 2 diabetes (42-47 mmol/mol or 5.7-6.4%) are classed as prediabetic. Normal levels are below 42 mmol/mol or 5.7%.

In some conditions such as if you're pregnant or have an uncommon form of hemoglobin (known as a hemoglobin variant) that can make the HbA1c test inaccurate, your doctor may decide to use an alternative test to diagnose diabetes. Usually one of the three following tests will be used in this situation:

1. A non-fasting (random) blood sugar test. A blood sample is taken at a random time and the sugar (glucose) concentration of plasma (the fluid part of the blood with the cells removed by centrifugation) or whole blood is measured. Blood glucose values are expressed in millimoles per liter (mmol/L) or milligrams per deciliter (mg/dL). A deciliter is one tenth of a liter or 100 milliliters. Regardless of when you last ate, a random blood sugar level of 11 mmol/L (200 mg/dL) or higher suggests diabetes, especially if any of the signs and symptoms of diabetes – such as often feeling thirsty and frequent urination – are present.

2. A fasting blood sugar test. For this test, you fast overnight, and a fasting blood sample is taken to measure your blood glucose level when you visit the physician in the morning. A fasting blood glucose level of 5.5 mmol/L (100 mg/dL) or less is normal. A fasting blood glucose level from 5.6 to 6.9 mmol/L (100 to 125 mg/dL) is considered to be characteristic of prediabetes. If it's 7.0 mmol/L (126 mg/dL) or higher you will be considered to have type 2 diabetes. Your physician may want to perform a repeat test on another occasion to confirm the diagnosis.

3. An **oral glucose tolerance test** (OGTT). For this test, you fast overnight, and the fasting blood sugar level is measured when you visit the physician in the morning. Then you drink a glucose solution that contains 75 g of glucose, and your blood glucose levels are tested periodically for the next two hours (this usually involves having a temporary cannula placed in a forearm vein so that blood can be sampled repeatedly – say every 15 minutes – without the need for multiple skin punctures). The typical results of such a test are shown in figure 2.2. For a normal healthy person the peak blood glucose value occurs after one hour and does not exceed the renal threshold (9.0-10.0 mmol/L or 160-180 mg/dL). The blood glucose level should return to its pre-test fasting value within 2-2.5 hours. The key diagnostic measurement for establishing the presence of type 2 diabetes in the OGTT is the blood glucose concentration two hours after consuming the drink. A reading of 11 mmol/L (200 mg/dL) or higher after two hours may indicate diabetes, whereas a reading of 7.8-10.9 mmol/L (140-199 mg/dL) indicates prediabetes. A blood glucose sugar level less than 7.8 mmol/L (140 mg/dL) is considered to be normal.

Table 2.1 Glycated hemoglobin (HbA1c) and blood glucose levels in the diagnosis of type 2 diabetes

	Normal range	Prediabetes	Type 2 diabetes
Hb1Ac mmol/mol (%)	30-41 (4.0-5.6)	42-47 (5.7-6.4)	≥48 (≥6.5)
Fasting glucose mmol/L (mg/dL)	4.0-5.5 (72-99)	5.6-6.9 (100-125)	≥7.0 (≥126)
Non-fasting glucose mmol/L (mg/dL)	4.5-7.7 (81-139)	7.8-10.9 (140-199)	≥11.0 (≥200)
OGTT 1-hour blood glucose mmol/L (mg/dL)	7.0-9.0 (126-162)	≥9.0 (≥162)	≥11.0 (≥200)
OGTT 2-hour blood glucose mmol/L (mg/dL)	4.5-7.7 (81-139)	7.8-10.9 (140-199)	≥11.0 (≥200)

dL: deciliter = 100 mL; mmol: millimoles; mol: moles; OGTT: oral glucose tolerance test; ≥ = equal to or more than

If you have diabetes, your physician will ask you to come in again so they can explain the test results and what will happen next. If you're diagnosed with diabetes, your physician (or a nurse specializing in diabetes) will explain to you what diabetes is, what your high blood sugar means for your health, what changes to your lifestyle behaviors you will need to make (e.g., changes to your diet, exercise, smoking, and alcohol intake), and what medication you may need either now or in the future.

WHAT HAPPENS AFTER THE DIAGNOSIS?

Usually, the following things happen after your diagnosis:

- You will probably be advised to make changes to your diet and be more active.

- You'll have to go for regular type 2 diabetes check-ups.

- You'll have to look out for certain signs to avoid other health problems.

- Your physician may prescribe medication or they may decide to delay this for a few years provided that you take the above steps to improve your condition which can be evaluated by regular monitoring of your weight, blood HbA1c, and other checks that are detailed in the next section of this chapter.

- If your physician does prescribe medication it may take some time to get used to the medication and to find the right dosage for you.

- Most people who are diagnosed with type 2 diabetes will start medication – usually in tablet form – after a few years. After a while, if this proves to be insufficient to keep blood glucose levels stable at an acceptable level, insulin therapy – by injection – will probably be prescribed.

TREATMENT OF TYPE 2 DIABETES

Type 2 diabetes is usually treated by medication and attempting to lose weight through changes to diet and lifestyle behavior. This often means changing what you eat, as well as how much you eat, and becoming more physically active.

MEDICATION

Some people who have type 2 diabetes can control their blood sugar levels and prevent their condition from getting worse by just changing their diet and doing more exercise, but many also need diabetes medications or insulin therapy. In fact, most people need medicine to control their type 2 diabetes. If you have Type 2 diabetes you may be prescribed medication to help manage your blood sugar levels and to prevent health problems. The most common tablet form is **metformin** which decreases liver glucose production, decreases intestinal **absorption** of glucose, and improves insulin sensitivity by increasing tissue glucose uptake. If your blood sugar levels aren't lower within a few months, you may need another medicine. There are numerous other types of medication available (see the sidebar) including **sulfonylurea** drugs which stimulate the pancreas to produce more insulin. Insulin (by injection) is not usually given in the first five years after diagnosis. Insulin is only needed when other medicines no longer work. Your physician or diabetes nurse will explain how to take your medicine and how to store it. If you need to inject insulin, they'll show you how. Once you start taking medication it is very likely that you'll have to take it for the rest of your life. Unfortunately, even with regular medication, diabetes usually gets worse over time, so your medicine or dose may need to change.

Medications used to treat type 2 diabetes

People who have type 2 diabetes need to try to keep their blood glucose levels within the normal range and avoid large spikes in blood glucose after consuming food and drinks. Particularly in the first few years after its diagnosis, some people with type 2 diabetes can achieve their target blood sugar levels with diet and exercise alone. However, after a few years most will also need diabetes medications or insulin therapy. The decision about which medications are the best ones to take depends on many factors, including your blood sugar level and any other health problems you have. Your doctor might prescribe just one drug to begin with or a combination of drugs from different classes to help you control your blood sugar in several different ways. Examples of possible treatments for type 2 diabetes include:

- *Metformin* (Glucophage, Glumetza, others). This is usually the first medication prescribed for the treatment of type 2 diabetes. It works by improving the sensitivity of your body tissues to insulin. That should mean that the insulin that your pancreas produces should work more effectively. Metformin also lowers glucose production in the liver which is not really needed as your blood sugar levels are higher than normal anyway.

- *Sulfonylureas* (glyburide [DiaBeta, Glynase], glipizide [Glucotrol] and glimepiride [Amaryl]). These medications help to stimulate your pancreas to produce and secrete more insulin which is needed to lower your blood glucose levels.

- *Meglitinides* (repaglinide [Prandin] and nateglinide [Starlix]). These medications also stimulate the pancreas to secrete more insulin, but are faster acting than the sulfonylureas, and the duration of their effect in the body is shorter.

- *Thiazolidinediones* (rosiglitazone [Avandia] and pioglitazone [Actos]). These medications have a similar action to that of metformin and make the body's tissues more sensitive to insulin. However, these drugs can have some serious side effects, such as an increased risk of heart failure and bone fractures, so are generally not prescribed unless some of the other medications that you have tried do not work for you.

- *DPP-4 inhibitors* (sitagliptin [Januvia], saxagliptin [Onglyza] and linagliptin [Tradjenta]). These drugs inhibit the action of dipeptidyl peptidase 4 (DPP-4), an enzyme which destroys the hormone incretin. Incretin helps the body produce more insulin when it is needed and reduces the amount of glucose being produced by the liver when it is not needed. These medications help reduce blood sugar levels but tend to have only a modest effect.

- *GLP-1 receptor agonists* (Exenatide [Byetta] and liraglutide [Victoza]). This class of medications can only be given by injection and they act to stimulate the glucagon-like peptide 1 (GLP-1) receptor to slow down digestion and help lower blood sugar levels, though not as much as sulfonylureas. Their actions mimic the effect of incretin and are normally prescribed for patients who have not been able to control their blood sugar level sufficiently well with tablet medication. In some situations they may be used as an additional therapy to one or more of the above medications.

- *SGLT2 inhibitors* (canagliflozin [Invokana] and dapagliflozin [Farxiga]). These are the newest diabetes drugs to become available. They work by inhibiting the **sodium-glucose cotransporter-2** (SGLT2) preventing the kidneys from reabsorbing glucose into the blood so some more of the excess glucose is excreted in the urine.

It is possible that your medicine(s) may cause some unpleasant side effects. These can include bloating, **diarrhea**, weight loss or gain, feeling sick, or getting swollen ankles.

With some medications the potential side effects, although relatively uncommon, can be more serious including heart failure, pancreatitis, and **urinary tract infections**. Not everyone has side effects. If you feel unwell after taking medicine or notice any side effects, speak to your physician or diabetes nurse as soon as possible but don't stop taking medication without getting their advice.

INSULIN THERAPY

Some people who have type 2 diabetes need insulin therapy in addition to some of the medications described above. Insulin therapy is not usually prescribed in the first few years after diagnosis, but it is commonly needed at some stage when the other forms of medication fail to maintain stable levels of blood sugar. This happens when the pancreatic β-cells stop producing enough insulin to counter insulin resistance. Insulin is a protein which means it would be denatured, digested, and destroyed by the enzymes in the stomach and gut if taken by mouth, so insulin can only work if it is given by injection. There are several different types of insulin formulations that can be taken, and it is common for your physician to prescribe two or more insulin types to use throughout the day and night. Initially it is common for people with type 2 diabetes to begin insulin therapy with just one long-acting shot that is administered during the evening. However, it is usual for diabetics to also need shorter-acting insulin injections before or after meals. Insulin injections involve using a fine needle and syringe (more generally administered by a health practitioner) or a pen injector containing a cartridge filled with insulin. These pen injectors are normally self-administered using easily accessible body sites such as the skin of the belly. The insulin does not need to be injected directly into a vein as it can work its way into the circulation when injected under the skin.

A variety of types of insulin are available that vary in dose, and speed, and duration of action. Some come as a slow release formulation and are used for controlling blood sugar levels over an extended period, such as while you are asleep at night. Others are fast acting (just like natural insulin) and are taken just before or after a meal with the aim of limiting the rise in the blood glucose concentration that will occur when your pancreas cannot produce sufficient insulin. You may have heard that it is also possible to take insulin by using an insulin pump which is a battery-operated device that gives you insulin regularly throughout the day. The pump is attached to a thin plastic tube that has a cannula (a soft thin plastic tube instead of needle) at the end through which insulin passes. This cannula is inserted under the skin, usually on the belly area, and is changed every two days. In many countries, insulin pumps are only available by prescription for people who have type 1 diabetes. However, ask your physician if this is something that could be considered for you as an alternative to injections that you administer yourself.

It is important to get the dosage and timing of insulin administration right, and you will be given instruction and advice on how to achieve this by your healthcare practitioner. An overdose of insulin can be fatal because it will cause your blood glucose level to drop too much, causing mental confusion, dizziness, fainting, and loss of consciousness. This could cause a serious injury (e.g., if you were to fall and hit your head), and if not corrected quickly it can lead to coma and death. Not taking your insulin when it is needed will lead to large rises in your blood sugar and increase your risk of the serious health complications in the near future. See the sidebar for more information on the different types of insulin and how to administer it yourself by injection.

More about how to safely inject insulin, and the different types of insulin

To inject insulin safely you'll need an insulin pen injector (photo 2.1) – this can be one that already has insulin in, which you throw away after it is empty, or, as is more common nowadays, a pen you can reuse by changing the insulin cartridge and needle yourself. For the reusable pen you will need a supply of disposable needles. Each needle is small and thin – much thinner and shorter than those used for taking blood from a vein or to administer a vaccination – as it only has to go just under the skin, not into a muscle or vein. These needles can only be used once and should be disposed of immediately after use in a sharps bin or needle clipper. You should carry out the following procedures to inject insulin using a reusable pen:

1. Wash your hands with soap and water and dry them using a clean towel or air dryer.

2. Choose the site where you're going to inject – you're looking for fatty tissue so the main sites are your abdomen (in a semi-circle under your belly button), sides of your thighs, and your bottom. It's vital that you select and use a different spot each time – at least one centimeter or half an inch from where you last injected. If not, hard lumps of scar tissue can appear that will stop your body absorbing and using the insulin properly.

3. Attach the needle to your reusable pen – removing the outer and inner caps – and dial up two units of insulin. Point your pen upwards and press the plunger until the insulin in a sterile liquid solution appears from the top of the needle. This is known as priming and helps regulate your dose by removing any air from the needle and cartridge.

4. Dial the dose that you need and make sure the spot you're injecting is clean, dry, and free of any spots or sores.

5. Insert the needle at a right angle (90-degree angle). It helps to gently pinch the skin on either side of the site you are injecting. After inserting the needle into your skin deliver the insulin (photo 2.2) by pressing the plunger until the dial goes back to 0.

6. You should then count to 10 slowly to give the insulin time to enter your body before removing the needle.

7. Dispose of the needle carefully using your sharps bin or needle clipper. Your healthcare team will instruct you how to get rid of the bin safely when it is full.

Types of insulin

There are five different types of insulin and they all work in slightly differently ways to help manage your diabetes and suit your daily routine. Which ones you take will be decided between you and your healthcare team.

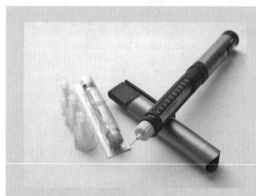 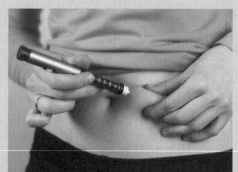

Photo 2.1: A reusable insulin pen injector with insulin cartridge and needle caps.

Photo 2.2: Injecting insulin.

- Rapid-acting insulin (sometimes known as fast-acting insulin) is taken shortly before or just after meals. It works very quickly, and it's usually taken alongside an intermediate-acting insulin or long-acting insulin. Your dose will depend on how much carbohydrate is in your meal.

- Short-acting insulin (sometimes known as bolus insulin) is similar to rapid-acting insulin but is slightly slower. Because it's slower, you need to take it around 20-30 minutes before you eat your meal.

- Mixed insulin is a combination of both short-acting and long-acting insulins. You still take it before meals, but you won't have to take a separate intermediate-acting or background insulin as well.

- Intermediate-acting insulin is also known as background insulin or basal insulin and is quite long lasting. This means it works throughout the day and it is only taken once or twice a day.

- Long-acting insulin is even slower than intermediate insulin and you usually take it just once – at the same time of day – every day. It's been shown to reduce the risk of hypoglycemia compared with intermediate-acting insulin.

CHANGES TO DIET AND LIFESTYLE BEHAVIOR

The best treatment is to reverse or get rid of type 2 diabetes by going on a diet to lose weight and doing more physical activity. As research shows that the longer you have type 2 diabetes the harder it is to reverse, it obviously makes sense to take action as soon as possible after you have been diagnosed with the condition. Going on a **very low energy diet** (only 800 calories per day compared with a typical average intake of 2,000 calories) for 20 weeks has recently been shown to be effective in reversing type 2 diabetes, but it takes a lot of willpower to stick to such a diet for a long time. Losing the excess body fat and weight by a combination of less severe dieting and exercise could theoretically achieve the same goal and is easier to stick to. These issues will be discussed in more detail later in this book. How you can live with type 2 diabetes and manage it effectively through healthy eating and exercise will first be covered in the next chapter.

Key Points

- Signs and symptoms of type 2 diabetes often develop slowly and usually don't make you feel ill. In fact, you can have prediabetes or type 2 diabetes for several years and not know it unless you happen to have a blood test.

- Symptoms of type 2 diabetes include increased thirst and frequent urination, increased hunger and appetite, fatigue, weight changes, blurred vision, frequent infections, slow wound healing, and patches of darkened skin in the folds and creases of the body.

- The presence of glucose in urine is an indicator that a person could be diabetic, and this is confirmed when a blood test reveals a glycated hemoglobin A1c concentration of 48 mmol/mol (or 6.5%) or higher.

- In some cases an oral glucose tolerance test may be used to confirm diagnosis of type 2 diabetes.

- Type 2 diabetes is usually treated by medication and losing weight through changes to diet, exercise habits, and other lifestyle behaviors.

- Medication may include drugs administered in tablet form or by injection and insulin therapy which can only be given by injection.

Chapter 3

How Is Type 2 Diabetes Monitored and Managed?

Objectives

After studying this chapter, you should:

- Understand why monitoring of people with type 2 diabetes is important.

- Know what will be monitored.

- Appreciate the importance of regular blood glucose monitoring.

- Know how type 2 diabetes is managed.

- Appreciate the importance of modifying your diet.

- Understand what a low glycemic index diet is.

- Appreciate the importance of practicing good hygiene.

- Appreciate the importance of doing more exercise.

Everyone living with type 2 diabetes or metabolic syndrome needs to have regular monitoring to keep their condition stable and delay the onset of health complications. Some of this monitoring can be self-administered, but some aspects require a 3-monthly, 6-monthly, or annual visit to see a physician or a diabetes nurse who will compare your test results to previous measurements and provide advice on any changes to your treatment or management of your condition that may be deemed necessary. You should always attend your check-up appointments because the sooner any issues or complications are identified, the easier it will be to resolve them, and it will be less likely that the problem will progress to something worse.

MONITORING OF PEOPLE WITH TYPE 2 DIABETES

Monitoring of type 2 diabetes involves regular visits to your local healthcare practitioners. They will collect blood and urine samples from you and conduct various tests and inspections that will help to evaluate your current condition and determine if there is a need for alterations to your treatment and lifestyle behavior. Your doctor or diabetes nurse is the person you should ask for advice about the management of your condition and for answers to any queries you may have. Do not rely on hearsay, or what you read in magazines, or see on the internet, unless it is from an established expert organization such as the American Diabetes Association, the UK National Health Service, or Diabetes UK. There are also some things you can monitor yourself at home. But let's begin with what to expect when you visit your local clinic.

MONITORING BY YOUR HEALTHCARE PRACTITIONER

When you visit your physician or diabetes nurse, they should ask you how you are feeling, and if you have had any health problems. It is very important to be absolutely honest about your health and how you are really feeling. Tell your healthcare practitioner if you have any concerns, if you are feeling tired and lethargic, or have developed any colds, sores, or ulcers. Be truthful when asked about your smoking, alcohol, and exercise habits.

Your blood HbA1c levels need to be checked at least once per year, and sometimes this is done up to four times per year (i.e., once every three months). Your target blood HbA1c level may vary depending on your age and other factors. However, for most people, the American Diabetes Association recommends that the blood HbA1c level is kept below 7.0% (54 mmol/mol). Ask your doctor or nurse what your blood HbA1c target is. Compared with repeated daily blood sugar tests which only indicate a single point in time, the HbA1c test is a better indicator of how well you are controlling your blood sugar level (remember that it gives an indication of your average blood glucose level over the past two to three months) and how well your diabetes treatment plan is working. An increase from your previous blood HbA1c level may signal the need for a change in your medication, diet, or physical activity level. In addition to the blood HbA1c test, your doctor or nurse will take blood and urine samples annually or periodically over the course of the year to check your cholesterol levels, thyroid function, liver function, and kidney function. The doctor or diabetes nurse will also assess your blood pressure. Regular eye and foot inspections are important as well. The following sidebar describes more detail about these checks, why they are done, and what the various levels mean.

What your annual or more frequent health checks will include

- *Body weight.* You will almost certainly have been advised to lose some weight so it is important that this is checked regularly using an accurate scale.

- *Blood pressure.* To check for early signs of hypertension which is a risk factor for coronary heart disease and stroke. If your systolic blood pressure (SBP) is over 140 mmHg you may be prescribed medication to bring it down.

- *Blood HbA1c.* To check how well your blood sugar is being controlled.

- *Serum cholesterol.* High levels of serum cholesterol can lead to cardiovascular disease. If your serum cholesterol is above 6.0 mmol/L you may be prescribed medication such as a daily statin tablet. Statins are drugs that reduce your body's production of cholesterol, and the good news is that these are usually very effective and side effects are rare.

- *Serum LDL and HDL.* Ideally you want your serum LDL (low-density lipoprotein) level to be below 2.0 mmol/L and your serum HDL (high-density lipoprotein) level to be above 1.0 mmol/L. A high LDL/HDL ratio (defined as 4.0 or more) is a risk factor for cardiovascular disease. LDL carries cholesterol to the cells that need it, but if there's too much cholesterol for the cells to use, it can build up in the artery walls. High levels of LDL cause fatty deposits (called plaques) to accumulate in your blood vessel walls which obstruct blood flow and are a major cause of heart attacks, so high levels of LDL are bad for your health. HDL actually removes such deposits and returns the fat to the liver, so a high level of HDL is good for your health.

- *Serum apolipoprotein B/apolipoprotein A-I* **(apoB/apoA-I)** *ratio.* This ratio of the two main types of **apolipoprotein** found in serum **lipoprotein** particles represents the balance of pro-**atherogenic** (plaque-forming) and anti-atherogenic lipoproteins and is now known to be superior to any of the cholesterol ratios in predicting risk of atherosclerosis and coronary heart disease.

- *Serum triglyceride.* Triglyceride is your normal storage form of fat, and it is found in meat and dairy products. Any excess of sugar in your diet and most of the alcohol that you drink tends to get converted into triglyceride. High levels of serum triglyceride are a risk factor for cardiovascular disease. Ideally you want your serum triglyceride level to be below 1.7 mmol/L.

- *Serum T3 and T4.* The thyroid hormones triiodothyronine (T3) and tetraiodothryronine (T4) (also known as thyroxin) are known to affect insulin action in adipose tissue, and the presence of thyroid dysfunction may affect diabetes control. Too little production of T3 and T4 is known as hypothyroidism and causes many metabolic abnormalities as well as multiple clinical symptoms. Some studies suggest that blood sugar may be affected in hypothyroidism and levels may increase. Indeed, it has been noted that patients with diabetes who also have hypothyroidism may have higher levels of HbA1c. Furthermore, a study in 2016, which examined over 8,400 people, reported that having too little thyroid hormone in the blood – even in the low-to-normal range – raises the risk of developing type 2 diabetes, especially in people with prediabetes.

- *Urine albumin/creatinine ratio.* This is used as an indicator of kidney function. **Albumin** is a serum protein that should not appear in your urine. **Creatinine** is a waste compound that is excreted in relatively constant daily amounts in your urine and is used as reference. A high albumin/creatinine ratio indicates that your kidneys are becoming "leaky" and suggests that you have some inflammation causing them to malfunction. In some cases, this might be a side effect of your medication and your doctor may prescribe an alternative drug to help with your blood pressure or blood glucose control.

- *Foot inspection.* This usually involves the nurse feeling for a pulse on the top of your foot, checking for any sores or cuts on your feet, and using a fine pointed needle to lightly prick the soles of your feet to test your sensation of pain. These tests can indicate the state of your circulation and nerve supply. Poor management of diabetes can cause poor circulation and nerve damage leading to reduced feeling in the feet and increased likeliness of foot sores and infections which are slow to heal and can develop into ulcers. You might think that it does not sound too serious but, if allowed to progress, such problems can lead to the need for amputation of your toes, foot, or lower limb.

- *Dilated eye examination.* This will probably be done in a separate appointment and be carried out by an eye specialist. Some drops are placed in your eye causing your pupil to dilate (i.e., open fully), allowing a clear photograph of the retina at the back of your eye to be taken. The healthcare practitioner who performs this test (called a retinal scan) will be looking for the presence of new small and fragile blood vessels in your retina which have a tendency to rupture leading to impaired or total loss of vision. People with type 2 diabetes are at increased risk of this condition which is called diabetic retinopathy. The presence of cataract, glaucoma, and optic nerve damage can also be assessed during this examination.

The various tests listed in the sidebar, apart from the dilated eye examination, will be done when you attend your regular appointments with your doctor or diabetes nurse and will usually take place at a local clinic or surgery. Your blood and urine samples will probably be sent to the local hospital's biochemistry or pathology laboratory for analysis, and you may have to wait a week or so for the results. This might mean that you have had to attend your local clinic or surgery around one week before so that a nurse or phlebotomist (a person who specializes in collecting blood samples) can take some blood (usually no more than 10 mL) from a vein in your arm. Most phlebotomists will choose the antecubital vein on the inner side of your elbow joint for this purpose, and the procedure is virtually painless. Once the blood results are in you can arrange to see your physician or diabetes nurse who will explain what the results mean and whether any adjustments to your treatment are needed. They will perform your body weight and blood pressure measurements and carry out the inspection of your feet at this time. Your retinal scan will usually be done on a separate occasion and may take place at your doctor's surgery, in the ophthalmology (eye) department of your local hospital, or at an optician's shop.

SELF-MONITORING AT HOME

In addition to the aforementioned monitoring procedures it is important that you carry out some self-monitoring at home. You can measure your nude body weight on a weekly basis using an electronic scale and record this in a diary or notebook. If your weight creeps up over three consecutive weeks, cut back on your food intake or do more exercise to get your weight back on track. If you have been told by your healthcare practitioner to lose some weight and have been given a target weight to aim for, try to achieve this over a period of months. Don't attempt a crash diet as you won't stick to it for long enough and will regain the weight fairly quickly when you start eating normally again. I will delve more deeply into the issue of weight loss later in this book.

You can also monitor your blood pressure on a weekly basis. For no more than 20-40 US dollars you should be able to purchase a battery operated digital blood pressure monitor (an inflatable cuff that gets wrapped around your upper arm and which is connected to a monitor device containing a pump and a digital display as shown in photo 3.1) from your local pharmacy. Full instructions are provided with these instruments, but if in doubt ask your pharmacist or your diabetes nurse for advice on how to use them correctly. Your diabetes nurse will be using a very similar device when your blood pressure is measured at the clinic. You should carry out this test in a relaxed state and in a sitting position (e.g., sit at the table in an upright dining chair and place the monitor on the table next to you). Write down your blood pressure readings. The **systolic** blood pressure (SBP) is the higher value. It should be around 110 to 140 mmHg (the mmHg is short for millimeters of mercury which is a unit of pressure) and represents the pressure in your arteries when the heart contracts and pumps blood into them. The lower value is your **diastolic** blood pressure (DBP) which should be about 70 to 90 mmHg and represents the pressure in your arteries when the heart is relaxed and refilling with blood prior to its next contraction or heartbeat. Most devices will also display your pulse or heart rate in beats per minute, and you should make a note of this also. For most people the resting heart rate will be about 60 to 100 beats per minute (bpm).

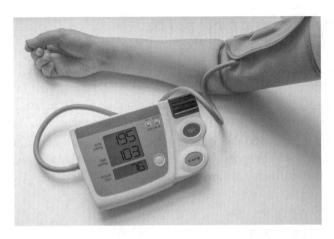

Photo 3.1: Measurement of blood pressure using a battery-operated digital blood pressure monitor.

It is also important to check your feet regularly. Diabetes affects the circulation and nerves in the feet causing you to lose some sensation of feeling and pain which means that some cuts, abrasions, blisters, and sores can go unnoticed. Diabetes also impairs your immune function meaning that the healing process can be rather slow and there is an increased likelihood of the damaged area becoming infected. Diabetics are also more susceptible to fungal infections between the toes (commonly known as athlete's foot). So check your feet every day for any signs of damage, and apply an antiseptic cream to any wounds. Visit your health practitioner if any damage persists without healing for more than a week. Be aware that even small infections can soon worsen, become ulcerated, and spread to affect larger areas of your feet (photo 3.2) and lower leg. Conditions such as **cellulitis** and **gangrene** can occur which are life-threatening and may lead to the need for surgical amputation of your toes, foot, or lower limb. Yet, with good diabetes healthcare and support, experts estimate that four out of five amputations could be prevented because 80% of cases begin as foot ulcers, which are largely avoidable and far more treatable if found early.

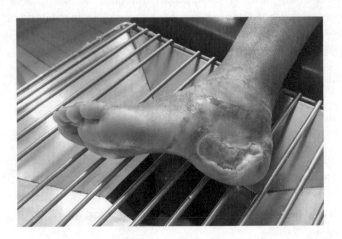

Photo 3.2: Foot ulcer in a person with type 2 diabetes.

MANAGEMENT OF TYPE 2 DIABETES

Other than taking any drugs you have been prescribed to help control your blood sugar, management of type 2 diabetes includes maintaining good care of your feet, practicing good personal hygiene, eating a healthy diet, and being more physically active. In some cases, and particularly for those on insulin therapy, there may be a need for regular blood glucose monitoring which can be done using a portable glucose monitor to measure your current blood glucose concentration from a tiny finger-prick sample. These steps will help keep your blood sugar level closer to normal, which can delay or prevent complications.

KEEPING YOUR FEET HEALTHY

Keeping your feet healthy is important for people with diabetes. Damage to nerves and circulation caused by diabetes leads to gradual loss of sensation and an increased risk of injury and infection that can lead to ulcers, cellulitis, gangrene, and amputation. Follow these ten actions to keep your feet clean and free of injury and infection:

1. Check your feet every day for cuts, abrasions, sores, blisters, swelling, or redness. Use a mirror to help you see the bottom of your feet.

2. Wash and moisturize your feet daily with soap and water. Wash between your toes using a gentle nonabrasive facecloth (use a separate one for your face).

3. Gently rub the soles of your feet with a pumice stone to file down any area of hard skin.

4. Dry your feet thoroughly especially between your toes.

5. If any areas of your skin are rough and dry, apply a moisturizing skin cream. Do not put any between your toes because moisture there can cause fungus growth.

6. Cut your toenails straight across using clippers designed for this purpose (invest in a fresh pair every six months). Follow the shape of the end of your toes but do not attempt to cut deep into the corners. Clippers are safer than using scissors. You probably cut your fingernails every one to two weeks, but only cut your toenails every six to eight weeks.

7. Put on fresh socks every day.

8. Always wear well-fitting shoes with socks.

9. Avoid wearing flip flops or sandals that may rub your toes or feet.

10. Test your toes and the soles of your feet by lightly touching them to check for any loss of sensation. Inform your healthcare practitioner if you notice any changes. Do not attempt to prick your own feet with a needle; leave this to your diabetes nurse who will very carefully use a fine sterile needle when you attend your regular clinic appointment.

PRACTICING GOOD PERSONAL HYGIENE

Diabetics have impaired immunity and are more prone to infection. Good personal hygiene practices can help to reduce the risk of picking up infections, including those that affect the mouth, nose, ears, eyes, respiratory tract, urinary tract, **gastrointestinal tract**, and skin. Pay attention to the following guidelines on personal hygiene to minimize your risk of infection:

- Wash your hands regularly (with the correct technique to ensure all parts of your hands are cleaned effectively) with soap and water which is effective against most **pathogens** (i.e., bacteria and viruses) but bear in mind that using soaps does not provide continuous protection. It is particularly important to wash your hands before meals and after direct contact with potentially contagious people, animals, blood, secretions, public places, and bathrooms. See the sidebar for details of how to effectively wash your hands.

- You can also use hand gels containing a minimum of 60% alcohol to disinfect effectively, but be aware that the protection they provide does not last more than a few minutes so they need to be applied frequently. For some people this frequent application can be a problem as it can cause skin drying and irritation. An alternative and more effective sanitization method is the use of non-alcohol based antimicrobial hand foams that contain cationic biocides and hydrophobic polymers which are claimed to disinfect hands for up to six hours. Carry antimicrobial foam/cream or alcohol-based hand-washing gel with you as both types of product are removed by hand washing and excessive sweating, and so really need to be reapplied every few hours.

- Wash your genitals regularly using water and a mild soap or shower gel to prevent the accumulation of dirt and germs in your genitalia that can potentially cause infection. Also be sure to wear clean underwear by changing them often.

- Avoid putting your fingers close to your eyes or rubbing your eyes with your hands as it increases the risk of eye infections such as conjunctivitis. Avoid people with this condition where possible as it is infectious. If you wear contact lenses clean them properly, and always wash your hands thoroughly before putting in or taking out your contact lenses. Make sure to disinfect contact lenses as instructed, and replace them as appropriate.

- Use disposable paper tissues to blow your nose, and do not hang on to them.

- Limit hand to mouth/nose/eye contact when suffering from symptoms of the common cold or gastrointestinal illness because putting your hands to your mouth/nose/eyes is a major route of viral self-inoculation.

- Keep your ears dry. Excess moisture can allow bacteria to enter and attack the ear canal. This can cause swimmer's ear or other types of ear infections, which can be dangerous for your hearing ability. Be sure you gently towel-dry your ears after bathing or swimming. If you can feel water in the ear, tilt your head to the side and tug lightly on the ear lobe to coax the water out. You can also ensure that your ears stay dry and healthy by using custom-fit swimmers' earplugs, which block water from entering the ear canal and have been shown to greatly reduce the risk of developing ear infections. Don't share your earplugs with anyone else.

- Don't use cotton swabs to dry or clean wax from your ears as this can cause abrasions in the inner lining of your ears which easily become infected.

- Maintain good oral hygiene. This encompasses everything you do to keep your mouth, teeth, and gums healthy. Brush your teeth regularly, ideally twice a day, and always brush before going to bed. Clean behind your teeth and gums, but take care to use only gentle pressure to prevent damaging your delicate gums; otherwise gum erosion, bleeding, and infection can occur. Use a toothpaste containing fluoride (1350-1500 ppm is most effective) which protects teeth against decay.

- Use the correct type of toothbrush. The American Dental Association recommends using a brush that has soft bristles and changing the brush every three months. An electronic toothbrush with a round head can be more effective for efficient removal of **dental plaque** which is a biofilm or mass of bacteria that grows on surfaces within the mouth. These dental biofilms may become acidic causing demineralization of the teeth (also known as **dental caries**) or harden into dental calculus (also known as tartar). It is also important to keep your oral care equipment clean. Rinse off your toothbrush after use and store it in an upright position inside your medicine cabinet. Do not cover the brush head as this can lead to bacterial and fungal growth.

- Do not use floss tape or string as it can be too harsh on gums, and most dentists now agree that its regular use poses too great a risk to the health of your gums. Dentists can repair damage to teeth caused by decay, but they cannot restore the health of your gums if they become damaged and infected. As we become older, the health of our gums is paramount; without healthy gums we risk losing our teeth, and the underlying bones can become infected as well. A safer, gentler alternative to string or tape flosses are interdental brushes which come in a variety of sizes to suit the size of the gaps between your teeth. An oral water flosser or irrigator which sends a pulsed water jet to clean both in-between teeth and below the gum-line is another safer but effective option.

- Use an antibacterial therapeutic mouthwash. A therapeutic mouthwash does more than mask bad breath. It can help reduce plaque, inflammation of the gums (**gingivitis**), cavities, and bad breath.

- Visit your dentist regularly, at least twice per year. Regular trips to your dentist for a comprehensive oral exam can pinpoint any problems and keep them from getting worse. Your dentist or the dental hygienist will remove tartar, plaque, and make recommendations about how you can improve the care of your teeth and gums.

- Avoid all tobacco products as not only does tobacco stain your teeth and cause bad breath, it can lead to oral cancer, gum disease (gingivitis), and abscesses. Of course, smoking tobacco has many other undesirable effects on your overall health including damaging vital organs like your lungs and heart.

How to wash your hands effectively

Keeping hands clean is one of the most important steps we can take to avoid getting sick and spreading pathogens (disease-causing microbes or germs) to others. Many diseases and conditions are spread by unclean hands. The following guidelines which are derived from the UK National Health Service and US Center for Disease Control and Prevention websites will help you to clean your hands in an effective way to avoid getting infections and passing germs to people you come into contact with.

- *Recommendation:* Wet your hands with clean, running water (warm or cold as the temperature of the water does not appear to affect microbe removal), and apply liquid or solid soap to the palms of your hands. *Why?:* Because hands could become recontaminated with microbes if placed in a basin of standing water that has been contaminated through previous use. Clean running water should always be used. Using soap to wash hands is more effective than using water alone because the surfactants in soap, lift soil and microbes from the surface of the skin, and people tend to scrub hands more thoroughly when using soap, which further removes germs. Common "antibacterial" soaps with special additives don't tend to be any more effective than non-antibacterial soap and water.

- *Recommendation:* Lather your hands by rubbing them together with the soap. Be sure to lather the palms of your hands, the backs of your hands, between your fingers (by interlacing them), your thumbs, the tips of your fingers (rub with back of the fingers to opposing palms with fingers interlocked), and under your nails. *Why?:* Lathering and scrubbing hands creates friction, which helps lift dirt, grease, and microbes from the skin. Microbes are present on all surfaces of the hand, often in particularly high concentration on the tips of fingers and under the nails, so the entire hand should be cleaned.

- *Recommendation:* Scrub your hands for at least 20 seconds. *Why?:* Although determining the optimal length of time for handwashing is difficult because few studies about the health impacts of altering handwashing times have been done, the available evidence suggests that washing hands for about 15-30 seconds removes more germs from hands than washing for shorter periods.

- *Recommendation:* Rinse your hands well under clean, running water. *Why?:* Rinsing the hands gets rid of the dirt, grease, and microbes that have been removed from the skin surface and prevents recontamination. Rinsing the soap away also minimizes the risk of skin irritation. Effectively washing and rinsing your hands should take about 30 seconds in total.

- *Recommendation:* Dry your hands using a clean dry towel, single-use disposable paper towel, or an air drier. *Why?:* Germs can be transferred more easily to and from wet hands; therefore, hands should be dried after washing. Using a clean towel, a single-use paper towel, or an air drier minimizes the risk of recontamination. Dirty towels are a haven for germs. See figure 3.1 for an illustration of the handwashing techniques mentioned here. The figure legend provides a brief summary of what to do.

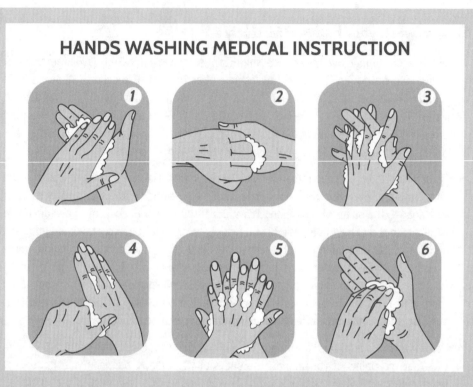

Figure 3.1 The best way to wash your hands to ensure all skin surfaces are cleared of dirt, grease, and germs. This is the technique that medics use: 1. After first wetting your hands with clean running water apply plenty of soap and create lather by rubbing your palms together. 2. Clean the upper parts of your fingers by rubbing with the back of your fingers to the opposing palms with fingers interlocked. 3. Clean between your fingers by interlacing them and moving up and down. 4. Clean your thumbs by clasping your thumb in the opposite hand and making rotational movements. 5. Clean the back of your hand with the opposite palm and interlacing your fingers. 6. Clean the tips of your fingers and under your fingernails by rubbing them into the opposite palm. The whole washing procedure should take about 30 seconds. Now rinse your hands with clear running water and dry them with a clean towel or air drier.

In addition, there are few other things that you can do to minimize your contact with the germs that cause infections. Employ the strategies listed below to reduce your risk of picking up infections:

- Minimize contact with infected people, young children, animals, and contagious objects.

- Avoid crowded areas and shaking hands.

- Keep at distance to people who are coughing, sneezing, or have a "runny nose", and when appropriate wear (or ask them to wear) a disposable mask.

- Protect your airways from being directly exposed to both very cold (below 0 °C) and dry air during outdoor exercise by using a facial mask.

- Do not share drinking bottles, cups, cutlery, towels, etc. with other people.

- When abroad, choose cold beverages from sealed bottles, avoid raw vegetables and undercooked meat. Wash and peel fruit before eating.

- Individuals should be updated on all vaccines needed at home and for foreign travel.

- For diabetic people it is particularly important to have an annual flu vaccine because there is a higher risk of complications such as life-threatening **pneumonia**, particularly in the over 60s. Being vaccinated is our best defense against flu. This has to be done every year (usually in the autumn as the vaccine takes 5-7 weeks to work) because different strains of flu virus become prevalent during winter from year to year. Having the flu vaccine protects you against the flu, and it also helps to protect your own family and the wider community. Typically the flu vaccine will offer protection to 30-60% of the people who have it (in adults it is usually administered by injection). But don't get vaccinated if you are currently suffering from any symptoms of illness; wait until you have recovered.

PRACTICING GOOD FOOD HYGIENE

Another important issue with regard to hygiene is taking care in how you store, prepare, and cook your food. Gastrointestinal infections can be very nasty and may cause bloating, abdominal discomfort, vomiting, and diarrhea that can last for days. These infections are caused primarily by eating food that has become contaminated with bacteria. This can be avoided by applying good hygiene practice. There are four main things to consider: cross-contamination, cleaning, chilling, and cooking. These are known as the 4'Cs and further details, including useful guidance documents and hygiene training videos, can be found on the UK Food Standards Agency website (https://www.food.gov.uk/business-industry/food-hygiene).

CHANGING YOUR DIET AND EATING LESS

Contrary to what many people think, there is no specific recommended diet for the management of type 2 diabetes. Diabetes is not simply caused by eating too much sugar, but rather just too many calories than we actually need. So it is not necessary to cut out all sugar from the diet, although it is best to avoid **sugar-sweetened beverage**s like soft drinks, energy drinks, and sports drinks, as well as candy, cakes, and cookies which generally provide lots of sugar and calories but hardly any useful **nutrient**s. There is also no need to cut out whole **food groups** or **macronutrients**. It is very important to get sufficient protein, **vitamins**, **minerals**, and **phytonutrients**; fat contains some **essential nutrients** including the four fat soluble vitamins (A, D, E, and K) and two **essential fatty acids (linoleic acid** and α-**linolenic acid**) so you should not avoid fat-containing foods altogether. However, it's best to limit your intake of **saturated fat** and – according to some sources of nutritional advice – cholesterol (see the sidebar for more on this issue). This means choosing lean cuts of meat or poultry, grilling or oven roasting them rather than frying them, and cutting down on fried and fatty foods in general. Choose low-fat versions of spreads (or use those that contain **unsaturated fats**), yogurt, and milk (i.e., used skimmed or semi-skimmed milk rather than whole milk). Oily fish are a good healthy source of essential fatty acids and vitamin D so try to include salmon, mackerel, sardines, tuna, or herring on your menu once or twice per week.

People should also cut down on their intake of **salt**. Although salt is not directly related to the risk of type 2 diabetes, a high intake is a known risk factor for high blood pressure and other cardiovascular diseases which are some of the health consequences of type 2 diabetes. Salt is simply sodium chloride (NaCl), and consuming too much **sodium** increases **water retention**, blood volume, and, consequently, raises blood pressure, which is itself a risk factor for cardiovascular disease, including atherosclerosis, coronary heart disease, and stroke. However, salt should not be absent from the diet altogether because its constituents – sodium and chloride – are both essential nutrients, and their recommended daily intakes are 1.5 g of sodium and 2.3 g of chloride which equates to 3.8 g of salt per day. Salt is present as an additive in many processed foods, including bread, cheese, pizza, soups, sauces, canned vegetables, smoked and cured meats as well as in salted nuts, potato chips, and pretzels, and even in natural products including meat, poultry, fish, and seafood. As an upper limit healthy adults are generally advised to ingest no more than 6.0 g of salt (2.3 g sodium) per day, but most people currently consume, on average, about 8.5 g salt per day (3.4 g of sodium) which is equivalent to about one-and-a-half teaspoons of salt. People should choose foods with little salt, prepare food with minimal amounts of salt, and add no more than a pinch of table salt to their food on the plate. Even this can be cut out altogether, though, because you'll find that if you stop adding salt to your food, your taste buds will adapt to it, and soon you won't be missing it.

Is my blood cholesterol too high because my diet contains too much cholesterol?

Cholesterol is a type of fat found in the cell membranes of all animal tissues, and it is transported in the blood mostly in the form of lipoproteins. Cholesterol also aids in the manufacture of **bile** (which is stored in the gallbladder and helps digest fats), is important for the metabolism of fat soluble vitamins, and is the major precursor for the synthesis of vitamin D and various steroid hormones (e.g., cortisol, testosterone, estrogen) so it is something we need in the body. I see many diets that promote eating foods that do not contain any cholesterol, and the US Food and Nutrition Board recommends that we eat "as little as possible". The **daily value** (DV) for cholesterol on nutrition facts labels found on packaged foods indicate that the maximum we should consume is 300 mg per day, and some authorities recommend no more than 200 mg per day for people with diabetes. All this is based on the knowledge that high levels of cholesterol in the blood are bad for our arteries and heart. High levels of LDL-cholesterol in particular are associated with increased risk of coronary heart disease. While all this is true, the normal healthy level of serum total cholesterol is around 5 mmol/L (equivalent to approximately 2,000 mg/L) or less which means that even healthy people have around 6,000 mg (6 g) of cholesterol floating around in their circulation, and that is 20 times the recommended upper level of daily intake. In reality it is not the amount of cholesterol we consume in the diet that has the biggest influence on our blood cholesterol levels because most of the cholesterol in our bodies is actually synthesized in the liver with a relatively small proportion coming from the diet. Blood cholesterol is raised when we consume large amounts of saturated fat so that is the real culprit.

You might think that substituting carbohydrate for saturated fat in your diet might be the solution, but not necessarily so according to recent research. Higher carbohydrate intake is associated with lower serum total cholesterol, but it also lowers HDL-cholesterol (the so called "good cholesterol" that removes fatty deposits from blood vessel walls) which results in a higher total cholesterol/HDL-cholesterol ratio and higher serum triglyceride concentration. Furthermore, the apolipoprotein B (apoB)/apoA-I ratio (which represents the balance of pro-atherogenic and anti-atherogenic lipoproteins) is now known to be superior to any of the cholesterol ratios in predicting risk of coronary heart disease and the apoB/apoA-I ratio has shown to be increased (i.e., made worse) by diets that are very high in carbohydrate. Serum triglyceride, total and LDL cholesterol levels, and the apoB/apoA-I ratio can all be lowered best by changes to diet (i.e., reducing saturated fat and sugar intake, and replacing them with unsaturated fats while maintaining a moderate carbohydrate intake), together with regular aerobic exercise. For chronically high serum cholesterol levels medication with drugs called statins is very effective. These drugs inhibit the synthesis of cholesterol by the liver.

As for carbohydrate, try to choose high-**fiber** food sources such as wholegrain bread, cereals, brown rice, and non-starchy vegetables like lentils, broccoli, cauliflower, kale, and **gourd**s such as aubergine (eggplant), squash, and zucchini (courgette). Choose fruit with low-fat yogurt rather than puddings, pies, cake, and ice cream for dessert. Eat three regular meals per day, and try to avoid snacking as much as possible. Cut out cookies and sweets, as well as chips, salted nuts, pretzels, and other salty foods as too much salt in the diet (more than 6 g/day) is a risk factor for hypertension. If you really want a snack try a crispy vegetable instead like celery, cucumber, or carrot. Occasionally, but not more than twice per week, you can treat yourself to a few bites of dark chocolate.

A healthy diet is often referred to as a balanced diet that emphasizes the need for variety and moderation so that all the essential nutrients can be supplied in sufficient amounts to support normal or optimal functioning. But how do we achieve a balanced diet? Well, the answer comes from some simple and comprehensive food guides that have been developed and progressively evolved by various expert groups of nutritionists during the past 100 years. In the USA a food guide called **MyPlate** was introduced in 2011 (figure 3.2) and is an integral part of the latest 2015-2020 Dietary Guidelines for Americans produced by the US Department of Agriculture's Food and Nutrition Service. In the UK a somewhat more detailed guide called the **Eatwell Guide** became available in 2016 (figure 3.3).

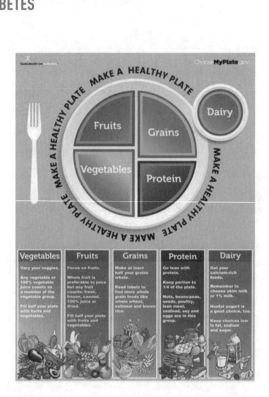

Figure 3.2 MyPlate *from the USA. From the US Department of Agriculture's Center for Nutrition Policy and Promotion.*

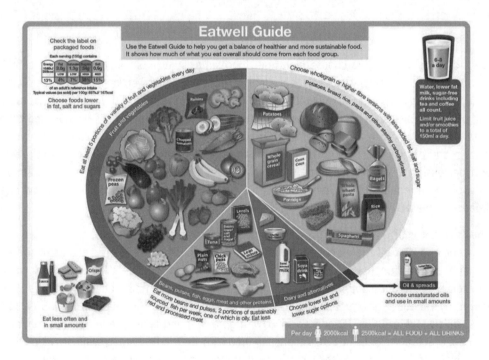

Figure 3.3 The Eatwell Guide *from the United Kingdom. © Crown copyright material is reproduced with the permission of the Controller of HMSO and Queen's Printer for Scotland.*

Some general guidelines for healthy eating based on these food
following sidebar. For further details see my book *Eat, Move, Sleep*
this topic in chapter 7.

Ten guidelines that summarize how to achieve a ba diet

1. Eat meals at regular times of the day. Don't skip breakfast, and don't eat snacks between meals.

2. Eat at least five portions of a variety of fruit and vegetables every day. Recently up to 10 portions per day has been shown to be associated with even lower risk of cardiovascular disease.

3. Try to choose a variety of different foods from the six basic food groups. That means including ones from the milk group (e.g., milk, cheese, yogurt), the meat group (e.g., meat, fish, poultry, and eggs, with dried legumes and nuts as alternatives), fruits, vegetables, and the breads and cereals group, and limited amounts of oils and fats.

4. The main source of energy for meals should come from potatoes, bread, rice, pasta, or other starchy carbohydrates. However, you should have only small to medium portions of these and choose wholegrain or higher fiber produce where possible.

5. Choose lower-fat and lower-sugar options where available for things like dairy products, coleslaw, yogurts, etc.

6. Eat some beans, pulses, fish, eggs, meat, and other high-protein foods. Aim for two portions of fish every week, one of which should be oily, such as salmon or mackerel.

7. Choose unsaturated oils and spreads, but only eat them in small amounts.

8. Drink plenty of fluids (six to eight cups or glasses per day are recommended), particularly water (plain, mineral, or soda), low calorie (diet or light) versions of popular beverages (e.g., cola, lemonade, and tonic water) and fruit juices with no added sugar. Tea and coffee are also fine in moderation, but if you like them to taste sweet use an artificial sweetener rather than sugar.

9. Limit your intake of alcohol by drinking no more than one 175 mL glass of wine or 350 mL beer with your main meal of the day, and on no more than five days of the week.

10. Try to limit foods and drinks that are high in fat, salt, and sugar by having these less often and in small amounts.

llow the guidelines and eat a healthy, balanced diet then supplements are usually cessary. However, there is no harm in taking a daily multivitamin tablet that contains all of e 13 essential vitamins and provides a dose equivalent to 100% of the **recommended dietary allowance** (RDA). One exception to this general rule is vitamin D. Vitamin D plays an important role in promoting immunity, helping the absorption of dietary calcium, and maintaining bone health. This is a concern as vitamin D insufficiency is common in people especially in situations where exposure to natural sunlight is limited (e.g., during the winter months or when living or working mostly indoors). Most of the vitamin D in our bodies is made in the skin and requires exposure to the ultraviolet (UV) rays from the sun; only about 10-20% of our vitamin D comes from the diet. I recommend a vitamin D3 supplement of 1,000 to 4,000 IU/day which is equivalent to 25-100 micrograms (µg)/day to optimize immune function from October to April in Northern hemisphere countries at latitudes of 48°North (equivalent to Paris in France and the USA-Canada border) and above since the skin is unable to form vitamin D between the months of October through to March because the sunlight is not strong enough.

CHOOSING LOW GLYCEMIC INDEX OR LOW GLYCEMIC LOAD FOODS

You may have heard that low glycemic index foods are a good choice for people with diabetes. It is true that low glycemic index foods may be helpful in the management of type 2 diabetes. The **glycemic index** (GI) is a measure of how quickly a food causes a rise in your blood sugar (figure 3.4). Foods with a high GI raise your blood sugar quickly. Low GI foods are digested and absorbed more slowly which helps you achieve a more stable level of blood sugar. Foods with a low GI typically are foods that are higher in fiber. Diets that are based on the low GI principle have also been linked to reduced risks for cancer, heart disease, and other conditions. A low GI diet is an eating plan based on how the foods you eat (in particular the items that are your main sources of carbohydrate) affect your blood sugar level. For this reason it is a good choice for managing type 2 diabetes, but it is not a diet plan that has been specifically designed for weight loss. There are much better diets available for losing body fat and body weight, and these will be discussed in detail later in this book.

The GI is a system of assigning a number to carbohydrate-containing foods according to how much each food increases your blood sugar. The GI values are based on experimental studies that have examined the impact of individual food items on the blood sugar level and how much it is increased over the two hours following a portion of the food item that contains 50 g carbohydrate compared with ingesting 50 g of pure glucose (which has the highest possible GI of 100). For example, boiled potato has an average GI of 80 relative to glucose, which means that the blood glucose response to the carbohydrate in a weight of potato containing 50 g carbohydrate (which will be in the form of starch) is 80% of the blood glucose response to the same amount of carbohydrate in pure glucose. In contrast, boiled chickpeas have an average GI of 28 relative to glucose. The GI itself is not a diet plan but a useful tool to guide food choices. The GI principle was in fact first developed as a strategy for guiding food choices for people with diabetes. An international GI database is maintained by Sydney University Glycemic Index Research Services in Sydney, Australia (available at https://www.researchdata.ands.org.au/international-glycemic-index-gi-database/11115). The

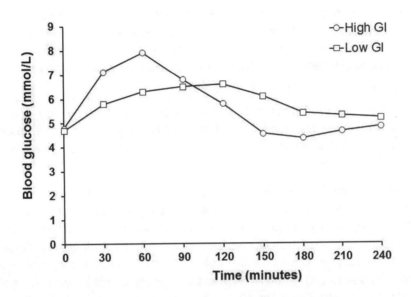

Figure 3.4 The blood glucose response to consuming a high or low glycemic index (GI) food containing 50 g carbohydrate. The GI is a measure of how quickly a food causes a rise in your blood sugar. Foods with a high GI raise your blood sugar quickly to relatively high levels. Low GI foods are digested and absorbed more slowly which results in a slower and smaller rise in blood sugar.

database contains the results of studies conducted there and at other research facilities around the world and provides an extensive list of foods and their GI values. In general, the GI value is based on how much a food item raises blood glucose levels compared with how much pure glucose raises blood glucose. GI values are generally divided into three categories:

- Low GI: 1 to 55.

- Medium GI: 56 to 69.

- High GI: 70 and higher up to a maximum of 100.

Obviously, foods that contain very little or no carbohydrate like meat, fish, poultry, nuts, oils, etc. have a zero GI value. Examples of foods with low, middle, and high GI values include the following:

- Low GI: Green vegetables, most fruits (including apple, cherries, grapefruit, grapes, orange, pear, plum, persimmon, strawberries), tomato, raw carrots, kidney beans, chickpeas, lentils, sweetcorn, milk, muesli, brown rice, spaghetti, and bran breakfast cereals.

- Medium GI: Couscous, muffin, fruit loaf, bananas, raw pineapple, raisins, cookies, oat breakfast cereals, and multigrain, oat bran, or rye bread.

- High GI: White rice, white bread, potatoes, pancakes, pizza, scones, cornflakes, watermelon, jellybeans, and candy.

People with type 2 diabetes should generally avoid foods in the high GI category or have only small portions of them that are consumed with low GI foods. All the low GI foods are good, and a selection of medium GI foods can also be consumed. Some of the foods in the medium GI category such as oat breakfast cereals (choose the no added sugar versions) can have other benefits like helping to lower your serum cholesterol.

The low GI diet is a specific diet plan that uses the index as the primary or only guide for meal planning. Comparing GI values, therefore, can help guide healthier food choices. For example, an English muffin made with white wheat flour has a GI value of 77 whereas a whole-wheat English muffin has a GI value of 45.

However, there are several limitations to GI values and probably the most important one is that they do not reflect the likely quantity you would eat of a particular food. In other words, the GI is based on the blood glucose response to consuming 50 g of carbohydrate. But typical portion sizes of many foods, including some high GI ones, contain far less carbohydrate than this and so, in reality, the blood glucose response will actually be rather small. For example, ripe watermelon has quite a high GI value of 75, which would put it in the category of food to avoid. But watermelon has relatively little digestible carbohydrate in a typical serving – a typical slice of watermelon (120 g or 4 oz) only contains 8 g of carbohydrate (most of watermelon is water). In other words, you have to eat a lot of watermelon (about 6 slices or more than a pound of watermelon in fact) to significantly raise your blood glucose level (figure 3.5) which is far more than the average person eats.

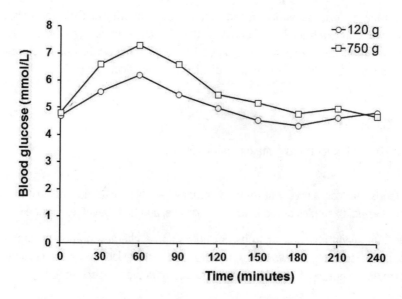

Figure 3.5 The blood glucose response to consuming a typical portion of watermelon (a 120 g slice) compared with consuming the amount of watermelon (about 750 g or 6 slices) that contains 50 g carbohydrate (the amount used to determine the GI).

To address this problem, nutrition scientists have developed the idea of **glycemic load (GL)**, a numerical value that indicates the change in blood glucose levels when you eat a typical serving of the food. Glycemic load is calculated by multiplying the grams of available carbohydrate in the food (for a typical serving size) by the food's GI and then dividing by 100. For example, a 120 g serving of watermelon has a GI value of 75 and a typical serving (one slice) contains 8 g carbohydrate so:

$$\text{GL of watermelon} = (\text{GI x g Carbohydrate})/100 = (75 \times 8)/100 = 6$$

A GL value of only 6 puts it in the healthy food choice category. Sydney University's table of GI values also includes GL values. The values are generally grouped in the following manner:

- Low GL: 1 to 10.

- Medium GL: 11 to 19.

- High GL: 20 or more.

Examples of foods with low, middle, and high GL values include the following:

- Low GL: Green vegetables, most fruits (including apple, cherries, grapefruit, grapes, orange, pear, plum, strawberries), raw carrots, kidney beans, chickpeas, lentils, pizza, milk, muesli, brown rice, fruit loaf, scones, watermelon, tomato, and bran breakfast cereals.

- Medium GL: White bread, boiled potato, sweet corn, couscous, muffin, doughnut, bananas, raw pineapple, persimmon, cookies, oat breakfast cereals, and multigrain, oat bran, or rye bread.

- High GL: White rice, baked potato, pancakes, raisins, cornflakes, spaghetti, jellybeans, and candy.

Because the GL takes into account the amount of carbohydrate consumed in a typical serving, it makes sense to use the GL in preference to the GI for diet planning. However, even when using the GL rather than the GI there are still several other important limitations:

- The GI or GL value tells us nothing about other nutritional information. For example, whole milk has a GI value of 31 and a GL value of 4 for a 250 mL serving. But because of its high-fat content, whole milk is not the best choice for weight loss or weight control; semi-skimmed or skimmed milk are better.

- The published GI database is not an exhaustive list of foods, but a list of those foods that have been studied. Many healthy foods with low GI values are not in the database.

- The GI value of any food item is affected by several factors, including how the food is prepared, how it is processed, and what other foods are eaten at the same time.

- Also, there can be a range in GI values for the same foods (depending for example on ripeness of fruits or different formulations by different manufacturers), and some nutritionists argue it makes it an unreliable guide to determine food choices.

Even with these limitations selecting foods based on their GI or GL value is a good choice for people with type 2 diabetes whose priority is trying to keep their blood glucose levels relatively low and stable. Choosing foods with low GI or GL may help you manage your weight because many foods that should be included in a well-balanced, low-fat, healthy diet with minimally processed foods – wholegrain products, fruits, vegetables, and low-fat dairy products – have low GI and GL values. Avoiding high GI and GL foods generally means eliminating candy, chocolate, sugar-sweetened beverages, most sauces, many processed foods, starchy vegetables like baked potato, as well as white rice and processed bread from your diet.

BECOMING MORE PHYSICALLY ACTIVE

Everyone needs regular aerobic exercise to achieve **optimal health** (i.e., having a state of health that is as good as it can be) and reduce their risk of developing cardiovascular disease, metabolic syndrome, **dementia**, and several forms of cancer – people who have type 2 diabetes are no exception. In fact, if you have this condition it is even more important that you do some exercise. Exercise is good for management of both type 1 and type 2 diabetes. Exercise has numerous benefits and the diabetic should take advantage of these benefits. People with type 1 or type 2 diabetes are capable of undertaking a wide array of exercise activities, and there are no contraindications to most sports for diabetic people. Indeed, competition at the highest level is possible. Examples of outstanding sportspeople with type 1 diabetes include Gary Hall Jr, Sir Steven Redgrave, and Pamela Fernandes. Hall is an American former competition swimmer who represented the United States at the 1996, 2000, and 2004 Olympics and won ten Olympic medals. He is a former world record-holder in two relay events. Redgrave is a retired British rower who won gold medals at five consecutive Olympic Games from 1984 to 2000. He has also won three Commonwealth Games gold medals and nine World Rowing Championships golds. He is the most successful male rower in Olympic history, and the only man to have won gold medals at five Olympic Games in an endurance sport. Pamela Fedrnandes is perhaps the most notable female athlete with diabetes. She was diagnosed with type 1 diabetes at the age of four and lost her sight by the time she was 18. A native of Connecticut, she won the gold medal at the 2000 Sydney Paralympic Games and amassed an impressive collection of medals and awards in her nine years of competing in elite Paralympic sport.

As you can imagine there are very few, if any, real athletes who are type 2 diabetics, simply because there are not many sports where being overweight helps. One possible exception is sumo wrestling. Some professional boxers tend to balloon in weight in between fights, and some of the older ones may well be type 2 diabetic or will soon become diabetic when they retire. It is common to see several top players of the games of darts, pool, and snooker looking decidedly overweight and probably several of the older competitors/former competitors in these non-athletic sports are type 2 diabetics. However, apart from sumo wrestling, being overweight is not actually a requirement for success in these sports!

So what sort of exercise should you do? I recommend that you choose activities that you know you will enjoy, such as walking, dancing, swimming, and cycling. What's most important is making physical activity part of your daily routine. Take the opportunities for activity that arise during

everyday life. Cycle or walk to your place of work if po
minutes' walk away and do the rest on foot. In the m
rather than the escalator or lift. Aim for at least 30
the week. Remember that all forms of physical activi
movement (e.g., walking around the house, climbin
chores, etc.) in addition to any sport or organize
don't need to do the 30 minutes all in one go;
over the course of the day. Stretching and stre..
research indicates that a combination of exercises – aero..
on most days, combined with resistance training, such as weightii..
per week – often helps control blood sugar more effectively than either ty
And you don't have to go to the gym to lift weights or do resistance exercise. Th
incorporated into your normal routine. For example, you could add some weight to your vacu..
cleaner or lawn mower to work out your arms, carry a basket around the department store rather
than using a trolley, or perform arm movements for a few minutes while holding a two to five
kilogram weight in the comfort of your house or garden.

Exercise is good for type 2 diabetics because physical activity lowers blood sugar and exercise
is known to improve **insulin sensitivity** independent of weight loss. This is because when the
muscles contract, their uptake of glucose from the blood increases several fold and, unlike at rest,
this uptake does not require the action of insulin. In fact, exercise increases glucose uptake via an
insulin-independent mechanism involving the rise in the intracellular calcium ion concentration
that initiates every single muscle contraction (figure 3.6). The repeated increases in calcium ions
in the muscle stimulate glucose transporters (called GLUT4) to become inserted into the muscle
fiber membrane, and these transport glucose molecules from the blood into the cell to be used
as a fuel for exercise.

Furthermore, after a single bout of moderate-intensity aerobic exercise, the muscle's sensitivity to
insulin is increased for several hours. Performing regular exercise (that's three or more times per
week) results in adaptations which further increase insulin sensitivity in the resting state. And
there's more: Exercise also burns fat and some of this fat comes from the breakdown of fat that
is stored in the belly region. Expending energy (calories) with exercise helps with weight loss or
maintenance. Regular light to moderate-intensity exercise also confers with other health benefits
that are listed in the following sidebar.

Regular exercise can also help to reduce blood pressure in people suffering from hypertension,
a common condition in type 2 diabetics. Research suggests that the best mode of exercise for
people with high blood pressure is swimming. Lying on your back (supine for backstroke) or front
(prone for crawl and breaststroke) and the buoyancy that water gives you allows your heart rate
to increase as in other forms of aerobic (cardio) exercise but your blood pressure does not increase
like it does in most other modes of exercise (e.g., running, cycling). Hence, people who suffer
from hypertension can swim at an appropriate moderate intensity that will provide excellent
health benefits (figure 3.7). However, people should also include some weight-bearing exercise
and resistance exercise into their weekly routine to help maintain their bone density as swimming
does not help with this aspect of health.

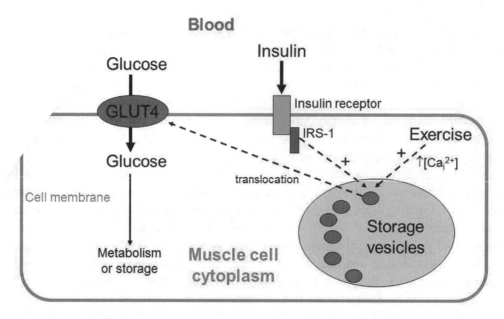

Figure 3.6 Glucose uptake from blood into muscle is stimulated by insulin at rest but exercise itself stimulates glucose uptake via a calcium mediated mechanism that does not require the presence of insulin. Both insulin and calcium ions, independently, stimulate the movement of GLUT4 glucose transporter proteins to move from intracellular vesicles to the cell membrane which allows glucose transport to take place. IRS-1: Insulin receptor substrate 1.

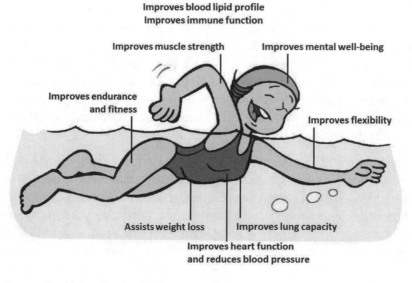

Figure 3.7 The many health benefits of swimming.

Check with your doctor that it is OK for you to start doing more exercise. If you haven't been active for a while, start slowly and build up gradually. Check your blood sugar level before any activity. You might need to eat a snack before exercising to help prevent low blood sugar if you take diabetes medications (including insulin) that lower your blood sugar.

Other reasons why exercise is good for your overall health

- In both healthy people and those with type 2 diabetes, high levels of physical activity are associated with a reduced risk of coronary heart disease and all-cause mortality.

- Regular physical activity can favorably modify cardiovascular disease risk factors including the apoB/apoA-I ratio, LDL/HDL ratio, serum cholesterol, and triglyceride, hypertension, and obesity.

- High levels of physical activity reduce the risk of stroke.

- Regular physical activity can lower but not necessarily normalize blood pressure in individuals who suffer from hypertension.

- High levels of physical activity are associated with lower risk of **colon** and breast cancer.

- Exercise is known to be good for mental health. High levels of physical activity are associated with a lower risk of depression, cognitive decline, and dementia in older adults.

- Regular moderate physical activity improves some aspects of immune function and is associated with reduced incidence of respiratory infection such as the common cold. Physical activity improves vaccination responses in the elderly.

- Physical activity enhances physical function and improves quality of life in those suffering from chronic heart failure, **chronic obstructive pulmonary disease**, depression, intermittent claudication (narrowing or blockage in the main arteries taking blood to the legs), **osteoarthritis**, and **osteoporosis**.

Buying a step counter or fitness tracker is a good idea and a good target to aim for is 10,000 steps per day. If you achieve that you will have covered around 7 kilometers (4.5 miles) and burned about 500 calories. You can keep a record of the number of steps you do each day in a diary or notebook.

BLOOD GLUCOSE SELF-MONITORING

One of the major health risks for diabetics is having high blood sugar levels. Knowing what your blood sugar levels are by occasionally testing your blood can help to manage your diabetes and reduces your risk of having serious complications – now and in the future. You can check your blood glucose concentration yourself by collecting a drop of blood from a fingertip and placing it onto a test strip that you place into a portable glucose monitor. Alternatively you can use a flash glucose monitor which is a sensor that you wear on your skin to measure the concentration of glucose in the **interstitial fluid** surrounding your cells. This gives an approximation of the concentration of glucose in your blood but it's not 100% accurate, so you'll still need to do a finger-prick test every now and again. For some people a more expensive continuous glucose monitor may be advised if your physician thinks it is necessary. You can do a blood glucose test several times each day to keep an eye on your levels as you go about your life and to help you work out what and when to eat and how much medication or insulin to take. Not everyone with type 2 diabetes needs to check their levels like this, but you will need to do so if you are on insulin therapy and certain other forms of diabetes medication such as sulfonylureas. Your healthcare team will advise you on whether to check your blood glucose levels, how to do this safely, and how often.

Regular checks of your current blood glucose concentration can help you know when you your levels might be starting to get too low (hypoglycemia or just hypo for short) or too high (hyperglycemia or hyper). If you make a note of your results in a diary or a chart it can help both you and your healthcare team spot patterns in the daily changes of your blood sugar which might allow suggestions as to how to improve your blood sugar stability. But more importantly, it will help you stay healthy and markedly reduce your risk of serious diabetes complications (described in chapter 1) developing in the near future. The higher your blood glucose levels are and the longer they're high for, the more at risk you are of the nasty consequences such as sight loss, limb amputation, stroke, kidney, and heart disease. Nobody likes the thought of having to do regular blood sampling, but don't worry: it is safe and virtually painless if you do it correctly as described in the following sidebar.

Fingertip blood sampling and using a blood glucose monitor

Measuring your blood glucose concentration with a drop of blood taken from a fingertip gives you an indication of your blood sugar level at that particular moment in time. It's a snapshot. Your diabetic nurse or another member of your healthcare team will show you how to do the test and it's important that you learn how to do it properly – otherwise you could get the wrong results. For most people, finger-prick testing isn't a problem and it quickly becomes part of their normal routine. For some people it can be a stressful experience, and that's totally understandable, but usually it's the initial thought of having to do it that puts people off, and when they have done it a few times the worries and stress go away.

In order to do the test you will need a blood glucose testing meter, a finger-prick device, a disposable lancet (a very short, fine needle), some test strips, and a sharps bin, so you can safely dispose of the lancet (which you should only use once).

How to do a finger-prick blood glucose test

Your diabetic nurse or healthcare assistant will show you how to do a fingertip blood glucose test correctly and safely the first time, but the key steps in the process follow:

1. Wash your hands with soap and warm water and dry them with a clean towel, paper tissue, or air blower. Make sure your hands are warm as it will be easier to get blood and won't hurt as much.

2. Take a test strip (these usually come in batches of 50 and must work with the type of meter you're using) and slot it into the meter to turn it on. Some meters have tests strips built in.

3. Remove the cap from your finger-prick device and put in a new lancet (a fine needle that will be used to prick your finger so that a drop of blood can be taken for testing). You can adjust the device to change how far it goes into the skin. The setting will depend on the thickness of your skin. Lancets come in different sizes and thicknesses (or gauges). A higher-gauge lancet is thinner so is normally less painful, but it might not always give you enough blood. You'll soon know which is best for you.

4. Replace the cap and set the device by pulling or clicking the plunger. Choose which finger to prick, but it is best to avoid your thumb or index finger and don't prick too close to a fingernail. Place the device against the side of your finger and press the plunger (photo 3.3). Use a different finger each time and a different area.

5. Touch the drop of blood on the tip of your finger to the test strip, and place it in the meter which should beep if the test strip has been sufficiently filled (photo 3.4).

6. It will take a few seconds for the meter to display your blood glucose reading so while you are waiting check your finger and use a clean tissue to stop any bleeding; then use it to take out the lancet and dispose of it in your sharps bin.

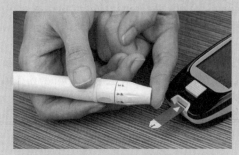

Photo 3.3: Collecting a fingertip blood sample using a finger-prick device containing a lancet.

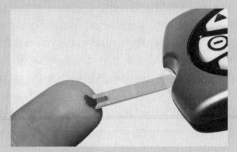

Photo 3.4: Transferring blood from a fingertip to a test strip that has been inserted into a blood glucose meter.

- When your meter shows the result in millimoles per liter (usually abbreviated as mmol/L or mM), write it down.

- Now remove the used test strip (they can only be used once) and dispose of it. Taking out the strip will usually turn the meter off.

Keep a record of your readings in a diary, a notebook, or a chart, or store it in the memory of your meter if it is one that lets you do this. There are now some diabetes apps that you can download to your mobile phone or tablet to make a record of your blood glucose measurements. If you keep a regular up-to-date record of your readings you can show it to your healthcare professional, and they will be able to see if you need to adjust your treatment. Everyone will have a particular target range which will be set by your healthcare advisor, but as a general guide for someone with type 2 diabetes your blood glucose concentration should be between 4.0 and 7.0 mmol/L before meals and be less than 9.0 mmol/L two hours after a meal. You can also use your blood sugar level to establish whether you need to eat something before bedtime, before you do some exercise, before going out or for a drive in your car.

WILL I GET BETTER?

If you take the medication prescribed by your doctor exactly as instructed, attend your regular monitoring appointments, carry out self-monitoring by measuring your blood pressure and inspecting your feet, and manage your type 2 diabetes by practicing good personal hygiene, eating a healthier diet, and doing more exercise – you will not get better. I'll hazard a guess that that is not what you expecting to hear. Taking your diabetes medication, doing the monitoring, and improving your diet and lifestyle will slow the progress of your disease but will not make it go away. These changes will help to delay a worsening of your condition and will, to some degree, reduce your risk of developing the awful potential complications of coronary heart disease, stroke, blindness, and foot amputation that are likely to affect the untreated diabetic a few years down the line. But the changes you make will not cure your type 2 diabetes, and you will still be at considerably higher risk than the nondiabetic for these complications. For example, remember that in chapter 1 it was mentioned that the relative risk of coronary heart disease, kidney disease, blindness, and foot amputation was 2, 3, 5 and 13 times more likely for the type 2 diabetic than the nondiabetic? Well those figures are based on all type 2 diabetics and include those who are not good at managing their blood glucose as well as those that are.

Feeling down and depressed about that? If your answer is yes and you want to do something about it, there is a solution that recent research has shown can work for many people with type 2 diabetes. And it's simple. The solution is weight loss. In the 1990s several studies of weight loss (bariatric) surgery carried out on morbidly obese people with type 2 diabetes showed that their elevated blood sugar levels dropped dramatically (though still stayed above normal) within days of the surgery. Subsequent dramatic weight loss over the following months resulted in further falls in blood sugar levels and many of them were able to come off their diabetic medication. Clearly there is a link between being overweight through overeating and type 2 diabetes that can be reversed by weight loss and reduced dietary energy intake. Now, I am not advocating weight loss surgery for everyone with type 2 diabetes; that is really only for people who are extremely obese and any form of major surgery has a risk of death due to shock, sepsis, or infection. For the vast majority, sufficient weight loss can be achieved through dieting or a combination of dieting and doing more exercise. For many people with type 2 diabetes, sufficient weight loss will mean losing 5-15 kg of body fat.

So if you aim to lose a substantial amount of that accumulation of body fat that has been the main cause of your condition – you can get better and rid yourself of type 2 diabetes. It will take willpower because you will have to reduce your calorie intake for quite some time (we are talking several months here) to achieve sufficient weight loss and, of course, how much weight each person will have to lose will very much depend on what their current weight is. Weight loss can be achieved by dieting alone, but research indicates that a combination of decreasing food energy intake through dieting and increasing energy intake by exercising is more effective. Exercise has other advantages as well. The other health benefits have already been mentioned in this chapter but doing exercise will also help maintain your muscle mass and **resting metabolic rate** during a period of energy deficit making it easier to stop the weight being put back on when you stop dieting. How to achieve this weight loss and beat type 2 diabetes is covered in chapters 8 and 9. Before we get to that, in the next chapter I'll explain the likely reasons you developed type 2 diabetes in the first place.

Key Points

- Everyone living with type 2 diabetes or metabolic syndrome needs to have regular monitoring to keep their condition stable and delay the onset of health complications. Some of this monitoring can be self-administered, but some aspects require a 3-monthly, 6-monthly, or annual visit to see a physician or a diabetes nurse.

- Monitoring involves analysis of a sample of your blood to measure levels of HbA1c, cholesterol, lipoproteins, triglycerides, thyroid function, liver function, and kidney function. The doctor or nurse will also assess your blood pressure and the condition of your feet. You will also undergo a retinal scan by an eye specialist.

- Self-monitoring can include regularly measuring your body weight and blood pressure and inspecting your feet.

- Other than taking prescribed drugs to help control your blood sugar, management of type 2 diabetes includes maintaining good care of your feet, practicing good personal hygiene, eating a healthy diet, and being more physically active.

- Eating a healthier diet is often advised for people with type 2 diabetes. A healthy diet is a balanced diet that emphasizes the need for variety and moderation so that all the essential nutrients can be supplied in sufficient amounts to support normal or optimal functioning. A healthy diet includes an emphasis on high-fiber foods (i.e., fruit and vegetables) and a limited intake of saturated fats, sugar, starchy vegetables, and salt.

- Carbohydrate food sources with a low glycemic index or (better still) low glycemic load can assist the type 2 diabetic in maintaining a more stable blood sugar level, but there are more effective diets if the goal is weight loss.

- Regular aerobic exercise can also help with blood glucose control as exercise increases muscle glucose uptake and increases insulin sensitivity. Exercise also burns fat and reduces the risk of other diseases including coronary heart disease, hypertension, stroke, dementia, and some cancers.

Chapter 4

What Causes Type 2 Diabetes?

Objectives

After studying this chapter, you should:

- Understand some of the suggested causes of type 2 diabetes.

- Appreciate the differences between insulin resistance and impaired insulin secretion and know why both must occur in the development of type 2 diabetes.

- Know what the main risk factors are for developing type 2 diabetes.

- Appreciate which of these risk factors are modifiable by changes to diet, exercise, and other lifestyle behaviors.

Type 2 diabetes is associated with two physiological defects: insulin resistance and impaired insulin secretion. However, the disease is not static and evolves over many years and progresses through multiple stages (figure 4.1). Although there is some controversy about the precise sequence of events in the natural progression of type 2 diabetes, the most common scenario is that peripheral insulin resistance develops relatively early in the course of the disease. The first tissue to develop insulin resistance is skeletal muscle, particularly in people who are not physically active. So long as the pancreatic β-cells retain sufficient functional reserve, plasma insulin levels will rise to compensate for the insulin resistance so that blood glucose remains relatively normal. Nevertheless, the compensation may not be complete, and some people may develop an elevated fasting glucose concentration (hyperglycemia).

While your muscles develop more insulin resistance and take up less glucose, more of the sugar is taken up by adipose tissue and you get fatter still. Later there is a progressive development of insulin resistance in adipose tissue and finally the liver. As the disease continues to evolve, impairment in the ability of the β-cells to secrete insulin reaches the point where the impaired β-cell function can no longer compensate for the preexisting insulin resistance. In part, this fall in insulin secretion is thought to be due to an accumulation of fat in the pancreas itself. This is usually when prediabetes becomes full-blown type 2 diabetes. Ultimately, it is the liver's glucose production and release that determines the magnitude of the elevation in fasting plasma glucose. Thus, in the final stage in the evolution of type 2 diabetes, the liver becomes insulin resistant, and this (combined with peripheral insulin resistance plus impaired insulin secretion) results in severe hyperglycemia and an inability to resolve the problem without resort to medication. The proportion of insulin resistance versus β-cell dysfunction differs among individuals, with some type 2 diabetics having primarily insulin resistance and only a minor defect in insulin secretion, and others with slight insulin resistance and primarily a lack of insulin secretion. This is one of the reasons why different medications and doses vary from one diabetic person to another.

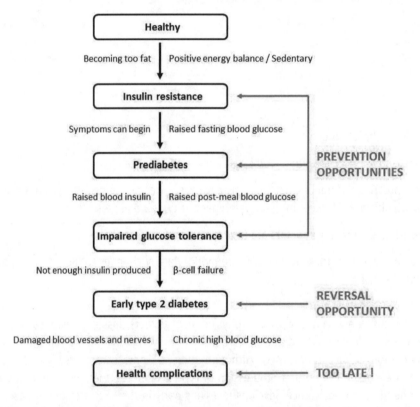

Figure 4.1 Progression from good health to type 2 diabetes via several stages showing the various opportunities for intervention to prevent or reverse the development of full-blown type 2 diabetes and the inevitable serious health consequences that would follow.

When we ask, "What causes type 2 diabetes?" we can attempt to answer this question in two ways: We can consider the factors that are known to increase the risk of diabetes, or we can examine what actually happens in the body, as a mechanism, before a diagnosis of type 2 diabetes is made. In this chapter we will look at both these approaches, starting with the possible mechanisms.

Much research time and money has been devoted to trying to discover the molecular mechanisms involved in development of type 2 diabetes, and in particular what actually causes the initial increase in peripheral tissue insulin resistance and the later reduction in pancreatic insulin secretion. Knowing the answers to these important questions would allow the development of more targeted and effective medication, but at present the answers remain elusive, although several theories are currently under intense investigation. The following section describes some of the popular current theories in simplified terms.

POSSIBLE MECHANISMS LEADING TO INSULIN RESISTANCE IN PREDIABETES AND TYPE 2 DIABETES

The molecular causes of type 2 diabetes are not well understood. The causes of type 2 diabetes are complex, and it is likely that several different mechanisms are responsible for the development of the disease. The condition results from a combination of lifestyle and genetic factors, some of which have not yet been identified. Both type 1 diabetes and type 2 diabetes are characterized by impaired insulin signaling and hyperglycemia which are thought to be the main culprits of the disease's damage to blood vessels, nerves, and organs. Some of the theories about the cause of insulin resistance that have received the most attention are summarized in figure 4.2 and described in detail next. The consequences of insulin resistance are described in the sidebar.

REDUCED NUMBERS OF INSULIN RECEPTORS IN TARGET TISSUES

Repeated large elevations of plasma insulin (known as **hyperinsulinemia**), due to consuming too many starchy and sugary foods and sugar-sweetened beverages, results in decreased expression of insulin receptors in the target tissues (a phenomenon known as receptor "**downregulation**") making the tissues less responsive to insulin. When insulin binds to its receptor on the target cell membrane, the cell internalizes the complex, digesting the attached insulin and recycling most of the receptors to the membrane surface. At chronically high insulin levels, this recycling can exhaust the receptors, such that very few remain on the cell surface to respond to further increases in insulin.

INHIBITION OF INSULIN ACTION RESULTING FROM INFLAMMATION IN ADIPOSE TISSUE

Most patients with type 2 diabetes are obese, and the increase in adiposity is believed to be an important causal factor in the development of insulin resistance. In people who are not overweight the amount of adipose tissue is relatively small and contains small adipocytes and some anti-inflammatory cells such as **T-regulatory lymphocytes** and **M2 macrophages**. Physical inactivity and positive energy balance lead to an accumulation of adipose tissue (particularly **visceral fat stores**) with expanded adipocytes which become infiltrated by pro-inflammatory immune cells called **M1 macrophages** and activated T lymphocytes. Adipose tissue then becomes inflamed and releases pro-inflammatory chemical messengers called **cytokines** (or **adipokines**) such as **tumor necrosis factor alpha** (TNF-α) and **interleukin-8** (IL-8) that lead to a state of persistent low-grade systemic inflammation which inhibits insulin action. This promotes the development of insulin resistance. TNF-α levels are increased in adipose tissue and in the circulation, in obese and insulin-resistant states. TNF-α inhibits the activation of an important molecule in the insulin signaling cascade called insulin receptor substrate 1 (IRS-1), which decreases insulin signaling in adipose tissue and skeletal muscle leading to decreased insulin sensitivity (i.e., insulin resistance).

DECREASED PRODUCTION OF ADIPONECTIN

The development of an inflamed state in adipose tissue also decreases the secretion of anti-inflammatory adipokines like **adiponectin**. Adiponectin is a hormone-like protein which is produced by adipose tissue and is involved in regulating blood glucose levels as well as fatty acid breakdown. The actions of adiponectin increase insulin sensitivity by promoting fatty acid oxidation and inhibiting of liver glucose production. These actions lower circulating fatty acid and glucose levels, respectively.

ELEVATED LEVELS OF PLASMA FREE FATTY ACIDS

The increase in adipose tissue in overweight people is also associated with an increase in plasma free fatty acid levels. This increase in levels promotes glucose production by the liver and inhibits the uptake and utilization of glucose by tissues (causing insulin resistance). Free fatty acids also stimulate **toll-like receptors** that are located on the cell membranes of monocytes and macrophages (types of white blood cells or **leukocytes** found, respectively, in the blood and tissues) which initiate inflammation and promote the production of cytokines such as TNF-α which inhibits insulin action.

ELEVATED LEVELS OF PLASMA TRIGLYCERIDES

High-fat diets are known to induce obesity and insulin resistance in both animals and humans. Obesity is accompanied by elevated levels of circulating triglycerides and free fatty acids that come from increased adipose tissue mass. Triglycerides stored in fat cells (adipocytes) are broken down into fatty acids, and these are taken up into the pancreatic β-cells, where they generate signals to increase insulin secretion, resulting in elevated blood insulin levels. This signaling cascade is initiated within the cytoplasm of the β-cell by the attachment of **coenzyme A** (CoA) to the fatty acids, forming long-chain acyl-CoA. Acyl-CoA itself is a potent signaling molecule and is also the precursor of other important signaling molecules such as **diglycerides**. In pancreatic β-cells, acyl-CoA has been shown to directly stimulate insulin secretion.

To explore the importance of long-chain acyl-CoA in the development of diabetes, researchers studying rodent models have replaced dietary long-chain triglycerides with medium-chain triglycerides, which are rapidly oxidized in the **mitochondria** and thus do not generate cytoplasmic acyl-CoAs to stimulate insulin release. When this dietary modification was applied in mice, the animals had lower fasting insulin secretion, improved insulin sensitivity, reduced food intake, no weight gain or increased fat mass, and they did not suffer from insulin resistance which typically accompanies a high-fat diet. Furthermore, in another study in high-fat-diet fed rodents in which increased fat burning was induced by a drug called fenofibrate, the plasma levels of fatty acids and triglycerides were reduced and both hyperinsulinemia and hyperglycemia were reversed. These findings point to high blood fat levels (probably in addition to regular spikes in blood sugar) as a driving force in the development of type 2 diabetes. By reducing levels of circulating fats, researchers have successfully stunted the development of diabetes in animal models.

CHRONIC HIGH LEVELS OF PLASMA INSULIN

There is also evidence that a sustained high level of plasma insulin (hyperinsulinemia) resulting from eating too many sugary and fatty foods is the initiating defect that leads to obesity, **hyperlipidemia**, and insulin resistance. Studies conducted in Pima Indians, one of the ethnic groups prone to obesity, have found that hyperinsulinemia precedes and predicts the development of type 2 diabetes. This concurs with several previous studies of people in other ethnic groups prone to obesity (such as Hispanic Americans and Pacific Islanders) that also concluded hyperinsulinemia precedes and predicts diabetes.

ELEVATED LEVELS OF METHYLGLYOXAL

There is evidence that several of the characteristics of type 2 diabetes, including insulin resistance, can be caused by a glucose metabolite called **methylglyoxal** (MG), the levels of which are elevated in response to hyperglycemia and are higher in type 2 diabetics. Insulin resistance and hyperglycemia are thought to also play causal roles in the disease consequences of type 2 diabetes. However, recent clinical studies have found that type 2 diabetes patients who received drugs to maintain blood glucose levels below the diabetes definition threshold (i.e., blood HbA1c less than 6.5%) still develop diabetic complications such as nerve and kidney damage. This suggests that type 2 diabetes might in fact have molecular causes that are not just directly related to insulin and glucose. In type 2 diabetics high levels of MG have been observed, and since MG can cause damage to proteins it could well be one of the culprits in causing typical diabetic damage.

Recent research has shown that when rats are given MG with their food, they develop many typical signs of diabetes, including insulin resistance. To investigate the effects of long-term elevated MG concentrations, researchers in Germany chose fruit flies as a model for this purpose. Although flies and humans are not very closely related, they have many metabolic pathways in common (because energy metabolism developed very early on in evolution) so results are usually be translated to humans. Using genetic engineering, the researchers ... that breaks down MG in flies. The glucose metabolite MG subsequently ... bodies. The flies soon developed insulin resistance. Later, they became ... blood glucose levels. The scientists concluded that it appears to be sufficient ... level to trigger insulin resistance and typical diabetic metabolic disturbances. In other words, the evidence suggests that elevated MG could constitute one root cause of type 2 diabetes, suggesting that the molecular causes of elevated MG warrant further study. It might be possible that using drugs to lower MG levels will be an effective therapy for type 2 diabetes, but much more research on this is needed.

The consequences of getting fatter and developing insulin resistance

When your tissues start to develop resistance to insulin, bad things happen:

- Your fat cells become larger and stretched. This seems to be interpreted by your **immune system** as a signal that the tissue is being damaged so white blood cells infiltrate adipose tissue and cause inflammation. When the adipocytes become full of stored fat and inflamed – as your body tries to cram more and more energy into them – you reach the point of exceeding your "personal fat threshold" (i.e., the maximum amount of fat that our adipose tissue cells can store). As there is no space left to store fat safely, it begins to be stored in your internal organs, such as your spleen, pancreas, and liver. This makes the liver even more resistant to the actions of insulin. Actually this is how foie gras – the famous goose liver pâté – is made. Geese are fed so much starchy maize that their livers become full of fat giving the foie gras its characteristic creamy texture. The same happens to your liver when you become obese. An individual's personal fat threshold depends on their sex (men have a greater tendency to accumulate fat in the belly region) and genetics. Your personal fat threshold determines how much fat you can accumulate – particularly in the abdomen – before it starts to overflow into your liver and pancreas. The accumulation of this visceral fat is very bad for your health as it is strongly associated with the development of coronary heart disease and the metabolic syndrome. High liver fat levels promote further insulin resistance and also result in higher levels of harmful lipoproteins, triglycerides, and cholesterol in the blood. High levels of fat in the pancreas may start to interfere with insulin production.

- Despite having all this excess body fat, you feel hungry all the time. That's because you now have high insulin levels, which encourage continuous fat storage and inhibit fat breakdown and burning. The peripheral tissue insulin resistance also means that your tissues cannot access the high levels of glucose that are in your blood, so essentially that means your tissues are surrounded by potential fuels but cannot use them. Your tissues are said to be "starving in the face of plenty". This lack of access to fuel stimulates your brain to generate hunger signals, encouraging you to eat more and more. So you do tend to eat more which only makes you fatter still; it's a vicious cycle that is very hard to get out of. What's more is that your hunger is still not satisfied, so the situation just gets worse and worse.

- High levels of insulin, glucose, and fats in the blood contribute to the development of many other diseases including breast and bowel cancer, dementia, hypertension, peripheral vascular disease, coronary heart disease, retinopathy, and nerve damage, as well as impaired immunity, poor wound healing, and reduced fertility.

POSSIBLE MECHANISMS LEADING TO IMPAIRED INSULIN SECRETION IN TYPE 2 DIABETES

As mentioned previously, type 2 diabetes occurs when insulin resistance and impaired insulin secretion occur simultaneously. The degree of both these defects can vary with some diabetics having strong insulin resistance and slightly impaired insulin secretion while in others insulin resistance may be moderate with a more pronounced impairment of insulin secretion when blood sugar levels rise. There are two main theories to explain the development of impaired insulin secretion in type 2 diabetes – β-cell exhaustion and genetic factors – and these are explained below:

β-CELL EXHAUSTION

The major theory about the cause of impaired insulin secretion in most type 2 diabetics is that the β-cells become "exhausted" by the sustained high levels of insulin secretion that are needed to attempt to overcome target tissue insulin resistance. The initial **hypersecretion** of insulin that occurs as the target tissues become less and less responsive to insulin can deplete the insulin reserves of the pancreatic β-cells. This leaves the β-cells unable to fully respond to a surge in glucose – a precursor to β-cell failure. In addition, the diabetic state leads to a vicious cycle in which insulin deficiency and hyperglycemia both further exacerbate insulin resistance.

GENETIC FACTORS

Genetic factors may also play a role as most of the **genes** that are known to be linked to a higher risk of developing type 2 diabetes are involved in β-cell functions, and many affected individuals have at least one close family member, such as a parent or sibling, with the disease. Studies have identified at least 40 genes and over 150 variations in **deoxyribonucleic acid** (DNA) coding that are associated with the risk of developing type 2 diabetes. Most of these changes occur in the genome of both people with diabetes and those without but each individual has some variations that increase risk and others that reduce risk. It is the balance of these changes that helps determine a person's likelihood of developing the disease when unfavorable lifestyle factors are present such as eating too much and not being physically active.

As well as influencing pancreatic β-cell functions, some of the genetic variations associated with type 2 diabetes act by changing the target tissue cells' sensitivity to the effects of insulin. However, for many of the DNA variations that have been associated with type 2 diabetes, the mechanisms by which they contribute to disease risk remains unknown. There are also some rare cases of type 2 diabetes that arise due to an abnormality in a single gene. These are known as monogenic forms of diabetes. Examples include maturity onset diabetes of the young, which accounts for about 5% of all cases of diabetes in young people; Donohue syndrome; and Rabson–Mendenhall syndrome. The vast majority of cases of diabetes in people below the age of 30 are due, as you would expect, to type 1 diabetes although in recent years the incidence of type 2 diabetes among adolescents and young adults has been on the increase.

Genetic variations likely act together with health and lifestyle factors to influence an individual's overall risk of type 2 diabetes. All of these risk factors are related, directly or indirectly, to the body's ability to produce and respond to insulin. Genes can also increase the risk of type 2 diabetes by increasing a person's tendency to become overweight or obese (this issue will be covered in more detail in chapter 5). By far the biggest risk factors for type 2 diabetes involve lifestyle choices: What and how much we eat, and how much exercise we do. These and other risk factors are described in the next section of this chapter.

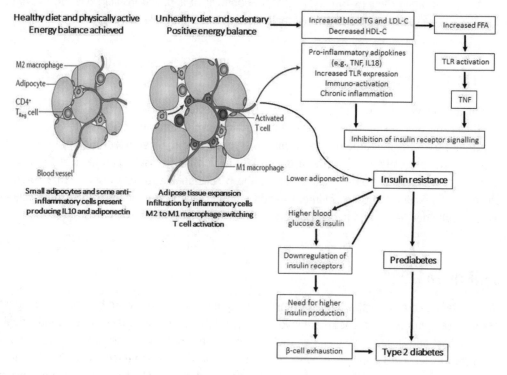

Figure 4.2 Possible mechanisms leading to insulin resistance and the subsequent development of prediabetes and type 2 diabetes. See text for details. FFA: free fatty acids; HDL-C: high density lipoprotein cholesterol; IL-18: interleukin 18; LDL-C: low density lipoprotein cholesterol; TG: triglyceride; TLR: toll-like receptor; TNF: tumor necrosis factor.

RISK FACTORS FOR TYPE 2 DIABETES

Your chances of developing type 2 diabetes depend on a number of risk factors such as your genes, diet, and lifestyle (figure 4.3). Some of these risk factors can't be altered such as family history, age, or ethnicity, but the risk factors related to lifestyle can be changed. These modifiable lifestyle risk factors include your diet, physical activity, and body weight. Making changes for the better – eating a healthier diet, doing more exercise, and losing some excess body fat – can strongly diminish your chances of developing type 2 diabetes. Taking action on the factors it is possible to change can help you delay the onset of type 2 diabetes or prevent it altogether.

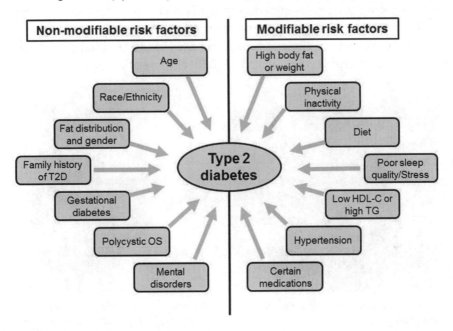

Figure 4.3 Risk factors for the development of type 2 diabetes.

You are more likely to develop type 2 diabetes if you are not physically active and are overweight or obese. Extra weight sometimes causes insulin resistance and is common in people with type 2 diabetes. The location of body fat also makes a difference. Extra belly fat is linked to insulin resistance, type 2 diabetes, and heart and blood vessel disease. The following factors increase the risk of developing type 2 diabetes:

- *High body fat or body weight.* Being overweight is the single most important risk factor for type 2 diabetes. The more adipose tissue you have, especially if it is in the belly region, the more resistant your cells become to insulin. Obesity (defined as having a BMI of 30 kg/m² or more) contributes as much as 80-85% to the risk of developing type 2 diabetes in the general population. However, you don't have to be overweight to that degree to develop type 2 diabetes. Excess body fat is associated with 30% of cases in those of Chinese and Japanese descent, 60–80% of cases in those of European and African descent, and 100% of cases in

Pima Indians and Pacific Islanders. Among those with type 2 diabetes who are not obese (i.e., those with a BMI of 25-29 kg/m²) carrying some excess fat in the belly region is common.

- *Fat distribution and gender.* If your body stores fat mainly in your belly region (abdomen), your risk of type 2 diabetes is greater than if your body stores fat in other areas, such as your hips and thighs. As men tend to store most of their fat in the abdominal area (photo 4.1), this increases their risk above that of women who have more fat stored under the skin and on the hips and thighs (photo 4.2). Men aged 35-54 are almost twice as likely to have type 2 diabetes compared to their female counterparts. However, women tend to develop the condition later in life, and the risk of death from heart disease associated with Type 2 diabetes is about 50% greater in women than it is in men. Key statistics on diabetes show that 2.4% (around 93,000) of men in England aged 35-44 have diabetes compared to 1.2% (around 47,000) of women of the same age, and 6% (around 197,000) of men aged 45-54 have diabetes compared to 3.6% (around 121,000) of women their age.

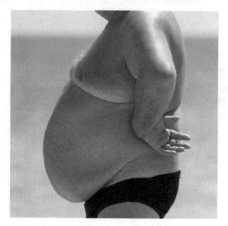
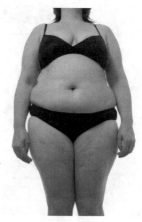

Photo 4.1: Men tend to store most of their fat in the abdominal area.

Photo 4.2: Women tend to store most of their fat under the skin and on the hips and thighs as well as in the abdominal area.

- *Being sedentary.* The less physical activity you do, the greater your risk of type 2 diabetes. Exercise helps you control your weight, burns fat and glucose as energy, and makes your cells more sensitive to insulin. A lack of exercise is believed to cause 7% of cases of type 2 diabetes.

- *Family history and genes.* The risk of type 2 diabetes is higher if your parent or sibling has type 2 diabetes. In fact you are two to six times more likely to get type 2 diabetes if you have a parent, brother, or sister with diabetes. Most cases of diabetes involve many genes, with each making a small contribution to an increased probability of becoming a type 2 diabetic. Genetic factors are often confirmed by studies examining identical and non-identical twins, and these studies indicate that if one identical twin has diabetes, the chance of the other developing diabetes within his or her lifetime is greater than 90%. For non-identical siblings the expected chance is something like 25-50%.

- *Race or ethnicity.* Type 2 diabetes tends to run in families and occurs more frequently in certain racial/ethnic groups such as those of African or Asian descent who live in North

America, the UK, and Europe, as well as Hispanics/Latinos, Native Hawaiians, and Pacific Islanders. Type 2 diabetes is two to four times more likely in people of South Asian descent and African-Caribbean or Black African descent than in white people.

- *Age.* The risk of developing type 2 diabetes increases with age, especially after age 45. This seems to be mostly associated with the tendency to gain weight and body fat as we get older. Compared with our younger years we tend to do less exercise, and even small daily excesses of calorie intake start to accumulate so that we gain body fat and body weight. We also tend to lose some muscle mass (a natural process of aging that the clinicians call **sarcopenia**) which means that our resting metabolic rate decreases a little whereas our energy intake does not. Although type 2 diabetes is still far more common in older people, a worrying trend has developed over the past two decades – namely that the incidence of type 2 diabetes has increased dramatically among children, adolescents, and younger adults. This appears to be closely associated with more and more young people being overweight or obese due to eating too much and not doing enough exercise.

- *Diet.* What you eat and drink as well as how many calories you consume also influences the risk of developing type 2 diabetes. For example, drinking above average volumes of sugar-sweetened beverages or eating large amounts of white rice are both associated with an increased risk of type 2 diabetes in people who are not highly physically active. The type of fats in your diet are important too, with saturated fats and trans **fatty acids** increasing the risk, and **polyunsaturated** and **monounsaturated** fats decreasing the risk.

- *Prediabetes.* Prediabetes is a condition in which your blood glucose level is higher than normal, but not quite high enough to be classified as type 2 diabetes. If you have prediabetes then, not surprisingly, you are at high risk of developing type 2 diabetes. When it is left untreated, prediabetes often progresses to type 2 diabetes. The trouble is that many people are not actually aware that they have prediabetes and consequently don't do anything about it.

- *Gestational diabetes.* Women who had gestational diabetes when they were pregnant have an increased risk of developing type 2 diabetes. The risk is also higher for women who gave birth to a baby weighing more than 4 kg (9 lbs).

- *High blood pressure.* A large-scale cohort study and meta-analysis published in 2015 assessed the link between increased blood pressure and risk of type 2 diabetes, and found an increase of 20 mmHg in systolic blood pressure raised the risk of type 2 diabetes by 58%.

- *Low serum HDL-cholesterol.* People with low serum levels of high-density lipoprotein (HDL) cholesterol, the "good" cholesterol, have a higher risk of type 2 diabetes. Having high levels of serum triglyceride is also a risk factor for type 2 diabetes.

- *Polycystic ovarian syndrome.* Suffering from **polycystic ovarian syndrome** – a common condition affecting women of child-bearing age that is characterized by irregular menstrual periods, excess hair growth, and obesity – increases the risk of diabetes.

- *Stress.* Stressful events or periods of time in people's lives (e.g., bereavement, divorce, moving home, redundancy, money problems) and stress at work that can cause negative emotions such as anger, frustration, anxiety, fear, worry, and sadness are also known to induce hyperglycemia and can therefore contribute to the development of type 2 diabetes. Blood sugar rises when we get stressed mentally or physically due to the release of so-called stress hormones like epinephrine (adrenaline) and cortisol which promote glucose release from the liver as part of the "fight or flight" response, even though the state of psychological stress does not require it.

- *Mental disorders.* People who suffer from certain mental disorders including schizophrenia, bipolar illness, depression, or are receiving treatment with antipsychotic medication are at increased risk of developing type 2 diabetes.

- *Certain medications.* Unfortunately, some prescription medications that are taken to treat or prevent other diseases may, if continued for more than a few years, result in some people developing type 2 diabetes. These medications include beta blockers and thiazides (used to treat high blood pressure), corticosteroids (used to limit the effects of autoimmune diseases like asthma and rheumatoid arthritis), and statins (used to lower serum cholesterol). Statins inhibit the liver's production of cholesterol which has the effect of reducing serum LDL-cholesterol and so reduce the risk of coronary heart disease and stroke. For this reason, the strong benefits of taking statins outweigh the slightly higher risk that you could develop diabetes.

- *Poor sleep quality.* People who complain of chronic **insomnia** and shortened sleep have an increased incidence of type 2 diabetes, hypertension, and cardiovascular disease. The latest evidence suggests that extremes of sleep duration (too little – less than 7 hours, or too much – more than 9 hours) alter circulating hormone levels and circadian rhythms, which contribute to weight gain and other risk factors for the development of chronic disease such as type 2 diabetes and cardiovascular disease. These influences may begin in childhood and have impacts throughout the course of our lives.

SEX DIFFERENCES IN TYPE 2 DIABETES AND ITS RELATION TO BODY FAT MASS AND DISTRIBUTION

In the first half of the 20th century the prevalence of type 2 diabetes was higher among women than among men, but this trend has now reversed; today more men than women are diagnosed with type 2 diabetes. This change is thought to have arisen mainly from a drop in physical activity levels particularly among men, resulting in increased obesity. However, men also tend to develop type 2 diabetes at a lower degree of obesity (i.e., lower percentage body fat and lower BMI) than women.

Obesity or just being overweight is by far the biggest risk factor for type 2 diabetes. An accumulation of abdominal visceral fat is particularly associated with increased risk of type 2 diabetes, and in general men have more abdominal fat, whereas women have more peripheral fat. Within the abdominal cavity (the belly region) men tend to have more visceral fat and store more fat in their livers than women, whereas women have more fat just beneath the skin (subcutaneous fat) than men (figure 4.4). Visceral and liver fat accumulation is much more strongly associated with insulin resistance than subcutaneous fat stores. Therefore, it seems that the reason men develop type 2 diabetes at a lower BMI and fat mass than women can be explained by the fact that men have more visceral fat for a given BMI than women.

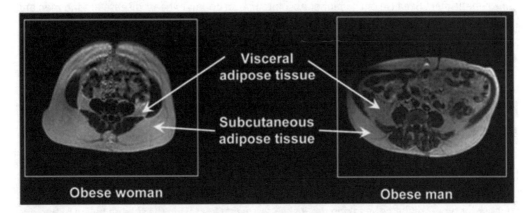

Figure 4.4: Cross-sectional abdominal magnetic resonance image (MRI) of an obese woman and an obese man. From Geer E B and Shen W. (2009). Gender differences in insulin resistance, body composition, and energy balance. Gend Med 6 Suppl 1: 60-75.

SEX DIFFERENCES IN INSULIN RESISTANCE AND BLOOD GLUCOSE LEVELS

The sex differences in body fat distribution are closely related to sex differences in insulin resistance. Men are in general more insulin resistant than women, which can be explained by their higher proportion of visceral fat. This is reflected in the finding that more men than women have elevated fasting glucose levels. In contrast, more women than men have elevated 2-hour glucose concentrations in the oral glucose tolerance test, but this is probably related to the fact that, in general, women have a smaller body mass than men, which means it may take them longer to metabolize the 75 g of glucose given during a standard oral glucose tolerance test. On the other hand, the sex differences in fasting blood glucose concentrations are likely to be caused by differences in the types and levels of the sex hormones in the two sexes (i.e., predominantly testosterone in men and estrogen and progesterone in women). After the menopause in women, insulin sensitivity declines, indicating that estrogen may exert beneficial effects on insulin sensitivity in women. Estrogen has also a beneficial effect on adipose tissue distribution. The preferential deposition of adipose tissue in the subcutaneous areas in women compared with the abdominal region in men seems to be related to the higher estrogen levels in women compared with men. In contrast, testosterone levels are significantly associated with abdominal visceral fat accumulation in both men and women.

SEX DIFFERENCES IN RISK OF CARDIOVASCULAR DISEASE

In general, men have higher absolute risk of coronary heart disease than women. However, the relative risk of coronary heart disease in people diagnosed with type 2 diabetes is greater in women than in men, indicating that type 2 diabetes exerts a greater adverse effect on cardiovascular risk in women compared with men. This suggestion is supported by the finding that cardiovascular risk factors differ more between women with and without diabetes than between diabetic and non-diabetic men. Because of the higher absolute risk for coronary heart disease among men and the higher relative risk among diabetic women, the absolute risk for coronary heart disease is similar between men and women with diabetes.

HOW TO EVALUATE YOUR OWN DIABETES RISK BASED ON YOUR PERSONAL DETAILS AND THE KNOWN RISK FACTORS

If you are someone who has not yet been diagnosed as either prediabetic or a type 2 diabetic but suspect that you may be one of the millions at risk of developing these conditions, you can evaluate your risk for type 2 diabetes by taking the *Risk Assessment Quiz* test in the sidebar below to find out.

Type 2 Diabetes Risk Assessment Quiz

(Adapted from the American Diabetes Association's Diabetes Risk Test.)

Select the correct answer for each of the following seven questions and then add up your total points score.

1. How old are you?
   a. Less than 40 years (0 points)
   b. 40–49 years (1 point)
   c. 50–59 years (2 points)
   d. 60 years or older (3 points)

2. Are you a man or a woman?
   a. Man (1 point)
   b. Woman (0 points)

3. Are you a woman who has ever been diagnosed with gestational diabetes or given birth to a baby weighing 4 kg (9 lbs) or more?
   a. Yes (1 point)
   b. No (0 points)

4. Do you have a mother, father, sister, or brother with diabetes?
   a. Yes (1 point)
   b. No (0 points)

5. Have you ever been diagnosed with high blood pressure?
   a. Yes (1 point)
   b. No (0 points)

6. Are you physically active (i.e., on average do you do more than 30 minutes of exercise per day on at least three days per week)?
   a. Yes (0 points)
   b. No (1 point)

7. What is your weight status? (see figure 4.5 to determine your score according to your weight and height)
   a. 1 Point
   b. 2 Points
   c. 3 Points
   d. If you weigh less than the amount in the left-hand column you score 0 points

Height	Weight					
	lbs.	kilos	lbs.	kilos	lbs.	kilos
4'10"	119–142	54.0–64.4	143–190	64.9–86.2	191+	86.6+
4'11"	124–147	56.2–66.7	148–197	67.1–89.3	198+	89.8+
5'0"	128–152	58.1–68.9	153–203	69.4–92.1	204+	92.5+
5'1"	132–157	59.9–71.2	158–210	71.7–95.3	211+	95.7+
5'2"	136–163	61.7–73.9	164–217	74.4–98.4	218+	98.9+
5'3"	141–168	64.0–76.2	169–224	76.7–101.6	225+	102.1+
5'4"	145–173	65.8–78.5	174–231	78.9–104.8	232+	105.2+
5'5"	150–179	68.0–81.2	180–239	81.6–108.4	240+	108.9+
5'6"	155–185	70.3–83.9	186–246	84.4–111.6	247+	112.0+
5'7"	159–190	72.1–86.2	191–254	86.6–115.2	255+	115.7+
5'8"	164–196	74.4–88.9	197–261	89.4–118.4	262+	118.8+
5'9"	169–202	76.7–91.6	203–269	92.1–122.0	270+	122.5+
5'10"	174–208	78.9–94.3	209–277	94.8–125.6	278+	126.1+
5'11"	179–214	81.2–97.1	215–285	97.5–129.3	286+	129.7+
6'0"	184–220	83.5–99.8	221–293	100.2–132.9	294+	133.4+
6'1"	189–226	85.7–102.5	227–301	103.0–136.5	302+	137.0+
6'2"	194–232	88.0–105.2	233–310	105.7–140.6	311+	141.1+
6'3"	200–239	90.7–108.4	240–318	108.9–144.2	319+	144.7+
6'4"	205–245	93.0–111.1	246–327	111.6–148.3	328+	148.8+
	(1 Point)		(2 Points)		(3 Points)	
	You weigh less than the amount in the left column (0 points)					

Figure 4.5 Height and body weight chart that can be used to assess your points score for weight status (question 7) in the diabetes risk assessment quiz.

The higher your score in the quiz shown in the previous sidebar, the higher your risk for getting type 2 diabetes. If you scored five points or more you have a high risk of developing diabetes. If you have not yet been diagnosed as diabetic, talk to your health care provider about simple blood tests to check for diabetes or prediabetes. Early diagnosis and treatment can prevent or delay heart attack, stroke, blindness, kidney disease, and other health problems.

Even if your points score was below five, you may be at increased risk of having prediabetes – blood sugar levels that are higher than normal but not high enough to be called diabetes. The good news for people with prediabetes is that you can lower your risk for type 2 diabetes. Talk to your healthcare team about getting tested, particularly if you are over 45, overweight, or have a family member with diabetes.

Find out about the small steps you can take to prevent or delay type 2 diabetes and live a long and healthy life by reading my book, *Eat, Move, Sleep, Repeat*.

Type 2 diabetes is more common in African Americans and people with African ancestry, Hispanics and Latinos, American Indians, Alaska Natives, Asian Americans, Native Hawaiians, and Pacific Islanders. The US National Diabetes Education Program (NDEP) has special information for these groups (see https://www.cdc.gov/diabetes/ndep/index.html). In European countries, the people who have origins in South Asia, Africa, and the Middle East are the ones most prone to developing type 2 diabetes.

Key Points

- The two key characteristics of type 2 diabetes are insulin resistance (which develops first) followed by impaired insulin secretion by the β-cells in the pancreas.

- When insulin resistance starts to develop the β-cells can compensate for this by increased secretion leading to chronically high plasma insulin levels (hyperinsulinemia). The condition called prediabetes now develops.

- The hyperinsulinemia can cause reduced expression of the insulin receptor molecules on the surface of the cells in the target tissues (liver, muscle, and adipose tissue) which further increases insulin resistance.

- After some time (typically a few years) the β-cells become exhausted and fail to produce enough insulin so that blood glucose levels become chronically high, even in the fasting state, and very high blood glucose concentration (up to 50 mmol/L) occurs following meals. When this point is reached full blown type 2 diabetes has developed.

- The initial cause of insulin resistance is still subject to much debate and there are several theories about why it occurs.

- The most popular current theory is that insulin resistance develops following expansion of adipose tissue mass (i.e., when we become overweight or obese) which then becomes inflamed and produces increased amounts of pro-inflammatory cytokines. At least one of these cytokines, tumor necrosis factor-alpha (TNF-α), is known to inhibit the insulin signalling pathway in target tissues. Furthermore, the production of adiponectin by adipose tissue is reduced in obesity and this cytokine is normally one that promotes insulin sensitivity.

- Other theories of insulin resistance are related to the effects of elevated levels of free fatty acids, triglycerides, and methylglyoxal.

- The most important risk factor for developing type 2 diabetes is being overweight. Other risk factors include a sedentary lifestyle, age (over 45), diet, genetics (family history), male gender, being of Asian, African, Hispanic/Latino, Pacific Island, or Middle-Eastern origin, having high blood pressure, having a low level of serum HDL ("good") cholesterol or a high level of triglycerides, having a history of gestational diabetes, having a history of heart disease or stroke, having polycystic ovary syndrome, and having poor sleep quality.

- Men have a higher risk of developing type 2 diabetes than women and men tend to become diabetic at a lower degree of adiposity. This is thought to be because men tend to store their fat as visceral fat in the abdomen whereas women have more subcutaneous fat stores. Visceral fat is more strongly associated with insulin resistance than fat stored in other areas of the body.

- You cannot control your gender, age, genetics or ethnicity, but you can modify some of the other risk factors including your diet, physical activity level, sleep quality and body weight.

Chapter 5

A Weighty Problem

Objectives

After studying this chapter, you should:

- Know the difference between being overweight and obese.

- Understand why obesity or being overweight is strongly linked to type 2 diabetes.

- Understand what causes obesity.

- Understand the concept of energy balance.

- Appreciate the roles of genetics, food addiction, sedentary behavior, and poor sleep quality in the development of obesity.

As mentioned in the previous chapter the biggest single risk factor for type 2 diabetes is being overweight or obese and most of the molecular mechanisms that have been suggested to cause insulin resistance to develop in the prediabetic stage of the condition are linked to increased adiposity. Obesity is defined by clinicians as having a BMI of 30 kg/m² or more or being overweight to the point where there are medical complications. For most adults, a BMI of 18.5 to 24.9 means you're a healthy weight, whereas 25 to 29.9 means you're overweight. 30 to 39.9 means you're obese, and 40 or above means you're severely or morbidly obese. Being overweight can mean anything from carrying a few extra kilograms of body fat to up to around 20 kg too much. People in the obese or **morbidly obese** category typically have 15-50 kg of additional fat that they don't need. Several largescale studies indicate that the average newly diagnosed type 2 diabetic is about 55 years of age, has a BMI of 33 kg/m², and is about 18 kg above their normal ideal healthy weight. When most people are first diagnosed as prediabetic or type 2 diabetic, they are probably not more than about 20 kg overweight, and many are actually only 5-15 kg overweight which is an amount of excess fat that could be lost within 10-20 weeks if a person is willing to cut down on their food intake and do more exercise. Doing just that has been shown to put type 2 diabetes into remission for a high proportion of people suffering from the condition. I'll deal with just how to do that in chapters 8 and 9, but for now let's examine just what causes us to become overweight or obese in the first place.

WHAT CAUSES OBESITY?

It's really rather simple: obesity is caused by overeating. Yes, I know that many people argue that socio-economic factors play a role but from a scientific standpoint consuming more calories from food and drink than we expend over a period of time is the thing that results in an accumulation of body fat and becoming overweight. For example, let's say a person eats, on average, 100 calories (kcal) per day more than they expend. That translates over time to 700 kcal per week, 3,000 kcal per month or 36,000 kcal per year. If all those extra calories were converted to fat it would result in a gain of about four kilograms (9 lbs) of fat. Hey presto, in five years you have gained 20 kg of fat from a relatively small daily energy excess.

The average adult expends about 1,700 kcal per day just to keep resting basal metabolism going. This represents the energy needed for essential processes such as membrane transport, nerve conduction, maintaining muscle tone, synthesis of new biomolecules and cells, and generally maintaining a constant internal environment in the body (called **homeostasis**). Heat is generated from the inefficiencies of metabolic reactions in the body but is needed to maintain the body temperature at a constant 37 °C (98 °F). The **basal metabolic rate** represents the energy expended at rest in the fasted state. We consume food to supply us with this energy but when we eat a meal there is an energy cost associated with the **digestion**, absorption, and storage of the nutrients which increases the metabolic rate by, on average, about 10% for a few hours. This is known as **diet-induced thermogenesis** (DIT) or the **thermic effect of food** (TEF) and adds about 200 kcal per day to the overall energy requirement. On top of that, even in a sedentary person, there is an additional energy cost of the essential movement that must be done to live a normal life. Even if it only involves getting dressed in the morning, going to the toilet, preparing and cooking food in the kitchen, doing some household chores, moving around the house and garden, etc., this additional energy need is usually at least 100 kcal per day. So the daily energy need of an average adult in the resting state adds up to 1,700 kcal (basal metabolism) + 200 kcal (diet-induced thermogenesis) + 100 kcal (essential movement) = 2,000 kcal. In other words this is the amount of energy expended each day and means we would have to consume 2,000 kcal in food and drink to match it and achieve what is called **energy balance** (when energy intake is exactly the same as **energy expenditure** – see the following sidebar for further explanation of this concept). In this context you can see that consuming an extra 100 kcal per day represents only a 5% increase above what is needed, yet it can be enough to gain an extra four kilograms of fat per year. That can be why many people gradually become overweight. Of course, there may be occasions when we rather overindulge in eating and drinking, perhaps adding an extra 500 kcal per day above normal, and all these indiscretions add to our positive energy balance. We tend to ignore this and don't compensate (or certainly don't compensate enough) by reducing our energy intake the next day or increasing our energy expenditure by doing some exercise to get our energy balance back to what it should be. Although overeating relative to our individual energy needs is undoubtedly the prime cause of becoming overweight or obese, there are other factors that can have a considerable influence on the rate at which we gain weight. Let's now look at these in turn after first examining the scale of the problem.

The concept of energy balance

Energy balance refers to the balance between energy intake and energy expenditure. Simply put, it is the difference between energy (i.e., calories) in and energy out. Energy intake comes from the energy we consume in food and drink. Energy expenditure is the sum of energy expended in resting metabolism (known as basal or resting metabolic rate) plus diet-induced thermogenesis/the thermic effect of food (the increase in metabolic rate that follows ingestion of food due to the energy cost of its digestion, absorption, and metabolism), plus the energy expended in physical activity (the **thermic effect of exercise**). Energy balance can be measured on a day-to-day basis, but it probably makes more sense to measure it over a period of several days or weeks. In order to remain weight-stable we need to achieve energy balance, and that means that over a period of time (say one week) our energy expenditure has to match our energy intake as illustrated in figure 5.1.

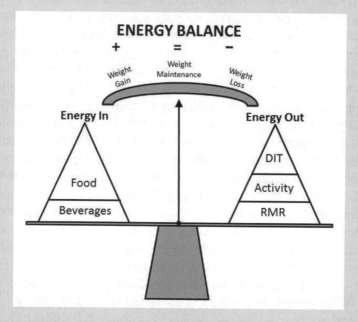

Figure 5.1 The concept of energy balance. DIT: diet-induced thermogenesis; RMR: resting metabolic rate.

When energy intake is greater than energy expenditure (i.e., when more calories come in than go out), the energy balance is said to be positive and weight gain will occur as most of the excess energy gets converted into body fat. When energy intake is below energy expenditure, the energy balance is negative and weight loss will result. Therefore, to maintain energy balance and a stable body weight, energy expenditure must match energy intake. Over the long-term, energy balance is maintained in weight-stable individuals even though this balance may be either positive or negative on a day-to-day basis. People who want to lose weight should increase energy expenditure relative to energy intake which can be achieved either by increasing energy expenditure (by exercising more) or reducing energy intake (by eating less) or a combination of both. There is no escaping this fact and there are no quick fix solutions to losing excess weight after it has been gained over a period of positive energy balance.

THE OBESITY PROBLEM

The obesity problem has now reached an epidemic scale in the populations living in many developed countries, with only the occasional exceptions such as Japan where a healthy diet is still the norm. However, even in Japan, the proportion of people who are overweight or obese has increased in the past two decades. In the USA two in three people are now classed as being overweight or obese; in fact, almost 38% of the adult population are classed as obese, a trend that has been growing for the past three decades. The UK has the highest proportion of obese people in Europe at 27%. Being obese or just overweight increases the risk of developing chronic metabolic and cardiovascular diseases and dying at an earlier age. Being overweight is the major cause of type 2 diabetes and is also an important risk factor for coronary heart disease, peripheral vascular disease, cancer, and dementia (figure 5.2). The latter may be due to the higher prevalence of type 2 diabetes in overweight people which is associated with numerous metabolic and circulatory defects that cause damage to blood vessels, potentially leading to reduced blood flow to the brain. One recent study found that being overweight in middle-age makes the brain age by 10 years. Human brains naturally shrink with age, but scientists are increasingly recognizing that obesity may also affect the onset and progression of brain aging.

As explained in chapter 1, the metabolic syndrome is a term used by clinicians and scientists to describe the co-occurrence of several known cardiovascular disease risk factors, including insulin resistance, obesity, high blood cholesterol, and high blood pressure (hypertension). All these risk factors are more prevalent in people who are carrying too much weight or an excess of fat, particularly around the waist. It is well known that some people have a lower metabolic rate than is average or are more metabolically efficient than others, increasing their tendency to put on fat when they eat. Indeed, it seems that many obese people use this as their "go to" excuse for their condition. Everyone seems to know someone else who can eat "as much as they like" without seemingly putting on any weight, and it does appear there is some truth to this and that our genetics may play a role in determining how efficient we are at putting on weight when we are in positive energy balance. Even so, there is no denying the fact that you have to be in positive energy balance (i.e., consuming more dietary energy than you need to meet your daily energy requirement) to put on weight.

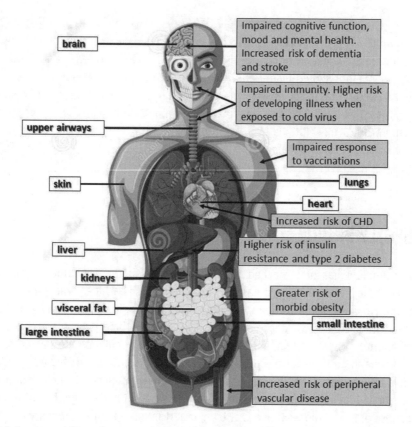

Figure 5.2 Being overweight or obese – particularly with an accumulation of visceral fat in the abdomen – increases the risk of developing several chronic diseases including type 2 diabetes. CHD: Coronary heart disease.

THE ROLE OF GENETICS

Again I will reiterate for emphasis that our tendency to put on weight is mostly due to our behaviors with regard to eating too much, exercising too little, and – as recent research seems to indicate – not getting good quality sleep. We know that at least some of the variation in body-fat levels between individuals is genetically determined, though not quite as much as you might think. Perhaps 25% to 40% of the fat stored in our body is the result of our genes that influence both our metabolic efficiency and, at least to some degree, our preferred behaviors (e.g., how much we like to eat to feel satisfied, whether we enjoy or hate performing exercise, whether we need relatively little or lots of sleep to function well, and whether we are "night owls" or "morning people"). Genetic factors also determine the susceptibility to gaining body fat in response to excess dietary energy intake, and also, to some degree, where in the body that extra fat gets deposited.

Several classic early studies have demonstrated a genetic factor in the development of obesity. In one such study, identical (monozygotic) twins were submitted to an energy surplus of 1,000 kcal per day for six days per week for 100 days (see the sidebar for a definition of calories, kcal, and other units of energy). The excess energy intake over the entire period was 84,000 kcal. The average gain in body mass was 8.1 kg – which just goes to show how much weight you can put on when a considerable excess energy intake is sustained over a few months – but considerable variation between individuals was evident. The range of weight gain was 4.3 to 13.3 kg, and the variation between 12 different pairs of twins was more than three times greater than the variation within pairs (which averaged 1.8 kg), suggesting an important genetic component (figure 5.3). The variation between pairs was even greater for changes in visceral fat, indicating that the site of storage is also partly genetically determined.

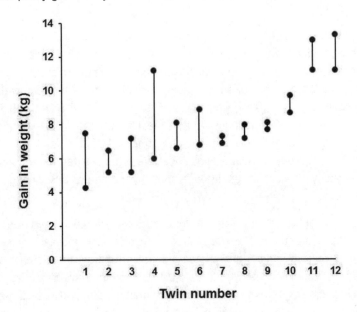

Figure 5.3 Changes in body mass in identical twins after overfeeding of 1,000 calories (kcal) per day for six days per week for 100 days. Considerably more variation occurred between pairs than within pairs, strongly suggesting a genetic component in the regulation of body mass. Data from Bouchard et al. (1990).

This link has been confirmed by large scale studies that have analyzed the contribution of potential genetic and environmental risk factors, identified at the molecular level, to the patterns and causes of obesity in defined populations (known as **molecular epidemiology studies**) and now more than 250 genes are believed to have the potential to influence body fatness. Several of the risk factors that are known to be associated with weight gain, such as a low resting metabolic rate, high reliance on carbohydrate metabolism, and a lower level of spontaneous physical activity, almost certainly have a genetic basis. But the relative contribution of genetic versus environmental (lifestyle-related) factors is still a subject of debate.

You can't do anything to modify your genes, but you can decide to adopt behaviors that will reduce your risk of becoming overweight. These behaviors include your eating, exercising, and sleeping habits. Eating a healthy diet, avoiding weight gain by maintaining an equal balance between energy intake and energy expenditure, and participating in some form of regular exercise are the most important things you can do to reduce your risk of accumulating excess body fat and developing chronic health conditions like type 2 diabetes, heart disease, cancer, and dementia. Not smoking tobacco products and avoiding drinking too much alcohol are other important behavioral factors in reducing your risk of chronic disease. Getting sufficient amounts of good quality sleep is also now recognized as having an important influence on our eating habits, our risk of chronic diseases, as well as our mood and mental health.

Units of energy

Energy is often expressed in calories (the Imperial system and what most people will be familiar with in relation to the energy content of foods) or joules (the **Systeme Internationale (SI) or** metric system which is the one that most scientists now use). One calorie expresses the quantity of energy (heat) needed to raise the temperature of 1 g (1 mL) of water by 1 °C (1.8 °F) (from 14.5 °C to 15.5 °C [58.1 °F to 59.9 °F]). One **kilocalorie** is equal to 1,000 calories. Thus, a meal containing 1,000 kilocalories (kcal) has enough energy potential to raise the temperature of 1,000 mL (or 1 liter) of water by 1 °C (1.8 °F). In everyday language, kilocalories are often referred to as Calories (which should be written with a capital C, although on many food items this is not done and the energy is listed as calories).

The SI (International System of Units) unit for energy is the **joule**, named after the British scientist Sir Prescott Joule (1818–1889). One joule of energy moves a mass of 1 g at a velocity of 1 m/s. A joule is not a large amount of energy; therefore, **kilojoule**s are more often used; one kilojoule (kJ) equals 1,000 joules. To convert calories to joules or kilocalories to kilojoules, the calorie value must be multiplied by 4.184. Because joules are not yet part of everyday language, both units are often mentioned on food labels, and in this book kcal will be used.

WHY WHAT WE EAT IS IMPORTANT

In order to maintain a healthy weight, we should aim to eat a healthy diet in appropriate amounts – that is enough to meet but not exceed our daily energy needs. After all, you can take in calories from food and beverages much faster than you can burn them off with metabolism and exercise! The US Office of Disease Prevention and Health Promotion recommends eating a variety of fruits and vegetables, wholegrains, low-fat dairy, and lean sources of protein, while limiting our intake of sodium (salt), added sugars, alcohol, and fats (particularly saturated fats and *trans* fats). This is sound advice, but what are the reasons behind it? Let's briefly examine what we know about the components of our diet that have an influence on our risk of becoming overweight or diabetic.

Carbohydrate Intake and Risk of Obesity and Type 2 Diabetes

The carbohydrate in our diet comes mostly from plant food sources that contain starch which is a glucose polymer (you can think of it as the plant form of glycogen which is only found in animals) and simple sugars like sucrose (cane and beet sugar). Plant foods that contain abundant amounts of starch include potatoes, sweet potatoes, rice, corn, cereal products including bread and pasta, and fruits like banana, apple, and pear. Foods that contain large amounts of simple sugars include soft drinks, fruit juices, energy drinks, candy, cake, cookies, sauces, and ready meals. The other main form of carbohydrate that we consume is fiber (which is mostly indigestible and abundant in cereals, grains, nuts, seeds, legumes, some fruits such as plums and berries, and vegetables such as green beans, broccoli, carrots, celery, and zucchini (courgette).

There is absolutely no doubt that both the quantity and quality of carbohydrate we regularly consume has important influences on the risk of developing obesity, cardiovascular disease, and type 2 diabetes. Studies show that refined carbohydrates lead to faster and bigger spikes in blood sugar, which leads to cravings and increased food intake. Refined carbohydrates tend to be very low in fiber, and they get digested and absorbed quickly. This results in more rapid and larger spikes in the blood glucose concentration meaning that they have a high glycemic index (GI), which is a measure of how quickly foods raise blood sugar. However, within one to two hours of eating a food that causes a rapid spike in blood sugar, the blood sugar levels fall below normal (known as the insulin rebound effect). When blood sugar levels drop it stimulates the appetite center in the **hypothalamus** of the brain and we get cravings for another high-carbohydrate snack. Indeed, studies show that people eat up to 80% more calories when given **ad libitum** (free to choose as much as desired) access to a high GI meal compared to a low GI meal.

Sugar consumption is a proven cause of weight gain, and obesity is strongly associated with increased risk of cardiovascular diseases, type 2 diabetes, and metabolic syndrome. In the Western diet, about half of the daily carbohydrate intake is in the form of sugars, especially sucrose and high-fructose corn syrups. Over the past century, the intake of simple sugars has increased dramatically to approximately 50 kg per person per year – 25 times more than 100 years ago. Added sugar intake averages 60 g/day and contributes 13% of total daily energy intake; this is highest among young people (figure 5.4). A substantial contributor to this increase is the high consumption of soft drinks, but candy, cookies, cakes, pies, sauces, ready meals, and other refined or processed foods have also contributed to the increase (figure 5.5).

Evidence is accumulating that the intake of large amounts of simple sugars is linked to increased risk of obesity, type 2 diabetes, and cardiovascular disease although considerable debate exists about this topic, because the results of studies to date are not conclusive, and the picture is often complicated by the fact that a higher sugar intake is often accompanied by higher saturated fat intake and higher energy intake as well. Therefore, sugar could just be a contributor and an indicator of an overall higher energy intake. A recent analysis of food availability data in the United States has confirmed that this is the case. It was found that between 1970 and 2014 the intake of all major food groups increased. Sugar intake increased, but so did the consumption of fats and oils; even fruit intake increased! Since the 1950s, Americans have been eating more and more. It may not be just increased intake of carbohydrate or sugar per se that is the problem, but this is very likely a contributor. However, it is fairly clear that generally, diets low in fiber and high in simple sugars are associated with weight gain and increased risk of obesity and type 2 diabetes.

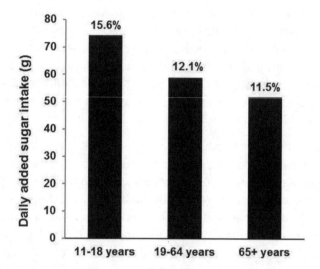

Figure 5.4 Daily added sugar intake (g) and its percentage contribution to daily energy intake by age group. Data from UK National Diet and Nutrition Survey Rolling Programme (2008/2009-2011/12), published 2014. Available at https://www.gov.uk/government/collections/national-diet-and-nutrition-survey.

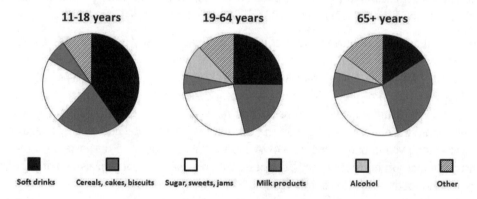

Figure 5.5 Sources of sugar intake in the Western diet: Where different age groups get their added sugar from. Data from UK National Diet and Nutrition Survey Rolling Programme (2008/2009-2011/12), published 2014. Available at https://www.gov.uk/government/collections/national-diet-and-nutrition-survey.

Although a dose response relationship (that is how the amount of an item – in this case sugar – is linked to the effect – in this case the incidence of obesity) between sugar consumption and obesity cannot be definitively determined at this time, the evidence was of sufficient strength and consistency for the World Health Organization (WHO) to officially launch guidelines in 2015 for sugar intake in adults and children. In these, they recommend adults and children reduce their daily intake of free sugars to less than 10% of their total energy intake, and they suggest that a further reduction to below 5% or roughly 25 g (6 teaspoons) per day would provide additional health benefits. In the UK, the Scientific Advisory Committee on Nutrition's recommendation of having no more than 5% of energy intake from free sugars has recently been adopted. The term "free sugars" includes any sugar added by the manufacturer or during cooking plus natural free sugars in honey, syrups, and fruit juices but excludes any natural sugars in fresh fruit.

Soft drink consumption in the Western world has increased considerably in the past two decades, particularly among children. On average, US adolescents and adults consume over 150 kcal/day from sugar-sweetened beverages (SSBs). During 2011-2014 in the US, on average, about 7% of children's and adults' total daily calories were obtained from SSBs. Globally there has been a steady upward trend in consumption of SSBs from 2005 to 2011. This is why some states (and also some countries such as the UK) are experimenting with sugar tax: adding tax to SSBs in an attempt to discourage sales.

Studies of SSB intake by children have shown regular consumption of these beverages results in larger weight gain compared with children who consume SSBs less often or rarely. This may relate to the lack of satiation (feeling of fullness) provided by these drinks as well as the calories they contain. Masking (i.e., hiding) replacement of SSBs with low or zero calorie beverages containing artificial sweeteners has been found to reduce weight gain in children. Several meta-analyses (large-scale statistical analyses based on data from numerous previously published studies) have suggested that SSBs are associated with weight gain and obesity in both children and adults and that the weight gain appears to be due to the increased energy consumption rather than any unique aspect of sugars themselves.

Another source of carbohydrate that has caused health concerns is the **monosaccharide** fructose which was only present in our diet in very small quantities up to a few hundred years ago but has now become a major constituent of our diet. Our main dietary sources of fructose are sugar in the form of the **disaccharide** sucrose (a combination of the monosaccharides glucose and fructose) from beet or cane, high fructose corn syrup, fruits, fruit juices, and honey. Fructose, like glucose, is a 6-carbon sugar but its metabolism differs markedly from that of glucose due to its almost complete uptake by the liver where it is converted into glucose, glycogen, or fat. High fructose intake has been shown to cause increased blood cholesterol and to impair liver insulin sensitivity. In large amounts, dietary fructose leads to greater adverse metabolic changes than equivalent amounts of glucose, although the extent to which fructose itself is contributing to many of the metabolic changes found in the obese, as distinct from the calories it provides, is still a matter of debate. Following feeding, fructose does not reduce levels of the appetite-stimulating hormone **ghrelin** as much as glucose, meaning that we will tend to want to eat more calories with fructose. Furthermore, fructose does not stimulate the **satiety** centers in the brain as strongly as glucose, which makes us want to eat for longer until we feel full. For these reasons, people, and especially those who are diagnosed as prediabetic or type 2 diabetic, should limit their intake of fructose which is found in table sugar and many processed foods, including frozen ready meals, candy, soft drinks, salad dressings, sauces, canned fruits, fruit juices, and some breakfast cereals.

Numerous studies indicate that dietary fiber has an important influence on satiety (the feeling of fullness after a meal that inhibits our desire to eat more), and that relatively high intakes of

...nt gain and also protect against cardiovascular disease and type ...ble (the kind found in cereals such as oatmeal, beans, and apples, ...p slow down the absorption of sugars and reduce dangerous visceral ...nt studies.

... fiber intake of at least 14 g per 1,000 kcal of dietary energy intake is ... people, this intake would equal 25 to 30 g of fiber per day. The typical fiber in... ...countries, however, is only about 15 g per day for females and 18 g per day for males. In An... countries, the intake of fiber is much higher, in fact as much as 40 to 150 g per day. A low fiber intake is associated with increased risk of cardiovascular disease and type 2 diabetes, whereas higher than average intakes of fiber from cereal, fruit, and vegetable sources are inversely associated with risk of cardiovascular diseases and type 2 diabetes.

Fat Intake and Risk of Obesity and Type 2 Diabetes

According to a large nutrition survey in the US called National Health and Nutrition Examination Survey (NHANES), fat intake has declined from 36.9% to 33.5% of total energy intake for men and from 36.1% to 33.9% for women in the period 1971 through 2004. Although at first sight that seems like a good thing, the actual amount of fat intake (in grams) increased slightly because of an increase in total daily energy intake. In the period 2004 through 2010 there has been a slight reduction in both total energy and fat intake. However, few people in Western countries have a fat intake below 20%. Most of our daily fat intake (over 95% in fact) is in the form of triglycerides which is the main storage form of fat in animals and humans. Triglyceride is also found in some plant foods such as avocado, but most of this is in the form of unsaturated fat which is healthier than the saturated fat that predominates in animals. The other fats such as **phospholipids**, fatty acids, cholesterol, and **plant sterols** make up the remainder of our daily fat intake. The daily triglyceride intake in the North American diet is about 100 to 150 g/day. The average person in the US consumes about a third of fat from plant origin (vegetables), and two-thirds from animal sources. Animal fat is higher in saturated fat than fat from plant sources (table 5.1), and saturated fat typically represents about 11% of the total energy intake.

Table 5.1 Comparison of the fat composition of a whole avocado weighing 200 grams and a 200-gram portion of pork belly

	Avocado (200 g)	Pork belly (200 g)
Total energy (kcal)	320	1,030
Total fat (g)	28	104
Saturated fat (g)	4.3	42
Polyunsaturated fat (g)	3.7	12
Monounsaturated fat (g)	20	50
Cholesterol (mg)	0	150

Research has shown that populations that consume diets high in saturated fats have relatively high levels of blood cholesterol and suffer a higher prevalence of type 2 diabetes and coronary heart disease. Some studies have suggested a correlation between high dietary fat intake and obesity, but currently the evidence that high-fat intake contributes to obesity is insufficient to make definitive recommendations for a very low-fat diet. Therefore, the 2015 *Dietary Guidelines for Americans* state that fat intake should be moderate (rather than low). In fact, a very low-fat, high-carbohydrate intake may have adverse health effects. Reducing dietary fat to below 20% of energy intake while replacing the calories from fat with those from carbohydrate results in elevated plasma triglycerides, increased LDL cholesterol, and decreased HDL cholesterol. These metabolic changes increase the risk of cardiovascular disease and predispose to type 2 diabetes and metabolic syndrome, particularly for those with a sedentary lifestyle.

A high intake of dietary cholesterol should also be avoided. Diabetics are generally advised to limit their daily cholesterol intake to no more than 200 mg. Foods that are relatively high in cholesterol and therefore should be eaten in only limited amounts or avoided altogether include lard, fatty cuts of meat, poultry skin, eggs, cream, whole milk, butter, cheese, saturated vegetable oils such as coconut and palm oil. One exception could be eggs which contain some cholesterol and saturated fat but also contain healthy nutrients such as unsaturated fats, protein, and many essential **micronutrients**. See the sidebar for more information on the debate surrounding this controversial issue.

Are eggs bad for type 2 diabetes?

Eggs are controversial for diabetes because they are high in cholesterol at about 190 mg per large-sized (50 g) chicken egg and also contain some saturated fat (though only 1.6 g). However, they are very low in carbohydrate (0.5 g), relatively low in calories (78 kcal), rich in essential minerals (e.g., potassium) and vitamins (e.g., biotin), a very good source of high quality protein (7 g), and also contain healthy carotenoids, polyunsaturated (0.7 g), and monounsaturated (2 g) fatty acids. In other words, eggs contain some nutrients that have been associated with an increased risk of type 2 diabetes (i.e., cholesterol and saturated fat), other nutrients that may confer a lower risk of type 2 diabetes (i.e., polyunsaturated fat), and have a high density of nutritious ingredients (i.e., protein and micronutrients).

There are limited and conflicting data from prospective population studies on the association between egg consumption and risk of type 2 diabetes. Studies based on US populations suggest an increased risk of type 2 diabetes with high egg consumption whereas studies in populations in other parts of the world generally indicate that eating four or more eggs per week is associated with a lower risk of developing type 2 diabetes. These differences may reflect residual confounding factors (e.g., high egg intake in the US could be associated with a high intake of fatty foods like bacon, burgers, and French fries) which might not be the case in other parts of the world. A recent 20-year study in Finland on over 2,300 middle-aged men found that, after adjustment for potential confounders,

(continued)

(continued)

those who had the highest compared with the lowest egg consumption had a 38% lower risk of type 2 diabetes and related metabolic risk markers such as fasting plasma glucose level and the serum concentration of C-reactive protein – an indicator of chronic low-level inflammation – but not with serum insulin. There were no positive associations between cholesterol intake and risk of type 2 diabetes, plasma glucose, serum insulin, and C-reactive protein, especially after accounting for egg consumption. In a related study the researchers found that men who ate, on average, one egg per day, had a certain lipid profile in their blood which is common among men who never develop type 2 diabetes.

Overall, it seems that eating up to seven eggs per week might have some moderate benefit in reducing the risk of type 2 diabetes. For those who are already diagnosed as diabetic and who may already have high serum LDL-cholesterol, several Diabetic Associations in the US and UK suggest that it is probably advisable to consume no more than three or four eggs per week. Choose boiled or poached eggs rather than fried to cut out other fats like oil or butter. For scrambled eggs, select pullet eggs which have only a small yolk or consider only using the egg whites, since this part of the egg contains virtually no cholesterol or saturated fat.

Alcohol Intake and Risk of Obesity and Type 2 Diabetes

Alcohol (also known as ethanol), is a nonessential nutrient that provides 7 kcal of energy per gram. Average alcohol intake in the USA is currently about 2 to 3% of daily energy intake. Alcohol is the most widely abused addictive drug, and, in the short term, causes intoxication which impairs mental function. In the longer term, regular drinking is known to cause damage to the liver and other organs. Alcohol is responsible for approximately 6% of deaths worldwide. However, alcohol may have health benefits when ingested in moderation. Moderate alcohol consumption reduces stress and raises levels of HDL cholesterol, which has a protective effect against cardiovascular diseases such as coronary heart disease and stroke. Moderate alcohol consumption also seems to help prevent type 2 diabetes. A meta-analysis (pulling together) of 20 studies concluded that moderate alcohol consumption was associated with a 30% reduced risk of developing type 2 diabetes in both men and women. Optimal alcohol consumption (compared with being tee-total) was 22 g/day for women and 24 g/day for men (20 g of alcohol is equivalent to one 175 mL glass of wine or a 330 mL bottle of beer). However, alcohol intake worsened the risk of type 2 diabetes when it exceeded 50 g/day for women and 60 g/day for men.

In contrast, a massive global study published in the Lancet in 2018 concluded that there is no safe level of drinking alcohol. In other words, even drinking one glass of wine or beer per day increases the risk of health problems such as cancer, injuries, and infectious diseases. But the overall increased risk to health of having just one alcoholic beverage per day is only 0.5% and this would probably not dissuade people from having a daily glass of wine with their meal. Specifically, for the risk of developing type 2 diabetes and cardiovascular disease, moderate alcohol consumption is actually beneficial and if you are aged over 50 this might be your major concern. Personally, I choose to drink one glass of red wine per day with my main meal of the day (e.g., evening dinner or Sunday lunch). However, I would emphasize that heavy consumption of alcohol, and in particular binge drinking, should be avoided altogether as it has numerous deleterious health effects and can be a significant contributor to the development of obesity. A 750 mL bottle of red wine contains about 600 kcal which is equivalent to two hamburgers, and a 500 mL bottle of beer contains around 220 kcal; despite this the energy content of alcoholic beverages is rarely shown on the bottle. Therefore, in the interests of health, alcohol should only be consumed in moderation and at appropriate times (i.e., not before driving or participating in sport or work). Furthermore, alcohol should be avoided during pregnancy.

THE PROBLEM WITH SNACKING

Probably not much more than 40 years ago most people believed that we should not "eat between meals". The idea was that you would get all your energy and nutrients from three main meals per day (i.e., breakfast, lunch, and dinner) and that eating between meals would spoil your appetite. Furthermore, most snack foods such as potato chips, cookies, cakes, and candy were (correctly) considered to be less nutritious than what you normally choose to eat for your main meals of the day. Back in the 1960s and 70s, before the modern-day obesity crisis had begun, the average adult would leave a window of about four and a half hours between meals. Nowadays that window is down to only three and a half hours for adults and that does not include any calorie-filled snacks and drinks (e.g., creamy, sugary coffees and shakes). The message about what (if anything) we should eat between meals has also subtly changed over time. "Not eating between meals" has now become "eat little and often"; in other words, consume maybe six or seven small meals over the course of a day. This has become known as a grazing pattern of eating. Breakfast, lunch, and dinner still exist (but are expected to be smaller) and our energy intake is bolstered by having mid-morning, mid-afternoon, and late evening snacks. The idea here is that if we eat little and often we are less likely to gorge on unhealthy junk foods as our hunger is kept at a low level throughout the day. However, the reality is that the opposite tends to happen, and we eat more junk foods that are high in calories but have low **nutrient density**, and we end up consuming more energy than we need. And who was mostly responsible for promoting this form of regular snacking? Not scientists or nutritionists, but (you guessed it) the snack food manufacturers! Studies have shown that this grazing pattern of eating has contributed to an increase of around 300 calories per day in what the average US person consumes now compared with 30 years ago. Around 180 calories of this extra energy intake come from snacks, but we also now consume about 120 calories more in our main meals. So snacking does not reduce our food intake at breakfast, lunch, and dinner at all. In fact, it seems that the more we snack, the more dietary energy we consume overall. Now, 300 extra calories per day represents an increase of about 15% compared with what we ate 30 years ago, and it is more than enough to make the average person overweight and obese within only a few years. Do the math: 300 calories per day is 2,100 calories per week (think of it as one extra day of eating per week), or 9,000 calories per month, or over 100,000 calories per year which would be predicted to cause weight gain of about 10-12 kg for the average person.

THE ROLE OF FOOD ADDICTION

For some people the development of a **food addiction** which triggers compulsive eating behavior can provide a fast track to becoming obese. Like addictive drugs, very tasty and enjoyable foods (that usually are rich in sugar, fat, and salt) activate the reward systems in the brain with the release of feel-good brain **neurotransmitters** such as **dopamine**. The experience of pleasure that results from increased dopamine transmission in the brain's reward pathway after eating a particular food item increases the desire to eat the same again in the near future. As a result, people keep on eating, simply for the pleasure it gives, even when they're not hungry. Taken to extreme this effect is called compulsive overeating. It is a type of behavioral addiction meaning that someone can become preoccupied with a behavior (such as eating, or gambling, or shopping) that triggers intense pleasure and becomes a pressing need to have on a regular basis. Psychological dependence has also been observed with this condition, meaning that withdrawal symptoms occur when consumption of these favorite foods stops or is replaced by foods low in sugar and fat. People with food addictions have essentially lost control over their eating behavior and find themselves obsessed with food and the thought of enjoying eating and the anticipation of doing so. As a result they become compulsive overeaters and can rapidly put on excess weight. Many people who have food addiction may also develop a kind of tolerance to their favorite food(s) just as drug addicts do with their drug(s) of choice. Food addicts may eat more and more, only to find that food satisfies them less and less, and their response is to eat even more! Overeating results in a daily positive energy balance (in some recorded cases daily energy intakes have exceeded 5,000 kcal) that can soon make a person become obese with all the associated health problems, including type 2 diabetes, that come with excess adiposity.

Many compulsive overeaters engage in frequent episodes of uncontrolled eating that could be called binge eating. The term "binge eating" means eating an excessive and unhealthy amount of food while feeling that one's sense of control has been lost. People who engage in binge eating may feel frenzied and consume a large number of calories before stopping. Food binges are often followed by feelings of guilt and depression, but unlike the condition known as **bulimia nervosa**, the binge eating episodes are not compensated for by so-called "purging behavior" to lose the extra calories such as vomiting, using laxatives, fasting for a prolonged period, or doing lots of exercise. When compulsive overeaters overeat through binge eating and experience feelings of guilt after their binges, they can be said to have **binge eating disorder**. In addition to binge eating, compulsive overeaters may also engage in "grazing" behavior, during which they continuously eat snacks (e.g., chips, cookies, cake, chocolate, and candy) throughout the day in addition to their regular meals. These actions result in an excessive overall number of calories consumed, even if the quantities eaten at any one time may not be particularly large.

It is thought that up to 20% of people may suffer from food addiction or addictive-like eating behavior, and this number is even higher among people with obesity (no doubt because it has already contributed to their excess fat accumulation). The take home message is that food addiction involves being addicted to food in the same way as drug addicts are addicted to drugs. It is really not that different to the alcoholic who is addicted to alcohol, or the smoker who is addicted to nicotine. People who have food addiction have effectively lost the ability to control their intake of certain foods. This does not apply to all foods because people don't just get addicted to any food. The addiction is usually for one or more specific food item or particular food type. In a recent study by researchers from the University of Michigan, the top ten most addictive foods were found to be pizza, chocolate, chips (known as crisps in the UK), cookies (known as biscuits in the UK), ice cream, French fries, cheeseburgers, sugary soft drinks, cake, cheese, and fried bacon/chicken. You can try using the simple quiz shown in the following sidebar to determine if you are a prime candidate for food addiction.

How to determine if you have a food addiction

Scientists at Yale University's Rudd Center for Food Science and Policy have developed a quiz to identify people with food addictions. Some of the questions used are listed below and you can answer these to determine if you have a food addiction. Simply answer yes or no.

Do you?:

1. End up eating more than planned when you start eating certain foods.

2. Keep eating certain foods even if you're no longer hungry.

3. Eat to the point of feeling ill.

4. Worry about not eating certain types of foods or worry about cutting down on certain types of foods.

5. Go out of your way to obtain certain foods when they aren't available when you want them.

6. Eat certain foods so often or in such large amounts that you start eating food instead of working, spending time with the family, or doing recreational activities.

7. Avoid professional or social situations where certain foods are available because of a fear of overeating.

8. Have problems functioning effectively at your job or college because of food and eating.

9. Have problems such as depression, anxiety, self-loathing, or guilt after eating food.

10. Need to eat more and more food to reduce negative emotions or increase pleasure.

11. Not gain the same amount of pleasure by eating food in the way you used to.

12. Have symptoms such as anxiety or agitation when you cut down on certain foods (excluding caffeinated and alcoholic beverages).

If you answered yes to five or more of the above questions you are likely to have a food addiction. The questionnaire and instructions can be found at www.midss.org/content/yale-food-addiction-scale-yfas.

(continued)

(continued)

> If you think you are addicted to a certain type of food or even only one specific food item, the only real way to end the addiction is to go "cold turkey" and cut out the food item from your diet completely for at least three weeks, and then reintroduce it sparingly, as a treat, perhaps only once or twice per week and stick to a reasonable amount that you have decided upon in advance. Unfortunately, successful recovery from a food addiction may be more complicated than recovery from some other kinds of addiction. Alcoholics, for example, can ultimately abstain from drinking alcohol altogether but people who are addicted to food still need to eat. In extreme cases of food addiction and compulsive overeating, a nutritionist, psychologist, or doctor who is educated about food addiction may be needed to help break the habit.

THE LINKS WITH SEDENTARY BEHAVIOR

Since the 1950s, participation in sports and levels of physical activity in general have declined among the majority, and many people now have sedentary lifestyle behaviors (e.g., occupations that involve minimal exercise, driving rather than walking or cycling, sitting watching television, playing computer games, spending lots of time texting and using social media platforms on tablets and mobile phones, etc.). It is easy to understand how the overall reduction in daily energy expenditure resulting from lack of exercise has contributed to the obesity epidemic. In 2014 researchers from Stanford University analyzed data from the National Health and Nutrition Examination Survey, a long-term project of the Centers for Disease Control and Prevention that collects information from surveys and from physical examinations to assess Americans' health. The researchers considered survey results from 17,430 participants from 1988 through 1994 and from approximately 5,000 participants each year from 1995 through 2010. Survey participants recorded the frequency, duration, and intensity of their exercise within the previous month. The team found that the percentage of women reporting no physical activity jumped from 19% to 52% between 1988 and 2010, and the percentage of inactive men rose from 11% to 43%. This was associated with the incidence of obesity over the same time period climbing from 25% to 35% in women, and from 20% to 35% in men. Waist circumference was also measured and increased significantly over time. Surprisingly, however, the number of calories consumed per day did not change significantly, although that doesn't mean that the number of calories consumed were optimal, and participants may have underreported their daily intakes. But these findings suggest it was the reduction in physical activity levels rather than diet that was the main contributor to the increased rates of obesity in both men and women. Some may think that many people do less exercise nowadays just because we have become lazier. However, that is not necessarily the case, and it might be that people just have less time or resources to do exercise. There are far more sedentary occupations than there were 50 years ago; people are expected to work longer hours; transport is more easily accessible and affordable; and there are increased numbers of single parents who are trying to balance work and childcare.

Engaging in regular physical activity can also help with eating well without going over the calorie limit that will weight. Exercise itself brings health benefits that will en the risk of many health problems and potential disabiliti Another problem with aging is that we tend to lose muscle which means that we become weaker and at some point independently (for example, you need a certain amount of armchair or the toilet!). Participating in regular exercise, anc exercise together with appropriate ingestion of dietary protei across the lifespan. In short, some regular moderate exercise can help you stay healthy, live longer, and be happier. Know _, ...ar types of exercise are best and understanding how your body adapts to exercise, how much is needed for health benefits, and just how many calories you are burning in different activities will allow you to decide what is best for you, and what is easiest to fit into your normal daily routine. These issues will be covered in more detail in chapter 7.

THE LINKS WITH POOR SLEEP QUALITY

A simple truth is what we eat can affect our sleep, and how we sleep can affect our food intake. The quality of the diet, and the consumption of certain foods and nutrients can influence regulatory hormonal pathways that can alter both the quantity and quality of sleep. In turn, the amount of sleep we get and its quality influence the intake of total energy, as well as of specific foods and nutrients, through both physiological and behavioral mechanisms. Research in this field has examined the effects of both short and long sleep duration on patterns of food intake and nutritional quality. The latest evidence suggests that extremes of sleep duration (too little or too much) alter circulating hormone levels and circadian rhythms, which contribute to weight gain and other risk factors for the development of type 2 diabetes (figure 5.6) and all-cause mortality (primarily cardiovascular events; figure 5.7). These influences may begin in childhood and have impacts throughout the course of our lives.

Short sleep duration has received more attention, and has been shown to be associated with an increased risk of obesity, type 2 diabetes, and cardiovascular disease, particularly among women. It has been suggested that this is due to interference with the body's restorative processes that occur during sleep, leading to biological and behavioral (including food choice) factors that increase our risk for chronic disease development.

Sleep influences the circulating levels of the appetite controlling hormones ghrelin and **leptin**. Ghrelin stimulates hunger, and leptin signals satiety. Sleep deprivation or insomnia causes relatively high levels of ghrelin and low levels of leptin which would be predicted to increase appetite and induce overeating behaviors. Furthermore, circulating levels of adiponectin (an anti-inflammatory chemical secreted from adipose tissue that is found in lower levels in the blood of individuals with obesity), were found to decrease following sleep restriction in Caucasian women and may be another mechanism by which reduced sleep duration promotes cardiovascular population. As explained in chapter 4, the development of chronic low-grade [...] a major risk factor for chronic metabolic and cardiovascular diseases.

[...]privation is associated with increased appetite and a higher motivation to consume [...]y-dense foods that are high in fat and sugar, leading to increased energy intakes and potential [...]ight gain. But that is not all. Having only a short sleep time increases the opportunities for eating, and can induce psychological distress, greater sensitivity to food reward, and disinhibited

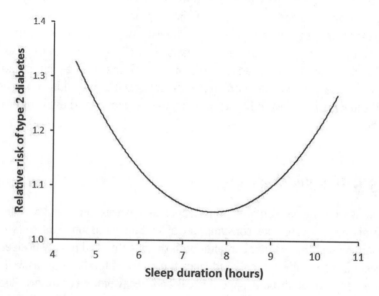

Figure 5.6 Association between sleep duration and relative risk of type 2 diabetes. Data from Shan et al. (2015).

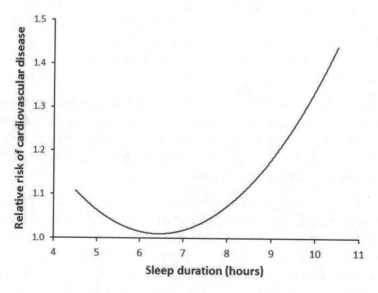

Figure 5.7 Relationship of sleep duration with all-cause mortality and cardiovascular events. Data from Yin et al. (2017).

eating. We tend to eat more for these reasons and because we need more energy to sustain extended wakefulness. Indeed, people who complain of short sleep duration are more prone to having irregular eating patterns, including more frequent consumption of energy-dense snacks outside of regular mealtimes, and higher total energy and fat intake. Other studies suggest that weight loss and weight maintenance through diet and lifestyle interventions can contribute to improvements in sleep quality.

It will come as no surprise to many parents that adolescents are at particularly high risk of short sleep duration, and the highest prevalence of insufficient sleep (69%) is reported for this age group. Their high use of electronic devices (television, computers, game stations, phones, tablets, etc.) as well as a tendency for unhealthy eating are among the behavioral risk factors that may account for this. Lack of sleep in adolescents is now known to be associated with a higher risk for obesity, decreased insulin sensitivity (predisposing to type 2 diabetes), and high blood pressure.

In recent years evidence has emerged indicating that overlong sleep duration, usually defined as more than nine hours of sleep, is also associated with higher risk of type 2 diabetes, obesity, cardiovascular disease, chronic kidney disease, and depression although at present the mechanisms for these relationships are not clear. It may be that long sleep duration is actually associated with more sleep disruptions, and indeed, the coexistence of poor sleep quality and longer sleep duration were shown to be associated with a higher incidence of coronary heart disease in one study. In summary, current evidence suggests that particularly short or long sleep durations are predictors of increased risk for unhealthy eating and weight gain and the subsequent development of several chronic cardiovascular and metabolic diseases including type 2 diabetes. But if you currently experience poor sleep quality (e.g., regular awakenings during the night, sleep lightly, or sleep for less than seven hours per night) don't despair; there are several things you can do to help you sleep better and these are explained in chapter 7.

SOCIO-ECONOMIC FACTORS IN THE DEVELOPMENT OF OBESITY

While obesity levels have been rising for all socioeconomic groups, some groups are more affected than others. Recent research highlights the complexity and variation in how socioeconomic status (SES) and obesity are related. A major global study that used data for 67 countries, representing all the regions of the world, examined how economic development, SES, and obesity were related. The researchers used self-reported height and weight to calculate BMI, and looked at the relationship between obesity, gross national product (as a measure of each country's economic status), and SES based on education, occupation, and income.

They found that obesity rose with a nation's economic development, but also that SES as it related to obesity changed. In high-income countries, those with higher SES were less likely to be obese. Conversely, in lower-income countries, people with higher SES were more likely to be obese. Why might this be so and what causes the SES influence to differ so markedly depending on the country's overall wealth? Well, it may be that in lower-income countries, higher SES leads to eating more and avoiding physically tough occupations. But in higher-income countries, individuals with higher SES may respond with healthier eating and participating in regular exercise. The implication is that while economic development improves health, problems of malnutrition affecting those with lower SES are replaced by problems of overconsumption of high-calorie foods. But some developing countries, such as India, exhibit continued high levels of malnutrition among the poor along with a rise in obesity among the relatively small population of the rich.

In North American and European countries, which are high-income nations, higher SES is beneficial for staying thin. One of the main reasons for this is the fact that most people living in high-income nations have more money so they can afford to go to the gym, afford to eat healthy foods (which are that much more expensive than unhealthy foods), don't have to work two jobs so have the time (and the money) to enjoy leisure time activities, such as attending cultural events, going to the movies, and do regular exercise. In other words, they can afford to be more "civilized" with the way they live and eat. The likelihood is that they've also come from more privileged backgrounds with childhoods full of healthier foods and eating patterns, and so on. In low SES groups in the US, selecting high-calorie food items, large plate size, uncontrolled eating, and eating at night were the main causes associated with increased obesity risk compared with those of high SES. This association between low SES and access to cheap energy-dense foods and subsequent obesity has been suggested to be because socioeconomic disadvantage increases psychological distress which, in turn, promotes maladaptive coping behaviors, such as emotional eating, and ultimately obesity. Indeed, recent research has shown that lower SES is associated with higher distress, higher distress is associated with higher emotional eating, and higher emotional eating is associated with higher BMI.

There are also subtle influences of gender and race that impact on the influence of SES on rates of obesity. For example, in the US, men with a middle-class upbringing and lifestyle who were presently working in lower-class jobs were almost as likely to be obese as those brought up in working-poor households. For women who were white, all SES groups had a greater risk of obesity compared with the most advantaged. In contrast, among black women, only those from working-poor households who had lower-status jobs were at increased obesity risk compared with the most advantaged group.

Overall, these studies show that factors that increase the risk of being obese affect SES groups differently, but that in developed, high-income countries like the US and UK, those with lower SES are more likely to be obese and subsequently suffer worse health and reduced longevity.

TOO MANY CALORIES INGESTED, OR TOO FEW EXPENDED?

Scientists continue to debate the relative importance of overeating and lack of exercise in the development of the global obesity epidemic. For some people, overeating may be the main issue while for others it may just be a lack of exercise that makes them put on weight. However, for the majority, the reasons for becoming overweight include both overeating and inactivity. What can be said with certainty is that consuming more calories than we need, as determined by our resting metabolic rate and the amount of exercise we do, is the root cause of weight gain. About 30-40 years ago the blame for the increasing prevalence of obesity was attributed to eating too much dietary fat. People used to think that eating an excess of fat made you fat, so the usual recommendation to lose weight was to cut down on their fat intake. But people would still get fat if they replaced the calories from fat with those from carbohydrate while their daily calorie intake exceeded their needs. More recently, the increasing incidence of obesity and type 2 diabetes in the past 10- 20 years has been attributed to consuming too much refined carbohydrate and sugary drinks which may have actually been promoted to some degree by our earlier obsession about cutting down on fat. However, the most important point is that we consume too much dietary energy overall. Whether it is too much fat, or too much carbohydrate, or both (which is probably closer to reality), we need to lose the excess body fat we have accumulated due to our overindulgence in food and drink if we want to live healthier lives and rid ourselves of type 2 diabetes.

Key Points

- Obesity is defined by clinicians as having a BMI of 30 kg/m² or more or being overweight to the point where there are medical complications. Overweight means having a BMI of 25-29 kg/m².

- The biggest single risk factor for type 2 diabetes is being overweight or obese, and most of the molecular mechanisms that it has been suggested cause insulin resistance to develop in the prediabetic stage of the condition are linked to increased adiposity.

- A number of factors including genetics, food choices, food addiction, sedentary behavior, poor sleep quality, and socioeconomic status are thought to contribute to the development of obesity.

- Excessive intakes of some nutrients (e.g., carbohydrates, fats) or certain subgroups (e.g., simple sugars, corn syrups, saturated fats, cholesterol) and other nonessential nutrients (e.g., alcohol) can have harmful effects on our health, particularly in the long-term, increasing our risk of developing obesity and the associated chronic metabolic and cardiovascular diseases, and cancer.

- Energy balance refers to the balance between energy intake and energy expenditure. Simply put, it is the difference between energy in and energy out. When energy intake is greater than energy expenditure (i.e., when more calories come in than go out), the energy balance is said to be positive and weight gain will occur as most of the excess energy gets converted into body fat.

- Although genetic factors may play some role there can be no doubt that a combination of eating too much and lack of exercise are the two main factors responsible for the obesity epidemic.

Chapter 6

How Do I Know If (or By How Much) I Am Overweight or Overfat?

Objectives

After studying this chapter, you should:

- Be aware of the possible risks and pitfalls of dieting.
- Understand how to tell if you are overweight.
- Understand how to tell if you are overfat.

If you have been diagnosed as prediabetic or type 2 diabetic, you are almost certainly overweight and carrying too much body fat. The only ways to improve your condition and reduce the risk of developing the serious health consequences that come with diabetes are to lose weight and do more exercise. Losing weight means changing your diet and eating less, and also trying to fit more exercise into your daily routine. Weight loss is desirable for the health reasons explained in chapter 2, but if it is not done correctly (e.g., eating insufficient protein, or cutting out major macronutrients or food groups from your diet) it can often be accompanied by a reduction in muscle mass and it may reduce liver and muscle glycogen stores as well which will make doing any exercise feel harder and make you feel more tired. Trying to lose too much weight too quickly can also result in chronic fatigue, irritability, and increased risk of injuries. Furthermore, too much emphasis on losing weight can lead to the development of micronutrient deficiencies and **eating disorders** such as **anorexia nervosa** and bulimia nervosa, which are harmful to health. Some elderly and illness-prone individuals may actually benefit from being slightly overweight rather than underweight in order to have an energy reserve when they become ill and are unable to eat properly. These are good reasons to (a) avoid extreme dieting and (b) learn how to lose weight effectively and safely with minimal disruption to your normal daily routine. How you can achieve this will be described in chapters 8 and 9.

For those who are determined to lose some weight, the first step in determining what target weight you should be aiming for is to know your current weight by measuring it in a normally hydrated state and obtaining a measure of your body composition. These measures can be used to determine how much body fat you should lose to put you back within an optimal range for health. For consistency it would be best to make these measurements in the morning, before you have breakfast and after you have gone to the toilet. Bear in mind that by emptying your bladder and taking a dump you can instantly lose, on average, around 0.5-1.0 kg!

NORMAL LEVELS OF BODY FAT

Body fat consists of **essential body fat** and storage fat. Essential body fat is present in all membranes, nerve tissues, bone marrow, and the vital organs, and we cannot lose this fat without compromising physiological function. Storage fat, on the other hand, is our main form of energy reserve, and it accumulates when more dietary energy than we need is consumed and decreases when more energy is expended than consumed. Essential body fat is approximately 3% of body mass for men and 12% of body mass for women. It is thought that the reason why women have more essential body fat than men is because of childbearing and hormonal functions. Women store more fat under the skin and on their hips, buttocks, and thighs than men who tend to deposit excess fat in the torso and particularly in the belly region. In general, the total healthy body-fat percentage (essential plus storage fat) is between 8% and 20% for young men and between 15% and 30% for young women (see table 6.1). As approximately 3% of body mass of males and 12% of body mass of females is essential body fat, no diet should ever aim to get rid of all fat from the body. For those aged over 40 years, the acceptable body fat percentages are a bit higher (table 6.2) because as we get older we tend to lose some lean muscle mass and – particularly in postmenopausal women – some bone mass.

Table 6.1 Body-fat percentages for men and women aged 18-40 and their classification

Men	Women	Classification
5–10%	8-15%	Athletic
11–14%	16-23%	Good
15–20%	24-30%	Acceptable
21–24%	31-36%	Overweight
Over 24%	Over 36%	Obese

Note that these are rough estimates. The "athletic" values are those found in elite sports persons such as distance runners, cyclists, soccer, and tennis players for whom low body fat is an advantage.

Table 6.2 Body-fat percentages for men and women aged 41-70 and their classification

Men	Women	Classification
8–13%	12-20%	Athletic
14–18%	21-27%	Good
19–22%	28-34%	Acceptable
23–28%	35-39%	Overweight
Over 28%	Over 40%	Obese

Note that these are rough estimates. The "athletic" values are those found in very fit people who participate regularly in sports or other strenuous physical activities.

HOW CAN I TELL IF I AM OVERWEIGHT OR OVERFAT?

In order to determine if you are overweight or overfat, a variety of measurements can be made, but bear in mind they all have some limitations. Body composition can be measured reasonably accurately by some methods, but these are generally found in a science lab or hospital (e.g., Dual Energy X-Ray Absorptiometry, Computed Tomography, Magnetic Resonance Imaging, Air Displacement Plethysmography) or require experience and expertise (e.g., using skinfold calipers, underwater weighing). Here I will only describe some methods that the general public can do for themselves. These can provide a rough estimate rather than a very accurate measure of body composition.

HEIGHT–WEIGHT RELATIONSHIP AND BODY MASS INDEX

Height-weight tables or charts, such as the one shown in figure 6.1, provide a normal range of body weights for any given height. Such charts and tables have limitations, however, especially when applied to people who have a large muscle mass. For instance, a muscular man who is 180 cm tall and weighs 100 kg may have low body fat but could be classified as overweight. In his case the "extra" weight is muscle, not body fat, which would lead to erroneous classification and possibly mistaken advice.

A rough but better measure than the height–weight tables is the body mass index (BMI), also known as the Quetelet index. Also derived from body mass and height, BMI in units of kg/m^2 is calculated by dividing the body mass in kg by the height in meters and then dividing again by the height in meters:

BMI = (body mass in kilograms ÷ height in meters) ÷ height in meters

Or BMI = body mass in kilograms ÷ (height in meters x height in meters)

Or BMI = body mass in kilograms ÷ $(\text{height in meters})^2$

You can also use the height-weight chart in figure 6.1 to determine your BMI if you prefer not to use a calculator. A person who is 1.75 m (5 ft 9 in) tall and weighs 75.0 kg (165 lbs) has a BMI of 75.0 ÷ $(1.75)^2$ = 75.0 ÷ 3.06 = 24.5 kg/m² (figure 6.2). The normal range is between 18.5 kg/m² and 25.0 kg/m². People with a BMI of 25-29 kg/m² are classified as overweight, people with a BMI of 30 kg/m² or higher are classified as obese, and people with a BMI of 40 kg/m² or higher are classified as morbidly obese. People with a BMI below 18.5 kg/m² are classified as underweight.

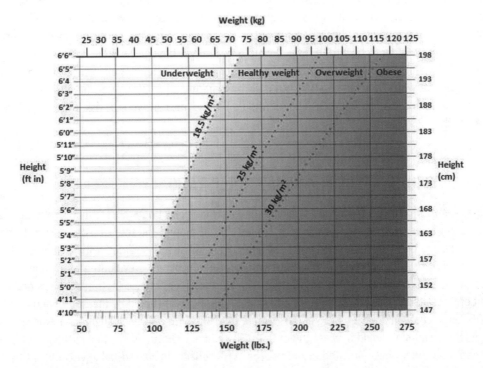

Figure 6.1 Relationship between height, weight, and body mass index (BMI) and criteria for underweight, normal (healthy), overweight, and obesity. BMI measures weight in relation to height (kg/m²). The BMI ranges shown are for adults and should not be applied to children. They are not exact ranges of healthy and unhealthy weights, but health risk increases at higher levels of overweight and obesity. Even within the healthy BMI range, weight gains can carry health risks for adults. Adapted from Dietary Guidelines for Americans (2000), https://www.health.gov/dietaryguidelines/dga2000/document/frontcover.htm.

Directions for using the BMI chart: Find your weight (unclothed) on the bottom (lbs) or top (kg) scale of the chart. Go straight up or down from that point until you come to the line that matches your height (without shoes). Then look to find your weight group.

Even when using BMI rather than just body weight, our muscular man weighing 100 kg and 1.80 m tall would be classified as overweight or even obese because the equation does not take into account body composition (his BMI = 100 ÷ $(1.80)^2$ = 30.9 kg/m²). In fact, it is quite possible that two individuals could have the same BMI but completely different body compositions. One could achieve his or her body weight with mainly muscle mass as a result of hard resistance training, whereas the other could achieve his or her body weight by fat deposition as a result of a sedentary lifestyle and overeating. Without information about body composition, they both might be classified as obese. In children and older people, the BMI is difficult to interpret because muscle and bone weights are changing in relationship to height.

The BMI, however, does provide useful information about risks for various diseases including type 2 diabetes and is used in many epidemiological and clinical studies. For example, BMI correlates with the incidence of type 2 diabetes and some other chronic diseases including hypertension, stroke, certain cancers, kidney disease, and dementia. The BMI, however, is best used for populations rather than individuals. When used for individual assessment, BMI needs to be used in coordination with other measurements such as waist circumference or body composition because it is possible to be within normal weight or BMI yet have unhealthily high levels of belly (visceral) fat. To see if your BMI puts you at risk for type 2 diabetes, find your BMI from figure 6.1. If you are white, your at-risk BMI is equal to or greater than 25 kg/m². If you are of Asian, African, Hispanic/Latino, Pacific Island, or Middle Eastern descent your at-risk BMI is equal to or greater than 23 kg/m².

WAIST CIRCUMFERENCE AND WAIST-TO-HIP RATIO

The **waist-to-hip ratio (WHR)** measurement gives an index of body-fat distribution (figure 6.2). Because it gives an indication of the body fat distributed around the torso, it can be used to help determine the degree of obesity. Excess fat around the waist is associated with increased risk of chronic disease including type 2 diabetes. The distribution of fat is evaluated by dividing waist size by hip size. A person with a 34 inch (86.5 cm) waist circumference (note that this is not your belt or trouser size – see the sidebar for an explanation of how it should be measured) and 42 inch (106.7 cm) hips would have a ratio of 0.81 (figure 6.2); one with a 40 inch (101.6 cm) waist and 41 inch (104.1 cm) hips would have a ratio of 0.98. The higher the ratio is, the higher the risk of heart disease and other obesity-related disorders. The WHR reflects increased belly (visceral) fat better than BMI. Females with a WHR greater than 0.80, and males with a WHR greater than 0.91, have a higher risk of developing type 2 diabetes, cardiovascular disease, and certain cancers. A WHR smaller than 0.73 for women and 0.85 for men indicates a low risk of developing chronic disease. WHR is also a better predictor of mortality in older people than waist circumference or BMI although some studies have found waist circumference alone to be a good indicator of cardiovascular risk factors, body fat distribution, and hypertension in people diagnosed with type 2 diabetes.

Waist circumference alone is also a useful and simple measurement that can give an idea of your risk of developing type 2 diabetes (if you don't already have it). See the sidebar for details on how to perform a waist circumference measurement correctly and how it should be used to assess your diabetes risk.

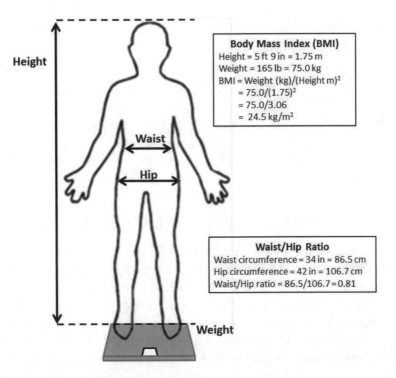

Body Mass Index (BMI)
Height = 5 ft 9 in = 1.75 m
Weight = 165 lb = 75.0 kg
BMI = Weight (kg)/(Height m)^2
= 75.0/(1.75)^2
= 75.0/3.06
= 24.5 kg/m^2

Waist/Hip Ratio
Waist circumference = 34 in = 86.5 cm
Hip circumference = 42 in = 106.7 cm
Waist/Hip ratio = 86.5/106.7 = 0.81

Figure 6.2 Waist-to-hip ratio and body mass index measurement

How to measure your waist circumference and its relationship to type 2 diabetes risk

Measuring your waist circumference is a simple and effective way of finding out whether you might be at risk of type 2 diabetes. Extra weight around your waist means fat can build up around organs, like your liver, gut, and pancreas. This build-up of belly fat is strongly associated with the development of insulin resistance which means the insulin your body produces doesn't work properly and that increases your chance of having high blood glucose. You should make sure your overall weight and BMI are healthy, but even if they are, you may still be at risk of type 2 diabetes if you have a large waist measurement.

Measuring your waist circumference takes less than a minute and all you need is a tape measure. You can always ask a friend or family member to help you as well if you can't do it on your own. It is important to understand that your waist size is often not the same as your jean size or belt size which is usually somewhat lower than our waist circumference measurement actually is. To measure your true waist circumference, find the top of your hip bone and the bottom of your ribcage. In the middle of these two points is where you need to measure. For many people, the belly button is a good guide, but this might not be the case for you, so it's best to find that midpoint between your ribcage and hip.

(continued)

A healthy waist circumference all depends on your gender and ethnicity. For a healthy measurement, with a low risk of type 2 diabetes, it should be less than:

80 cm (31.5 in) for all women

94 cm (37 in) for most men

90 cm (35 in) for black or South Asian men (because there is a higher risk of type 2 diabetes if you are of black or South Asian background).

ESTIMATING PERCENTAGE BODY FAT BY BIOELECTRICAL IMPEDANCE ANALYSIS

In scientific studies body fat percentage is usually estimated by indirect methods such as **dual energy X-ray absorptiometry** (DEXA), air displacement plethysmography (commonly known as Bodpod), or underwater weighing (used to determine body density which is related to percentage body fat), or is derived from skinfold caliper measurements made by a skilled technician at three or more body sites. However, the simplest way to measure body fat for most people who do not have access to a science lab is to use an electronic scale that incorporates a bioelectrical impedance device. **Bioelectrical impedance analysis (BIA)** is based on the principle that different tissues and substances have different impedance (resistance) to an electrical current. For example, impedance or conductivity is quite different for fat tissue and water. Adipose tissue – of which only 5% is water – has high resistance, or impedance, whereas muscle – of which up to 77% is water – has low resistance. A BIA device sends a small, safe electrical current through the body to measure impedance and so can be used to estimate percentage body fat. For consistency it is best to make these measurements in the morning, before you have breakfast and after you have gone to the toilet. Compare your body fat percentage measured by BIA with the values in table 6.1 or 6.2 depending on your age to see if you are overweight or obese.

Key Points

- If you have been diagnosed as prediabetic or type 2 diabetic you are almost certainly overweight and carrying too much body fat. The only ways to improve your condition and reduce the risk of developing the serious health consequences that come with diabetes are to lose weight and do more exercise.

- If you are determined to lose some weight the first step in determining what target weight you should be aiming for is to know your current weight by measuring it in a normally hydrated state and obtaining a measure of your body composition.

- Weight loss is desirable for health reasons but if it is not done correctly (e.g., eating insufficient protein or cutting out major macronutrients or food groups from your diet) it can often be accompanied by a reduction in muscle mass and it may reduce your glycogen stores as well which will make doing any exercise feel harder and make you feel more tired.

- Trying to lose too much weight too quickly can also be associated with chronic fatigue, irritability, and increased risk of injuries. Furthermore, too much emphasis on losing weight can lead to the development of micronutrient deficiencies and eating disorders which are harmful to health.

- In general, the total healthy body-fat percentage (essential plus storage fat) is 10-20% for young men and 15-30% for young women. For people aged over 40, the healthy ranges of body fat are 13-22% and 20-34% for men and women, respectively.

- As approximately 3% of body mass of males and 12% of body mass of females is essential body fat, no diet should ever aim to get rid of all fat from the body.

- Your body weight, height-weight relationship, and body mass index (BMI) provide a rough guide to whether you are overweight or not but do not indicate anything about your body composition.

- Waist circumference and waist-to-hip ratio provide a better indication than BMI of how fat you are.

- Bioelectrical impedance analysis using an electronic digital scale can give an estimate of percentage body fat but with limited accuracy. For consistency it is best to make these measurements in the morning, before you have breakfast, and after you have gone to the toilet.

Chapter 7

What Can I Do to Reduce My Risk of Complications If I Have Type 2 Diabetes?

Objectives

After studying this chapter, you should:

- Appreciate the very real dangers of serious health complications if you rely only on prescribed medication to treat type 2 diabetes.

- Know what you can do to reduce your risk of these complications and live well for longer.

- Understand how to eat a healthier diet.

- Understand why it is important to exercise more.

- Understand the importance of sleep and how to achieve better sleep quality.

- Appreciate that trying to lose body fat and weight is crucial for reducing the risk of diabetic complications.

If you are reading this chapter you are probably someone who has been diagnosed with prediabetes or type 2 diabetes. That means that you are likely to be over 45 years old, overweight, and not overly enthusiastic about exercise. Despite warnings about the complications, many diabetics choose to ignore them. Although they may take their medication regularly, they do not adopt the recommended changes to their diet and lifestyle or only make a token effort to do so. Diabetes is a progressive disease and the medications only delay the onset of complications; the drugs you take will not prevent the complications from happening. And it is these complications: disease of the heart, circulation, and kidneys, damage to the eyes and nerves, and serious life-threatening infections that are the real dangers of diabetes. Let's examine some statistics, using recent data from the UK as an example. In 2018 there were 4.7 million people with diabetes (90% of which were cases of type 2 diabetes) and an estimated further 13 million considered to be at risk. Diabetes is currently responsible for 26,000 early deaths per year (most commonly due to heart failure) alongside serious complications such as blindness, amputation, or stroke. Each year in the UK about 30,000 people living with diabetes suffer a heart attack, and more than 40,000 people with the illness have a stroke. The annual number of diabetes-related amputations is currently over 8,000. Around one third of people develop **diabetic retinopathy** within 10 years of being diagnosed as type 2 diabetic. Currently in the UK the cost to the NHS of prescribing drugs to treat type 2 diabetes is one billion pounds sterling per year, but it is estimated that the total cost to the NHS is over 10 billion pounds sterling per year, so the real price society has to pay for diabetes is not medications, but the devastating complications that require expensive treatment that may include surgery as well as additional medications and stays in hospital.

The rate of these serious, debilitating, and often life-changing or life-threatening complications could be markedly reduced if diabetics took more heed of the advice given to them by healthcare practitioners about their diet and lifestyle behaviors. The remainder of this chapter describes some of the things you can do to reduce your risk of these complications, improve your quality of life, maintain your independence, and live well for longer. This involves more than just the strategies employed to manage your condition which were described in chapter 3.

EAT A HEALTHIER DIET

As mentioned in chapter 4, a major contributor to the development of type 2 diabetes is eating too much in general, and also eating too many foods that are high in sugar, fat, and salt but low in important nutrients such as vitamins, phytonutrients, and fiber. In order to improve your diabetic condition and reduce your risk of nasty complications your diet needs to change for the better. Some advice on how to do this was given in chapter 3 where I described how diabetes could be managed by manipulation of diet, but more detail is provided here. Changing your diet to reduce your risk of cardiovascular, kidney, nerve, and eye problems in the years ahead is not as difficult as you may think it is. It really means changing your food choices and selecting more natural foods – fruits and vegetables in particular – rather than processed foods, ready meals, fast food, and takeaways. In fact, you will probably find that your food looks and tastes better, and it may well cost you less. The guidelines for healthy eating that follow apply to all adults who are above 18 years of age, and most of them are generally applicable to younger people from the age of four. In other words, although not the focus of this particular book, your children should be eating pretty much the same as the adult members of the family, but because the youngsters are smaller, they should be given smaller portions.

RECOMMENDATIONS FOR HEALTHY EATING

Here is an extensive list of evidence-based recommendations on how you can eat a healthier diet. I have put this together from information provided by the 2015-2020 *Dietary Guidelines for Americans*, the 2016 *Eatwell Guide* from the UK, and guidelines published by organizations and institutions in various other countries. In this bulleted list, the recommendation is first stated, and then the reason(s) why this recommendation is given is briefly summarized.

- *Recommendation:* Follow a healthy eating pattern across the lifespan. *Why?:* Healthy eating patterns (i.e., the combination of foods and drinks that a person eats over time) ensure a diet that is balanced, nutritious, and unlikely to be fattening. Such diets are an important contributor to health. Healthy eating patterns include a variety of nutritious foods like vegetables, fruits, grains, low-fat and fat-free dairy, lean meats, and other foods high in protein and plant-based oils (e.g., extra virgin olive oil), while limiting saturated fats, *trans* fats, added sugars, and salt. A healthy eating pattern can be tailored to meet a person's taste preferences, traditions, culture, and budget.

- *Recommendation:* Eat a wide variety of nutrient-rich or nutrient-dense foods. *Why?:* By eating a variety of foods from within each food group and between food groups, people will likely ingest adequate amounts of all essential nutrients. The term "**nutrient-dense**" indicates the essential nutrients and other beneficial substances in a food have not been "diluted" by the addition of calories from added solid fats, sugars, or refined starches, or by the solid fats that are naturally present in the food. Thus, nutrient-dense foods are those that provide vitamins, minerals, and other substances that contribute to adequate nutrient intakes or may have positive health effects, but contain little or no solid fats, added sugars, refined starches, and salt. Ideally, these foods should be in forms that retain naturally occurring healthy components, such as vitamins and dietary fiber. All vegetables, fruits, wholegrains, seafood, eggs, legumes (beans and peas), unsalted nuts and seeds, fat-free and low-fat dairy products, and lean meats and poultry can be considered to be nutrient-dense foods. These foods contribute to meeting food group recommendations within the desirable calorie and sodium limits. In contrast, many processed foods, sauces, pastries, and ready meals are not nutrient-dense because they contain substantial amounts of undesirable high calorie items and often include added sugars and salt.

- *Recommendation:* Eat a diet rich in vegetables, fruits, and wholegrain and high-fiber foods. People should eat at least five portions of fruit and vegetables daily. *Why?:* Consuming vegetables, fruits, and wholegrain and high-fiber foods will help to achieve the recommended carbohydrate intake and increase fiber intake which is good for digestive and cardiovascular health. In addition, these foods contain relatively large amounts of phytonutrients, which have some beneficial health effects. Epidemiological studies have generally shown that diets high in wholegrain products (bread and cereals), legumes (beans and peas), fruits, and vegetables, have significant health benefits.

- *Recommendation:* Eat a variety of healthy protein foods. *Why?:* Consuming a variety of high-protein food sources including seafood, lean meats and poultry, eggs, legumes, soy products, and nuts and seeds, that provides 10-15% of daily calories should ensure that daily protein requirements are met while avoiding excessive fat intake. Eating a diverse range of high protein foods gives your body other important nutrients, including iron, zinc, and other important minerals and vitamins (particularly B-group vitamins).

- *Recommendation:* Choose a diet moderate in total fat but low in saturated fat, *trans* fats, and cholesterol. *Why?:* Apart from the essential fatty acids linoleic and α-linolenic acid, there is no specific requirement for fats. Too much saturated and *trans* fat intake is linked to cardiovascular disease. But some fat is needed to help with the intake of the fat-soluble vitamins A, D, E, and K. Because most foods contain some fats, the intake of these vitamins is usually not a problem. To lower total fat intake, dairy products that are fat-free or low in fat (e.g., semi-skimmed milk; low-fat yogurt) are recommended. The standard recommendation (over the course of one week) is to have an intake of saturated fatty acids below 10% of total energy intake, limit cholesterol intake to 0.3 g or less per day and keep *trans* fat intake to a minimum.

- *Recommendation:* People should eat fewer commercially prepared processed foods, baked goods, and avoid fast foods. *Why?:* These foods are generally high in energy and fat and contain a significant amount of *trans* fatty acids which are harmful to cardiovascular health. Consumption of small amounts of oils is encouraged, including those from plants: canola, corn, olive, peanut, safflower, soybean, and sunflower. Oils also are naturally present in nuts, seeds, seafood, olives, and avocados.

- *Recommendation:* Cut back on beverages and foods high in calories and low in nutrition. *Why?:* Beverages such as soft drinks, and foods with added sugar contribute significantly to energy intake while not adding useful nutrients. High levels of added sugar intake are associated with high blood triglyceride concentrations, obesity, insulin resistance, and increased incidence of dental cavities. The US National Academy of Sciences has advised that added sugars should make up no more than 25% of the total daily energy intake but that reducing this to 10% may be a healthier alternative. Indeed, the 2015-2020 *Dietary Guidelines for Americans* recommends that less than 10% of daily calorie intake should come from added sugars, and in the UK this has been reduced to no more than 5%.

- *Recommendation:* Use less sodium and salt. *Why?:* Too much sodium raises blood pressure, a risk factor for cardiovascular disease. Healthy adults are generally advised to reduce sodium intake to 2.3 g of sodium (equivalent to 5.8 g salt) per day or less. Most people currently consume, on average, about 3.4 g of sodium (8.5 g salt) per day. One teaspoon or 5 g of salt contains 2.0 g of sodium. People should choose foods with little salt and prepare food with minimal amounts of salt. However, a small pinch of salt (about 0.2 g) can be added to food on the plate as a condiment, particularly if most of the food is plant-based as it has a lower sodium content than animal produce. At the same time, people should also consume potassium-rich foods, such as fruits and vegetables.

- *Recommendation:* Do not consume more than 500 g of red meat per week. It is also recommended to limit intake of processed meat. *Why?:* Evidence derived from numerous large scale prospective epidemiological studies and their meta-analyses shows that regularly consuming red meat (beef, lamb, and pork) and processed meat (including bacon, ham, and salami) increases colorectal cancer risk by 20-30%.

- *Recommendation:* Those who drink alcohol should drink in moderation. *Why?:* Alcohol is a non-nutrient but contains 7 kcal per gram. It can add significant energy to total daily intake without adding nutrients. Current evidence suggests that light to moderate alcohol intake (one standard drink per day) will cause no real risk for healthy adults and may be of benefit by reducing the risk of cardiovascular disease. During pregnancy, alcohol should be avoided.

Current guidelines recommend drinking up to one drink per day for women and up to two drinks per day for men. A standard drink is defined as 360 mL (12 fl oz) of regular strength beer (5% alcohol), 150 mL (5 fl oz) of wine (12% alcohol), or 45 mL (1.5 fl oz) of spirits (40% alcohol).

- *Recommendation:* Avoid excessive intake of questionable food additives and nutrition supplements. *Why?:* Although most food additives used in processed foods are safe, it is often recommended to avoid these additives. In addition, although nutritional supplements are often claimed to have various positive health effects or performance benefits, some negative effects may occur. Nutrition supplements are not under strict regulation and may contain substances that are not listed on the label, and therefore pose a greater risk to health.

- *Recommendation:* Practice food hygiene and safety. *Why?:* Food should be stored appropriately to avoid accumulation of bacteria. This practice often means refrigerating perishable foods and not storing foods for too long. Food should be cooked to a safe temperature to kill microorganisms, but people should be aware that excess grilling of meat can produce **carcinogenic** substances called heterocyclic amines. To avoid microbial food-borne illness, when preparing food it is important to have clean hands, cutlery, and work surfaces. Fruits and vegetables should be washed in cold running tap water, but meat and poultry should not be washed or rinsed. People should avoid raw or partially cooked eggs or foods containing raw eggs, raw or undercooked meat and poultry, unpasteurized juices and milk, or any products made from unpasteurized milk.

- *Recommendation:* Cook food in ways that preserve the integrity of nutrients and remove some of the fat. *Why?:* The way that we cook food influences its nutrient and energy content. Grilling or roasting meat, poultry, and fish and discarding the fat is better than pan-frying or deep fat frying. For example, a whole chicken weighing 2 kg contains about 400 g of fat which will be lost if you cook the bird in a roasting bag in a hot oven for two hours. Losing the fat by this method of cooking makes the meat much healthier to eat as it is now low in fat but still high in protein. Steaming rather than boiling vegetables will retain more of the vitamins and phytonutrients. Remember that some vegetables are good to eat raw such as grated carrot, diced onion, celery, cucumber, tomato, and salad leaves.

DIETS THAT ARE KNOWN TO BE VERY HEALTHY

There are several diets that are known to be good for health because they have been consumed by certain large populations for long periods of time who have been shown to have relatively low risk of major chronic illnesses such as type 2 diabetes, cardiovascular disease, and cancer. Two stand-out examples are the Mediterranean diet and the Japanese diet. You might not want to adopt these particular diets on a full-time basis, but you could try adding some of their typical meals into your regular eating plan. Both these diets contain foods that combat chronic inflammation which is thought to be a major contributor to the development and progression of type 2 diabetes. These anti-inflammatory foods include tomatoes, fresh fruit (e.g., strawberries, cherries, blueberries), nuts (e.g., almonds, pecan, walnuts), extra virgin olive oil, leafy greens (e.g., broccoli, kale, spinach), and oily fish (e.g., mackerel, salmon, tuna). The Mediterranean diet is particularly rich in these types of food while the Japanese diet includes lots of seafood, vegetables, and fruit but avoids most forms of refined and processed foods (e.g., bread, cake, fried foods, sugar, soft drinks, lard, and fatty or processed meat) which are the food types that promote inflammation.

The Mediterranean Diet

The Mediterranean diet (see photo 7.1) is the traditional diet that was eaten by many of the poorer people who lived in the Mediterranean region (particularly the southern parts of Spain, Italy, Sicily, Greece, and Crete) a generation ago. It does not include the pizzas and pasta favored by many in parts of southern Europe today. Research has shown that adopting a Mediterranean diet helps people become slimmer and much healthier and reduces the risk of a heart attack or stroke by 30%, together with a reduced risk of cognitive decline. For women, there is also a 50% reduced risk of breast cancer. Among people who are not already diabetic, a Mediterranean diet reduces the risk of developing type 2 diabetes by 60%. In order to enjoy the benefits of a Mediterranean diet, follow this list of the foods you should be aiming to eat and the foods you should avoid.

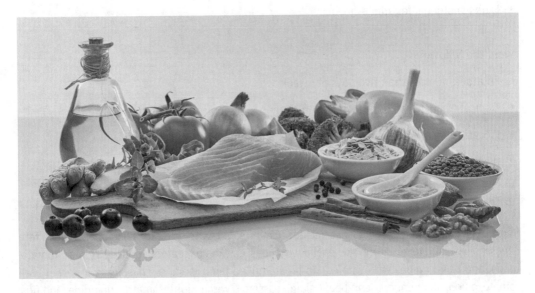

Photo 7.1: A selection of foods found in the Mediterranean diet.

Eat the following:

- Fresh, lean meat such as pork, chicken, turkey, and lamb; oven roasted, grilled, or fried with a little extra virgin olive oil.

- Fresh fish such as sardines, mackerel, and salmon; grilled or oven-baked.

- Eggs; poached, or boiled, or as an omelet.

- Wholegrain foods such as quinoa, whole rye, bulgur wheat, and pearl barley.

- Rice, preferably brown.

- Unsalted nuts such as walnuts, almonds, and cashews.

- Full-fat dairy products such as yogurt, milk, and feta cheese (but in small amounts).

- Legumes including beans, chickpeas, lentils, and peas.

- Olives, tomato, and onion.

- Gourds such as aubergine (eggplant), cucumber, marrow, squash, and zucchini.

- Fruits such as orange, lemon, grapes, persimmon, and watermelon.

- One glass of wine (preferably red) per day.

- Wholegrain, wholemeal, or rye bread.

- Raisins, grapes, or nuts make healthy snacks.

- Extra virgin olive oil (in small amounts) rather than vegetable oil or lard for frying.

- Herbs and garlic for added flavor.

Avoid the following:

- Potatoes on more than two days per week.

- Tropical fruit such as honeydew melon, mango, pineapple, and bananas.

- Processed meats like ham, bacon, sausage, and salami.

- White bread, pasta, and pizza.

- Processed foods, cakes, pastries, milk chocolate, and sweets.

Some typical Mediterranean dishes include Greek salad with tomato, cucumber, onion, feta cheese, olives, and lemon juice; rice paella with peas, chicken or seafood; grilled sardines, tomato, onion, and salad greens with wholegrain bread; grilled lamb, pork, or chicken on a skewer with tomato, onion, and peppers; lean beef or lamb casserole with onions, tomato, aubergine, and figs; chopped watermelon with grapes. For more meal ideas for the Mediterranean diet see chapter 10 and the BBC Good Food website (https://www.bbcgoodfood.com/recipes/collection/mediterranean).

The Japanese Diet

The Japanese people are known to have a relatively low incidence of type 2 diabetes, cardiovascular disease, and cancer. They also enjoy a long life expectancy, more than almost anywhere else in the world. So why is the Japanese diet so healthy and what does it consist of? The traditional

Japanese diet (see photo 7.2) is largely fresh and u[...]
major protein sources, with very little refined foo[...]
study published in the British Medical Journal four[...]
dietary guidelines – a diet high in grains and ve[...]
products (mainly fish and shellfish), fruit, and soy, b[...]
early and suffering from heart disease or stroke.

The Japanese also have the lowest rates of obesi[...]
life expectancy. Okinawa, in southernmost Japan, [...]
world as well as the lowest risk of age-related dise[...]
and **Alzheimer's disease**. This has partly been attri[...]
is low in calories and saturated fat, yet high in nu[...]
such as **carotenoids** and **polyphenols** (e.g., **flavono**[...], flavonones, and anthocyanins),
found in different colored vegetables and seasonal fruits. These also include phytoestrogens, or
plant-based estrogens, that may help protect against hormone-dependent cancers, such as breast
cancer. Fermented foods containing **probiotic** bacteria are also popular, and these can positively
influence the gut bacterial population (known as the **microbiota**) which is now recognized to
play an important role in health maintenance. The diet of the Okinawan people has been little
influenced by the dietary changes influenced by western culture, which have been seen in more
urban parts of Japan.

The traditional Japanese diet isn't that dissimilar to a traditional Chinese diet, with rice, noodles
made from wheat flour, cooked and pickled vegetables, fish, meat, and soy products being staple
choices. However, because Japan is actually a group of over 6,500 islands, its residents consume
a lot more fish and shellfish compared to other Asian countries. They also eat raw fish in sushi and
sashimi, plus a lot of pickled, fermented, and smoked foods. The main sources of carbohydrate
are rice and noodles made from rice or wheat. Bread, potatoes, and cookies are generally absent
from the Japanese diet.

Soybeans, usually in the form of tofu or fresh edamame, are another key part of the Japanese
diet, along with other beans such as aduki and various mushrooms. Increasingly, fermented foods
are being shown to support a healthy digestive system. Fermented soybean products such as
miso and natto are staples of the Japanese diet. Miso pastes (a traditional Japanese seasoning
produced by fermenting soybeans with salt and the fungus Aspergillus oryzae, known in Japanese
as kōjikin and in English as koji, and sometimes rice, barley, or other ingredients) are a popular
way of adding flavoring to food and can be categorized into red (akamiso), white (shiromiso),
or mixed (awase). The Japanese also consume a wide variety of vegetables, both land, and sea
vegetables such as seaweed, which is rich in minerals, and may help to reduce blood pressure.
Fruit is often consumed with breakfast or as a dessert, especially Fuji apples, tangerines, and
persimmons in preference to cakes, pastries, puddings, and sweets.

Alongside their diet, the Japanese like to drink green tea which is high in antioxidant compounds
called **catechins**, which have been linked to fighting cancer, viruses, and heart disease.
Furthermore, the Japanese tend to have a healthy attitude to food and eating. They have a
saying, "hara hachi bu", which means to eat until you are 80% full, and it is not uncommon to

BEATING TYPE 2 DIABETES

teach it to children from a[...]
characteristic contribu[...]
one large plate, th[...]
rice, a bowl of [...]
communally[...]
when it [...]
than [...]

young age. The way the Japanese serve their food is also an important
ting to their general avoidance of high calorie intake. Rather than having
often eat from a small bowl and several different dishes, usually a bowl of
miso, some fish or meat, and then two or three vegetables dishes, often served
and eaten in rotation. The Japanese are also strong believers of "flexible restraint"
omes to treats and snacks, enjoying them from time to time but in smaller portions. Other
he occasional beer and sake rice wine they are not great drinkers of alcoholic beverages.

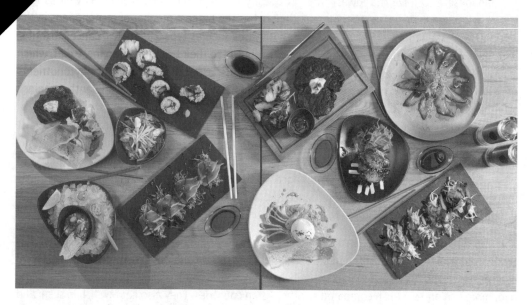

Photo 7.2: A selection of foods found in the Japanese diet, served as is usual in Japan, in small bowls or on plates.

Some typical Japanese dishes include miso chicken and rice soup; salmon and avocado rice; soba noodle and edamame salad with grilled tofu; Japanese salad with ginger soy dressing; chicken or beef teriyaki with white or brown rice. For more meal ideas for the Japanese diet see chapter 10 and the BBC Good Food website (https://www.bbcgoodfood.com/recipes/collection/japanese).

Vegetarian, Vegan, and Flexitarian Diets

Vegetarian and **vegan** diets are associated with lower health risks compared with diets containing meat. A vegetarian diet generally excludes meat and meat products with most food of vegetable or plant origin. Some versions of the diet allow the consumption of dairy products (e.g., milk, butter, cheese, yogurt) and/or eggs. A vegan diet is a very strict type of vegetarian diet in which no animal products are allowed. Research shows that a vegetarian diet can reduce a person's risk of heart disease, stroke, metabolic syndrome, and type 2 diabetes by about one third. This is probably because people who consume plant-based diets tend to have a lower BMI than meat eaters, their prevalence of obesity is lower, and they have higher intakes of phytonutrients and fiber. Overall cancer incidence is also 11% lower in vegetarians and 19% lower in vegans compared with meat eaters.

However, being vegetarian isn't always healthy; it depends on what types of plant foods are consumed and in what amounts. In fact it has been reported that some plant-based diets can actually raise the risk of heart disease. For example, a US study found a vegetarian diet based on less healthy food options, such as refined grains, starchy vegetables like potatoes, and foods with high sugar content increased the risk of heart disease whereas those eating a healthy plant-based diet high in wholegrains, fruits, vegetables, and healthy fats were less likely to get heart disease. Essentially, the diet advice for vegetarians is the same as it is for nonvegetarians: eat a balanced diet with at least five portions of fruit and vegetables per day, choose wholegrain carbohydrates where possible, and limit intake of sugar, salt, and saturated fat. Eating too many starchy vegetables (e.g., potatoes), dairy products (particularly cheese), and too much bread, can also be fattening and so should be avoided. For some meal ideas for the vegetarian diet see chapter 10 and the BBC Good Food website (https://www.bbcgoodfood.com/recipes/category/vegetarian).

A vegetarian diet may not reverse type 2 diabetes but should reduce the risk of health complications because it is low in saturated fat and high in phytonutrients and fiber. Vegetarian or vegan diets are fine for people with type 2 diabetes as long as high glycemic food items are restricted and care is taken to ensure adequate protein and iron intake. An appropriate selection of foods is important for vegetarians and vegans to avoid deficiencies of protein, vitamin B12 (which is only found in animal products although nowadays some foods (e.g., breakfast cereals and milk) are fortified with vitamin B12, calcium (if dairy products are not consumed), and iron (heme iron is only found in foods containing animal meat, heart, liver, kidney, and blood and the nonheme iron present in plants is not as readily absorbed). For vegans in particular a daily vitamin B12 supplement supplying 100% of the RDA is recommended.

Because meat, poultry, and fish are the most common sources of protein, vegetarians and vegans could be at risk for marginal protein intake. Vegetarians and vegans often compensate by eating more grains and legumes, which both are excellent protein sources. But grains and legumes do not contain all **essential amino acids**. Grains (e.g., wheat, rice, oats, cornmeal, barley) lack the essential amino acid lysine, and legumes (e.g., peas, beans, chickpeas, lentils) lack methionine. An exception may be well-processed soybean protein, which is a **high-quality protein** comparable in quality to protein from animal sources. The potential problem for vegetarians of missing essential amino acids can be solved by not eating grains and legumes in isolation but combining both grains and legumes in their meals (together with other protein sources such as cheese or egg. Good sources of iron in a vegetarian diet include tofu, legumes (lentils, dried peas, and beans), wholegrain cereals (in particular, iron-fortified breakfast cereals), green vegetables (broccoli, watercress, and kale), nuts, dairy products, and eggs. The absorption of nonheme iron can be enhanced by consuming a good source of vitamin C (e.g., orange juice) in the same meal. The intake of fat – particularly unhealthy saturated fat – will be lower in a vegetarian diet. When on such a diet, fat will be provided by margarine, salad dressing, vegetable oils, nuts, egg, and some dairy products.

Some people prefer to follow a semi-vegetarian diet – also called a **flexitarian diet** – which is primarily a plant-based diet but includes meat, dairy, eggs, poultry, and fish on occasion (e.g., two or three times per week) or in small quantities. This option can be a very healthy diet and is similar to the Mediterranean diet described previously. Another variation of this is the **pescatarian diet** which typically includes vegetables, grains, and pulses along with fish and other seafood, but generally excludes meat, poultry, and sometimes dairy products.

FOOD SHOPPING TIPS, AND HOW TO USE NUTRITION FACTS LABELS ON PACKAGED FOODS

Supermarkets and food manufacturers now highlight the energy, fat, saturated fat, sugar, and salt content on the front of the packaging, alongside the maximum daily recommended intake (called the **reference daily intake**) for each of these (see figures 7.1 and 7.2 for examples of labels found on US and UK packaged food items, respectively). Other products will show nutrition information on the back or side of packaging. You can use Nutrition Facts labels to help you choose a more balanced diet. If you're standing in the supermarket aisle looking at two similar products such as a ready meal, trying to decide which is the healthier choice, check to see if there's the relevant label on the pack, and then see how your choices stack up when it comes to the amount of energy, fat, saturated fat, sugars, and salt.

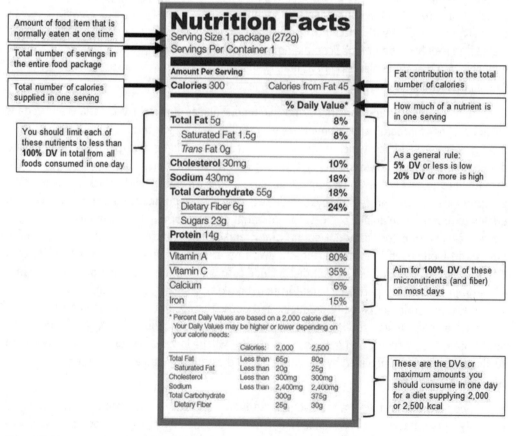

Figure 7.1 How to read a US Nutrition Facts label on packaged foods. Adapted from US Food and Drug Administration, https://www.accessdata.fda.gov/scripts/InteractiveNutritionFactsLabel/#whats-on-the-label

If the Nutrition Facts labels use color coding as introduced in the UK in 2013, and more recently in France, you will often find a mixture of traffic light colors: red, amber, and green (see photo 7.3 for an example). I suggest that you interpret these as follows: RED means STOP and think if you really want this product as it contains high amounts of fat, saturated fat, sugars, or salt. If just one of these is RED then maybe consider it but more than two is a definite no-no if you want to eat healthily. AMBER means BE PREPARED to consider choosing this product as it has medium amounts of fat, saturated fat, sugars, or salt. GREEN means GO AHEAD and buy the product as it has low amounts of fat, saturated fat, sugars, or salt. So, when you're choosing between similar products, try to go for more greens and ambers, and fewer reds, if you want to make a healthier choice. But remember, even some of the healthier ready meals may be higher in energy, fat, sugar, and salt than the homemade equivalent. If you make the meal yourself, you have full control of the ingredients, and you could save money, too!

Nutrition				
Typical values	100 g contains	Each slice (typically 44 g) contains	% RI*	RI for an average adult
Energy	985 kJ 235 kcal	435 kJ 105 kcal	5%	8400 kJ 2000 kcal
Fat	1.5 g	0.7 g	1%	70 g
of which saturates	0.3 g	0.1 g	1%	20 g
Carbohydrate	45.5 g	20.0 g		
of which sugars	3.8 g	1.7 g	2%	90 g
Fibre	2.8 g	1.2 g		
Protein	7.7 g	3.4 g		
Salt	1.0 g	0.4 g	7%	6 g
This pack contains 16 servings *Reference intake of an average adult (8400 kJ/2000 kcal)				

Figure 7.2 Example of a UK/EU Nutrition Facts label found on the side or back of packaged foods. In this example the food item is a loaf of sliced white bread.

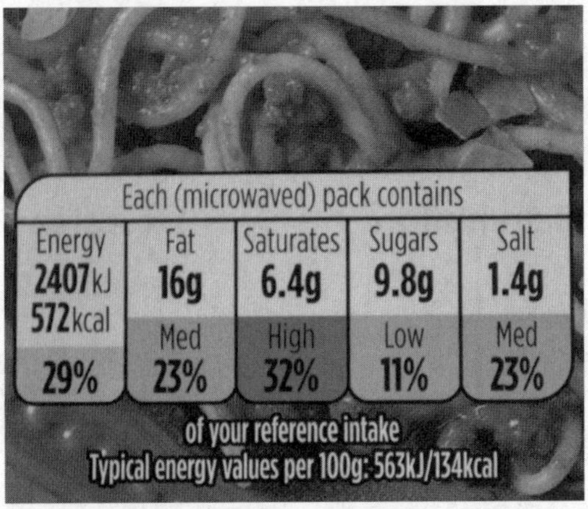

Photo 7.3: Example of a front-of-pack UK color-coded nutrition facts label. In this example the food item is a spaghetti Bolognese ready meal. Saturates are in RED, fat and salt in AMBER, and sugars in GREEN.

EXERCISE MORE

Becoming more physically active is recommended for all diabetics because it can help with weight loss or maintenance and has been shown to improve insulin sensitivity and help prevent cardiovascular disease, dementia, and some cancers, as well as having the added bonus of reducing infection risk. Doing exercise expends energy and for low to moderate-intensity exercise, fat is the predominant fuel that is burnt (oxidized) to provide this energy. Hence, if exercise is performed regularly it can help to decrease body fat stores and assist with weight loss. This in turn will start to dampen down the inflammation in adipose tissue that is one of the main triggers for increasing insulin resistance. Exercise itself causes the secretion of anti-inflammatory mediators including interleukins 6 and 10 and the **steroid** hormone cortisol which reduce the activation of white blood cells and inhibit the secretion and actions of pro-inflammatory cytokines produced in inflamed adipose tissue. It is this anti-inflammatory effect of exercise, in concert with its ability to reduce visceral fat stores by increasing fat mobilization and oxidation, that is thought to be responsible for decreasing the risk of chronic diseases such as type 2 diabetes (figure 7.3). As explained in chapter 3, both acute bouts of exercise and the training adaptations that occur in response to regular exercise increase insulin sensitivity which reduces the need for high levels of insulin secretion. In addition, regular exercise also imbues cardiovascular health benefits by reducing blood pressure and improving the blood lipid (fat) profile by decreasing the concentration of plasma triglycerides and LDL particles and by increasing the concentration of protective HDL particles. These beneficial alterations in plasma lipids are presumed to limit the development of atherosclerosis. Regular moderate exercise also improves fitness, strengthens bone, maintains mental function, improves immunity and vaccination responses, and reduces the risks of infectious illnesses such as the common cold and influenza.

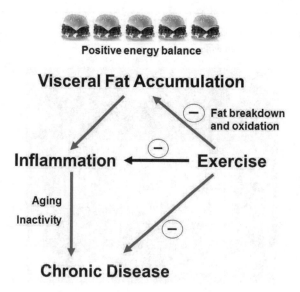

Figure 7.3 Exercise reduces the risk of chronic diseases like type 2 diabetes by reducing inflammation and increasing fat breakdown and oxidation.

RECOMMENDATIONS FOR PHYSICAL ACTIVITY

In the long-term, regular physical activity can protect against the health complications that develop in people with type 2 diabetes as well as having other benefits for health, functional capacity, and quality of life. For example, being regularly active also reduces the risk of falling and breaking bones in old age and helps people to remain independent. Here are some recommendations on what you need to do to obtain the health benefits of exercise. In this bulleted list, the recommendation is first stated and then the reason(s) why this recommendation is given is briefly summarized.

- *Recommendation:* Everyone who is capable should try to do some exercise on at least three days per week. *Why?:* The biggest reduction in chronic disease risk is between those who do no exercise whatsoever and those who do some exercise amounting to about 30 minutes of light-moderate-intensity exercise on a minimum of three days per week. Further improvements in health markers and reduced disease risk will come by doing more exercise than this, and a good target to aim for is about 45-60 minutes of moderate-intensity exercise on four or five days per week. Beyond that the benefits become increasingly smaller. The most important thing to realize is that doing some physical activity is far, far better than doing nothing at all.

- *Recommendation:* People should aim to do at least 30 minutes of physical activity on most, if not all, days of the week. *Why?:* This is the amount of exercise needed for the average healthy adult to maintain health and substantially reduce the risk of chronic disease. The American College of Sports Medicine (ACSM) and the American Heart Association (AHA) recommend moderately intense aerobic exercise for 30 minutes a day, five days a week, or vigorously intense aerobic exercise for 20 minutes a day, three days a week. Moderate-intensity physical activity means working hard enough to raise the heart rate and break a sweat yet still be able to carry on a conversation. Note that to lose weight or maintain weight loss, 60 to 90 minutes of physical activity per day may be necessary.

- *Recommendation:* People are advised to undertake a small volume of resistance exercise by performing several different strength training exercises designed to work all major muscle groups in the arms, shoulders, and legs at least twice a week. *Why?:* For ordinary people, improvements in muscle mass and strength may prove extremely useful in later life because as we get older we tend to get less fit and lose muscle mass (a phenomenon known as sarcopenia) which may compromise our ability to carry out everyday tasks such as walking to the shops, climbing a flight of stairs, or even getting off the toilet!

- *Recommendation:* If moderate-intensity exercise such as jogging or aerobics is too hard for you, try walking instead. *Why?:* You can achieve the same amount of work by exercising at a lower intensity (e.g., walking) for longer. If using a step counter or pedometer, you can aim for a target of 10,000 steps per day which is equivalent to about 7 km (4.5 miles) and will expend about 500 calories per day. The health benefits and improvements to your fitness will be better if you exercise at moderate rather than low-intensity and brisk walking is better than a gentle stroll, but the more exercise you do, the fitter you become, and the exercise feels easier than before which means you may then be capable of doing something a little harder.

- *Recommendation:* Try doing some forms of sociable activities that you know you are likely to enjoy like playing a round of golf, a game of doubles tennis or badminton, walking pace 5-a-side football, dancing, aerobics, cycle spinning, or swimming. *Why?:* Doing exercise that you enjoy, especially with family or friends, can be fun. You are more likely to be motivated to continue with regular exercise if you get to enjoy it and look forward to it.

SLEEP BETTER

Habitual lack of sleep or poor sleep quality (e.g., frequently waking up during the night) is called insomnia and is linked to poor mood, decreased quality of life, increased use of healthcare resources, poor food choices, and increased risk of obesity and chronic disease. Not getting enough sleep means that we do not feel refreshed in the morning, and consequently we feel more tired and listless throughout the day. Insomnia is a common problem thought to regularly affect around one in every four people in the USA and Europe and is particularly common in adolescents and the elderly. The medical literature shows that people who complain of chronic insomnia and shortened sleep have an increased incidence of type 2 diabetes, hypertension, and cardiovascular disease. They are also more susceptible to infectious illnesses such as the common cold. If you have insomnia, you may:

- Find it difficult to fall asleep.

- Lie awake for long periods at night.

- Wake up several times during the night.

- Wake up too early in the morning and not be able to get back to sleep.

- Not feel refreshed when you get up.

- Find it hard to nap during the day, despite feeling tired.

- Feel tired and irritable during the day and have difficulty concentrating.

- Be prone to picking up **upper respiratory tract infections**.

It's not always clear what triggers insomnia, but it can often be associated with stress and anxiety, a poor sleeping environment (e.g., an uncomfortable bed, or a bedroom that's too light, noisy, damp, hot, or cold), lifestyle factors (e.g., jet lag, exercising hard, or working rather than relaxing in the evening), watching television, looking at your phone or tablet, or playing computer games before bedtime. Night-time insomnia can also be due to napping during the day, drinking alcohol or **caffeine** (in coffee, cola, and energy drinks), smoking or eating a heavy meal just before going to bed, a poor diet, and/or micronutrient deficiencies (e.g., deficiencies of the B vitamins folate and thiamin, as well as the minerals iron, magnesium, phosphorus, selenium, and zinc are associated with shorter sleep duration).

Sleep loss, short sleep duration, and complaints of sleep disturbance are associated with increases in inflammation, which are thought to be due to the effects of sleep disruption on **sympathetic nervous system** activity that promotes inflammatory gene expression. This may be one of the mechanisms by which poor sleep quality and quantity put us at increased risk of cardiovascular disease and cancer. Good sleep quality is therefore something that people with type 2 diabetes would benefit from. The amount of sleep an individual actually needs varies (see sidebar) but is generally at least six hours, and maybe up to eight hours per night.

How much sleep do I actually need?

There are no official guidelines about how much sleep you should get each night because everyone is different. How much sleep we need and want is influenced by our genetics which explains why some people are "night owls" and some are "early birds". Some people seem to be able to cope well with as little as five hours of sleep per night but, on average, a "normal" amount of sleep for an adult is considered to be between seven and nine hours per night. Babies and young children may sleep for much longer than this, whereas older adults may sleep somewhat less. What's important is whether you feel you get enough sleep such that you don't feel tired or lethargic during the daytime, and whether your sleep is good quality and you feel refreshed after waking in the morning. You're probably not getting enough good-quality sleep if you constantly feel tired throughout the day and it's affecting your mood and ability to carry out the tasks of everyday life.

RECOMMENDATIONS FOR IMPROVED SLEEP QUALITY

By examining information provided by the US National Sleep Foundation, the American Academy of Sleep Medicine, and other relevant literature, I have identified a number of things you can try to do to help improve your sleep quality. Bear in mind that when you sleep there are three main things that happen: (1) your muscles become relaxed, (2) your heart rate slows, and (3) your body core temperature drops by a degree or so. Therefore, anything you do before bedtime to delay these effects may impair your ability to get off to sleep. On the other hand, if you spend the last hour or two before bedtime in a relaxed state, not getting excited, and in a comfortably warm but not hot room, you can get to sleep easier. Some people who have difficulty sleeping well find over-the-counter sleeping tablets helpful, but they don't address the underlying problem and can have troublesome side effects. The following practical guidelines should be followed to improve your sleep quality if it is not already good. Just as for diet and exercise each recommendation is first stated and then the reason(s) why this recommendation is given is briefly explained.

- *Recommendation:* The general recommendation is to aim to get 7-8 hours of sleep per night. *Why?:* Less than 6 and more than 9 hours of sleep are associated with higher risks of health problems.

- *Recommendation:* Set regular times for going to bed and waking up. Use an alarm clock so that you do not have to worry about waking up on time in the morning for work etc. Avoid oversleeping or having a long lie in at weekends. *Why?:* Your body will find it easier to relax and get to sleep more easily if you stick to a regular routine. Variable bedtimes and lie-ins disrupt your normal sleep schedule.

- *Recommendation:* Relax before bedtime – try taking a warm bath or listening to calming music. *Why?:* You go to sleep quicker if your mind and muscles are relaxed at bedtime.

- *Recommendation:* In the bedroom use thick curtains or blinds, and an eye mask and earplugs to stop you being woken up by light and noise if these are potential problems. Have a comfortable, warm bed and pillows. Good quality cotton is best for sheets and pillows and a duvet is cosier and lighter than blankets. *Why?:* If you are comfortable and undisturbed you will sleep better.

- *Recommendation:* Your bedroom temperature should be about 15-19 °C and you should have a selection of duvets to hand (e.g., 5, 10, and 13 tog) and use them according to the night-time bedroom temperature. In hot countries, an air conditioning system that does not create much noise is a must. *Why?:*A bedroom temperature of 15-19 °C is generally best for sleeping well. If you are too hot or too cold you will find it more difficult to relax and go to sleep.

- *Recommendation:* Avoid caffeine, nicotine, alcohol, heavy meals, and large volumes (over 200 mL) of fluid for at least a few hours before going to bed. *Why?:* Caffeine and nicotine are stimulants that will keep you awake. Coffee should be avoided by people with sleep problems as it is high in caffeine which stays in the circulation for a long time (after ingestion it takes about five hours for the blood caffeine concentration to fall by half). Alcohol in moderation may make you feel relaxed and tired, but it can disrupt sleep patterns by reducing the cycle of restorative rapid eye movement sleep. Furthermore, alcohol is a diuretic (a drug that increases urine production) which means that frequent trips to the bathroom are more likely which will disrupt your sleep. Having too much fluid to drink just before bedtime will make you want to go to the toilet to empty your bladder after a few hours.

- *Recommendation:* Don't do any exercise for at least a few hours before going to bed. *Why?:* Exercise may raise your core body temperature and activates your sympathetic nervous system which tends to keep you alert and wakeful.

- *Recommendation:* Try eating some cherries or kiwi fruits or drinking some milk a few hours before bedtime. *Why?:* The consumption of these foods in the hours before bedtime has been shown to improve sleep quantity and quality. Some of these foods have a relatively high content of tryptophan (an essential amino acid that is the precursor of the sleep-regulating hormone and neurotransmitter called **serotonin**) and this may be responsible for their sleep promoting effects. The intake of bread, pulses, fish, and shellfish appear to extend sleep duration so are a good choice for what to eat in the last meal before bedtime. Increases in tryptophan intake via protein ingestion in the evening have been shown to improve sleep in adults with sleep disturbances and result in enhanced alertness in the morning, most likely as a result of improved sleep quality.

- *Recommendation:* Don't watch television or use phones, tablets, or laptop computers in bed shortly before trying to go to sleep. *Why?:* The blue light emitted from electronic devices suppresses the secretion of **melatonin**, the hormone that controls our body clock. Reduced levels of melatonin make it harder to fall asleep and stay asleep during the night.

- *Recommendation:* Avoid napping during the day. *Why?:* It makes you less tired at bedtime and makes it more difficult to get good quality restorative sleep at night.

- *Recommendation:* Think of pleasant things when you are trying to get off to sleep. Try to ignore your worries, and ideas about how to solve them, before going to bed in order to help you forget about them until the morning. *Why?:* Your brain has to be in a relaxed state before you can sleep.

- *Recommendation:* If your partner is keeping you awake by snoring, do something to help them stop it or sleep in the spare room. *Why?:* You need peace and quiet to get off to sleep, and you don't want to be repeatedly awoken during the night.

- *Recommendation:* Lose some weight. *Why?:* Studies have shown that if you are overweight or obese, losing 5% of your body weight will help you sleep better. When you put on excess weight, the fat not only goes in your belly region but also around your neck. Having a fat neck means you are more likely to snore (which will keep your partner awake), and you are more likely to develop obstructive sleep apnea, a disorder which causes people to stop breathing while sleeping, resulting in disrupted sleep with frequent awakenings. A 2014 study found that people who lost 5% or more of their body weight got about 20 minutes more sleep, and it was better-quality sleep.

LOSE SOME WEIGHT

If you are diabetic the single most effective thing you can do to reduce your risk of complications and reverse or at least delay the progression of your disease is to lose some body fat and body weight. The first step in the process of losing weight should always be to define the goals: Is weight loss really required, and if so, how much, and over what period of time? With goals established, various strategies can be put in place to achieve the weight loss. In the process of attempting to achieve weight loss, several mistakes can be made so I will first explain what these are.

COMMON MISTAKES

When trying to lose weight, people often make at least one of the three following mistakes:

1. *Trying to lose weight too rapidly.* Most people are impatient about weight loss. They want to see results within a couple of weeks, but unfortunately this expectation is not

realistic. Although rapid weight loss is possible, the initial reduction of body weight on low-carbohydrate or very low energy diets is mostly **dehydration** as water that is combined with glycogen is lost as the body's carbohydrate reserves become depleted. Only a small part of the weight loss will be fat, and it will be restored as soon as normal eating resumes.

2. *Not eating breakfast.* A weight loss method that people often try is skipping breakfast, and sometimes even skipping lunch as well. Although this approach may work for some, it increases hunger feelings later in the day and one large evening meal can easily compensate for the daytime reduction in food intake. In addition, missing breakfast may make you feel tired during the day and less inclined to exercise later on after your occupational work has finished.

3. *Cutting down on protein intake as well as carbohydrate or fat.* When losing body weight (being in negative energy balance), you also risk losing muscle mass. Eating less protein than normal will accelerate this loss of muscle mass. You want to lose fat not lean tissue so you must consume sufficient amounts of protein. Indeed the proportion of protein in your diet should increase at the expense of carbohydrate or fat to assist with your weight loss and preserve muscle mass.

DEFINING GOALS

It is essential to decide on your weight loss goals right at the start. These goals should be thought out carefully and be realistically achievable. Goals also have to be defined with a time schedule in mind. How much weight must be lost and how soon? So decide on the target body weight you want to reach (I recommend that you do so in consultation with your healthcare practitioner), and stick to it. A realistic expectation is a weight loss of about 1 kg (2.2 lbs) every two weeks, so to lose 3 kg at least six weeks are needed.

Achieving this particular goal means generating, on average, a 500-kcal energy deficit per day. While this could be achieved by dieting alone, it is common for most people to find that weight loss becomes gradually more difficult due to the lowering of resting metabolic rate as your body adapts to the reduced daily energy intake. Therefore, it makes more sense to try to achieve the desired weight loss through a combination of dieting and exercise. This will give you scope to lose more weight, more quickly, and with a smaller impact on your appetite than with dieting alone, while maintaining your muscle mass and improving your fitness and overall health.

RECOMMENDATIONS FOR WEIGHT LOSS BY DIETING

The next step is to establish a strategy that will help you lose weight. The following general tips about losing weight by dieting will help you successfully achieve weight loss:

• Do not try to lose more than about 0.5-1.0 kg/week (about 1-2 lbs/week), and do not restrict dietary energy intake by more than 750 kcal/day on consecutive days.

- Eat more fruit and non-starchy vegetables to achieve a diet that has a low energy density – that is fewer calories per gram of food on your plate.

- Avoid snacking between your regular meals. If you really feel the need for a snack choose low-fat and low-carbohydrate food items; raw celery, spring onion, shredded carrots, and watermelon are excellent choices.

- Study food labels and try to find substitutes for high-fat foods. Look not only at fat content but also at the added sugar and energy content per serving.

- Limit fat add-ons such as sauces, sour cream, coleslaw, and high-fat salad dressings, or choose the low-fat versions of these products. Better still, use a sprinkle of dried mixed herbs to add extra flavor without the calories.

- Avoid drinking sugar-sweetened beverages; choose the low energy versions with artificial sweeteners and no added sugar.

- Try to structure your eating into three or four smaller meals each day.

- Avoid eating any extremely large meals. Try using a smaller diameter plate; for example use one that is 23 cm (9 inches) in diameter rather than the usual 28 cm (11 inches).

- Make sure that protein intake is the same or higher than normal, and consume a high-protein meal at breakfast and for your main meal in the evening. High-protein items (which can include beans, fish, and egg, as well as meat) should cover about one quarter of your plate.

- Limit your intake of bread and starchy vegetables like potatoes by serving these on only two or three days of the week.

- Use higher fiber carbohydrate sources like brown rice and legumes, and limit these to no more than one quarter of your plate. Fill half your plate with low energy density vegetables like gourds, carrots, broccoli, and leafy greens.

- Use only skimmed or semi-skimmed milk (or soya milk) and reduced fat versions of yogurt, coleslaw, etc.

- Add some beetroot, beansprouts, red cabbage, or sauerkraut to your main meals for added bulk, fiber, and flavor. These items are very low in calories.

- Add a sprinkle of dried herbs, chili bits, curry powder, ground pepper, garlic granules, or ginger to your meals to add flavor without calories. A pinch of salt can be added to the food on your plate as a condiment if desired when you are eating mostly plant-based and unprocessed foods with low sodium content.

- Eat slowly, savor your food, and begin your main meal by eating the high-protein and low energy density food items first. Finish with the higher carbohydrate items.

- Try to stop eating when you feel 80% rather than 100% full.

- Do you really want dessert? If you do have dessert, stick to fruit such as chopped apple, pear, persimmon, or melon, with one tablespoon of low-fat yogurt.

- Avoid drinking alcoholic beverages. If you don't want to cut out alcohol altogether, then compensate by doing more exercise: one small (125 mL) glass of wine or a half pint (235 mL) of beer both contain about 100 kcal and you will have to walk or jog one mile (1.6 km) to burn that off.

- A multivitamin and mineral supplement supplying no more than the RDA may be useful during periods of energy restriction to guard against possible deficiencies. This is the only supplement you will need apart from a vitamin D3 supplement in the winter months.

- Remember that to lose weight dieting is not the only answer. Increase your energy expenditure by doing more exercise. It will improve your fitness and health and help to maintain your muscle mass when you are in negative energy balance.

- Measure body weight weekly and obtain measurements of body fat regularly (every 1-2 months). Keep a record of the changes.

WAYS OF LOSING BODY FAT AND WEIGHT

The various ways to lose body fat and weight include pharmacological and surgical procedures (see the sidebar), increasing energy expenditure with exercise, and reducing dietary energy intake. Numerous different diets designed to promote weight loss exist, some of which have been commercialized. Some diets have proved to be effective, whereas others (probably the majority) have not and may be based on a list of erroneous assumptions and unjustified claims. Some diets (e.g., high-carbohydrate low-fat diets and ketogenic very low-carbohydrate diets) are not the most suitable diets for people with type 2 diabetes (see chapter 8 for the reasons why). For the individual wanting to lose some weight while remaining healthy, distinguishing between the facts and the fallacies is often difficult. It is important to appreciate that weight loss with dieting is mostly dependent on the size of the weekly energy deficit; that is, by how many calories you have reduced your energy intake, compared to when you are weight stable and in energy balance. Research indicates that an accumulated energy deficit of 3,500 kcal – which could be achieved by a daily energy deficit of 500 kcal/day for seven days – will normally result in a loss of 1 lb (0.46 kg) of body fat and a similar or slightly greater reduction in body weight.

Methods that can be used to achieve weight loss

Dietary methods:

- Energy restriction (moderate or severe).

- Fasting.

- Very low energy diet.

- Intermittent fasting diet (e.g., the 5:2 Fast diet).

- Very low-fat diet.

- Food-combining diet.

- Low Glycemic Index (GI) diet.

- High-protein diet.

- Zone diet.

- Paleo diet.

- Very low-carbohydrate ketogenic diet (e.g., Atkins diet, Sugar Busters).

- Low energy density diet.

- Calcium and dairy product diet.

- Mediterranean and Japanese diets.

- Vegetarian and vegan diets.

Exercise:

- Increased physical activity of any kind.

- Regular exercise (e.g., daily walking).

- Aerobic endurance exercise or cardio (e.g., jogging, cycling, swimming for 30 minutes or more).

- High-intensity interval exercise (repeated sprints with short recovery periods).

- Resistance exercise (e.g., weightlifting).

- Participation in sport.

Pharmacological methods:

- Drugs that stimulate metabolism or fat burning.

- Drugs that suppress appetite.

- Drugs that promote satiety.

- Drugs that make the stomach feel fuller.

- Drugs that reduce fat absorption.

(continued)

(continued)

Surgical procedures:

- Stomach (gastric) band – a band is placed around the stomach, so you don't need to eat as much to feel full.

- Stomach (gastric) bypass – the top part of the stomach is joined to the small intestine, so you feel fuller sooner and don't absorb as many calories from food.

- Sleeve gastrectomy – some of the stomach is removed, so you can't eat as much as you could before, and you'll feel full sooner.

- Intra-gastric balloon – a soft balloon filled with air or salt water that's placed into your stomach so that you won't need or be able to eat as much before you feel full.

- Removal of a section of the small intestine so that you are unable to digest and absorb food as effectively.

- Liposuction – Sucking out small areas of fat from areas of the body where deposits of fat tend to collect, such as the abdomen, buttocks, hips, and thighs.

IF YOU ARE A SMOKER, STOP SMOKING

Smoking any tobacco product markedly increases your risk of lung cancer and heart disease whether you are diabetic or not. Having just one cigarette per day has been reported to increase the risk of coronary heart disease by over 50%, and that should be interpreted as a very good reason for not smoking at all. In general, smokers are three to four times more likely to experience a fatal heart attack than non-smokers, and this risk is doubled if you are a diabetic. When you have diabetes, you are already at a much higher risk for cardiovascular problems and having a heart attack. People with diabetes who smoke, are three times as likely to suffer a heart attack as people with diabetes who don't smoke. Smoking can also lead to oral cancer, gum disease (gingivitis) and abscesses, in addition to staining your teeth and causing bad breath. Smoking is also bad for your eyes as it increases the risk of developing cataract, age-related macular degeneration, and optic nerve damage, all of which result in partial loss of vision and can lead to blindness. For diabetics, with an already increased risk of eye damage due to diabetic retinopathy, this is a serious concern. People who smoke are addicted to nicotine, and a safer alternative is to switch to vaping with electronic cigarettes (e-cigs) instead. Vaping liquids contain the nicotine that satisfies the cravings associated with addiction to cigarettes, but they are thought to be far less harmful to health.

THE TAKE HOME MESSAGE

In order to reduce the risk of the serious and life-threatening health complic
type 2 diabetes, there are several things that you can do. These are summar
key things are to modify your lifestyle by exercising more, eating a healthie
quality sleep, practicing good personal hygiene, taking care of your feet, and ...sing some weight.
Making these changes to your lifestyle will improve your quality of life and help you to maintain
your independence and live well for longer.

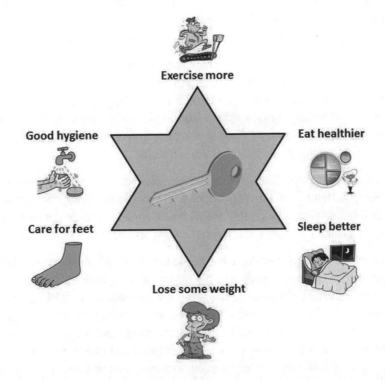

Figure 7.4 The key to reducing your risk of serious and life-threatening health complications that come with type 2 diabetes is to modify your lifestyle by exercising more, eating a healthier diet, getting better quality sleep, practicing good personal hygiene, taking care of your feet, and losing some weight. Plus, if you are a smoker, stop smoking or switch to vaping which is safer and satisfies your addiction to nicotine.

In the next chapter I will describe and comment on some of the most common dietary and exercise regimens that have been suggested for effective weight loss, with particular emphasis on what I consider to be the best ones for losing weight if you are a type 2 diabetic.

ʀoints

- Diabetes is a progressive disease and the medications only delay the onset of serious health complications such as cardiovascular disease, kidney disease, damage to the eyes and nerves, and serious life-threatening infections.

- The risk of these health complications can be reduced by eating a healthier diet, doing more exercise, improving sleep quality, and losing some excess weight.

- Even if we consume adequate amounts of essential nutrients, this in itself does not guarantee the absence of potentially harmful effects on our health in relation to the food that we consume. Deficiencies of some of the nonessential nutrients (e.g., fiber, phytonutrients) can also mean that our diets will not deliver what we need for optimal function and health.

- General guidelines for healthy eating include consuming a wide variety of nutrient-rich and nutrient-dense foods; eating a diet rich in vegetables, fruits, wholegrain foods, and high-fiber foods; selecting a diet that is moderate in total fat but low in saturated fat, *trans* fat, and cholesterol; cutting back on beverages and foods that are high in energy but low in nutrients; consuming less sugar and salt; drinking alcohol only in moderation; practicing food hygiene and safety; and avoiding processed foods when possible.

- Two well established healthy diets are the Mediterranean diet and the Japanese diet. Both are healthy, but for different reasons. Vegetarian diets can also be healthy and suitable for type 2 diabetics provided that appropriate food choices are made to avoid deficiencies of protein, vitamin B12, calcium, and iron, and lower fat options are chosen.

- The health benefits of regular exercise may be mediated via both a reduction in body fat mass (with a subsequent decreased release of pro-inflammatory cytokines from inflamed adipose tissue) and the induction of an anti-inflammatory environment with each bout of exercise that results from the exercise-induced secretion of interleukins 6 and 10 and the steroid hormone cortisol. Regular exercise also results in an improved blood lipid profile and increased insulin sensitivity. Regular moderate exercise improves fitness, strengthens bone, maintains mental function, improves immunity and vaccination responses, and reduces the risks of infectious illnesses such as the common cold and influenza.

- The minimum recommended amount of exercise to get significant health benefits is about 30 minutes of light to moderate-intensity on a minimum of three days per week. Further improvements in health markers and reduced disease risk will come by doing more exercise than this, and a good target to aim for is about 45-60 minutes of moderate-intensity exercise on four or five days per week. Beyond that the benefits become increasingly smaller.

- Doing some resistance exercise may help to maintain muscle strength which naturally decreases with aging. Improved leg strength can reduce the risk of falls and broken bones that can lead to loss of independence in later years.

- A lack of sleep and poor sleep quality (regular awakenings) in both healthy people and diabetics is often associated with stress and anxiety, a poor sleeping environment, inappropriate lifestyle habits (e.g., late evening work or exercise), use of electronic visual devices before bedtime, sleeping during the day, drinking alcohol or caffeine, smoking or eating a heavy meal just before going to bed, a poor diet and micronutrient deficiencies.

- There are a number of things you can try in order to help yourself get a good night's sleep if you have insomnia. These include having regular times for going to bed and waking up, relaxing before bed time, having a dark, quiet, warm sleeping environment and a comfortable bed, avoiding caffeine, nicotine, alcohol, heavy meals, large volumes of fluid, and exercise for a few hours before going to bed, and ignoring your worries.

- If you are diabetic, the single most effective thing you can do to reduce your risk of complications and reverse or at least delay the progression of your disease is to lose some body fat and body weight.

- The most effective and healthiest weight loss strategies include a combination of moderate reductions in daily dietary energy intake and regular moderate exercise that includes both aerobic and resistance exercise modes.

Chapter 8

What Can I Do to Beat Diabetes?

Objectives

After studying this chapter, you should:

- Appreciate that the key to getting your diabetes into remission is to lose a significant amount of body fat and weight.

- Know some reasons why calories from different foods are not the same when it comes to their influence on body weight.

- Know how your body's metabolism adapts to restriction of food intake.

- Know at least five different diets that have proven to be effective in achieving moderate weight loss and are suitable for people with type 2 diabetes.

- Understand how a diet with a low energy density can be achieved.

- Know how hunger can be abated when dieting.

- Understand why you need to exercise as well as restrict energy intake.

- Know what sort of exercise is best for body fat loss.

- Understand why fat burning is most effective at a moderate exercise intensity.

- Know the amount of calories burned when performing different activities or sports for one hour.

- Appreciate how much exercise is needed to achieve significant body fat and weight loss.

- Know why combining dieting and exercise is best for weight loss.

This chapter is all about how you can reverse and ultimately get rid of type 2 diabetes. As mentioned previously the biggest risk factor by far for developing prediabetes and type 2 diabetes is being overweight and having too much belly fat. Losing a little weight and being more physically active can help to slow the progression of your type 2 diabetes and risk of developing complications such as coronary heart disease and diabetic ret will not reverse your diabetes. In order to achieve this you need to lose a significan weight and body fat. Just how much will depend on your current body weight, percenta fat, the distribution of your body fat stores, how long you have had diabetes for, and your g

LOSING SUFFICIENT WEIGHT IS THE KEY TO REVERSING AND GETTING RID OF TYPE 2 DIABETES

For most people who have been diagnosed with type 2 diabetes in the past five years the amount of weight loss needed to stand a good (say 50%) chance of getting your diabetes into remission will probably be at least five kilograms and probably, for most people, maybe as much as 10-20 kilograms. This amount of weight loss is not easy to achieve but with determination, perseverance, and support from family and friends it can be done, and the health benefits will be tremendous.

Weight loss requires a negative energy balance which means that your daily dietary energy intake must be lower than your daily energy expenditure. The size of the average daily energy deficit over a period of time (i.e., days, weeks, or months) will be the major determinant of how much weight you lose. A commonly quoted estimate is that you can expect to lose 1 lb (0.46 kg) of body fat tissue for a 3,500-kcal energy deficit. This value is equal to the energy content of one pound of body fat tissue which is, on average, 87% fat, 10% water, and 3% protein by weight. An energy deficit of 3,500 kcal could be accumulated in one week if you were to have a daily energy deficit of 500 kcal. Adaptation to the energy deficit over time and differences in the macronutrient composition of your diet, and whether you are physically active or not will have some influence on how much weight you lose over several weeks or months, as well as how much of this is body fat rather than lean tissue and water. A negative energy balance can be achieved by dieting alone, exercising more instead of dieting, or a combination of both dieting and exercise.

Research that has been done in the past few decades has shown that if you lose sufficient body weight, your diabetes can be put into remission. For example, the findings of one non-randomized study (The 1991 Malmö Feasibility Study) showed that 54% of participants with early stage type 2 diabetes were in remission by the end of a 5-year diet and exercise intervention. The good news from more recent research is that similar results can be obtained within a much shorter time frame, maybe as little as 20 weeks. In a recent UK-conducted landmark study for people diagnosed with type 2 diabetes called DiRECT (short for Diabetes Remission Clinical Trial), it was shown that losing weight and body fat by sticking with a very low energy diet (VLED) for 20 weeks could reverse and essentially cure the condition in many people. In the UK study about 300 people diagnosed with type 2 diabetes were either put on a VLED (800 kcal/day) or remained on conventional care and were followed for up to one year. On average, those on the VLED lost 10 kg (22 lbs) and 50% of them had put their diabetes into remission (defined as their blood HbA1c level dropping below 6.5% or 48 mmol/mol, the cut off for diagnosis of type 2 diabetes). Those getting conventional care lost 1 kg (2 lbs) and only 6% went into remission.

...ould reduce your
...pathy, but it
...amount of
...e body
...nes.

f this important study see the sidebar. A typical average
in energy balance is 2,000 kcal/day, so an 800 kcal/day
00 kcal/day. Going on a VLED for 20 weeks takes a lot of
nd participants in this study received regular counselling
ers to help them stick to the weight loss plan and not
et weight had been lost. Losing the excess body fat and
ieting and exercise could theoretically achieve the same
itional health benefits. It is that approach I recommend
r.

Details of the 2018 DiRECT UK study showing that a very low energy diet can put type 2 diabetes into remission

Lead authors: Professors Michael Lean and Richard Taylor

Paper details: Primary care-led weight management for remission of type 2 diabetes (DiRECT): an open-label, cluster-randomized trial. *The Lancet*, February 2018, 391(10120):541-551.

Study aim: To assess whether intensive weight management (specifically going on a very low energy diet) within routine primary care would achieve remission of type 2 diabetes.

Study methods: The study was conducted at 49 primary care practices in Scotland and the Tyneside region of England. Practices were randomly assigned to provide either a weight management program (intervention) or best-practice care by guidelines (control). The participants were individuals aged 20-65 years who had been diagnosed with type 2 diabetes within the past 6 years, had a BMI of 27-45 kg/m², and were not receiving insulin. The intervention comprised withdrawal of antidiabetic and antihypertensive drugs, total diet replacement (825-853 kcal/day formula diet for 3-5 months), followed by stepped food reintroduction (for 2-8 weeks) with structured support for long-term weight loss maintenance.

Main study findings: Between 2014 and 2017, 306 individuals were recruited from 49 intervention (n=23) and control (n=26) general practices with 149 participants in each group. At 12 months, a weight loss of 15 kg or more was recorded in 36 (24%) participants in the intervention group and no participants in the control group. Diabetes remission (defined as blood glycated hemoglobin HbA1c of less than 6·5% after at least 2 months off all antidiabetic medications, from baseline to 12 months) was achieved in 68 (46%) participants in the intervention group and six (4%) participants in the control group. Remission varied with weight loss in the whole study population, with achievement in none of 76 participants who gained weight, six (7%) of 89 participants who maintained 0-5 kg weight loss, 19 (34%) of 56 participants with 5-10 kg loss, 16 (57%) of 28 participants with 10-15 kg loss, and 31 (86%) of 36 participants who lost 15 kg or more. Mean body weight fell by 10·0 kg in the intervention group and 1·0 kg in the control group. Quality of life, as measured by a validated visual analogue scale, improved by 7 points in the intervention group, and decreased by 3 points in the control group.

Study conclusion: At 12 months, almost half of participants achieved remission to a non-diabetic state and off antidiabetic drugs. Remission of type 2 diabetes by diet-induced weight loss is a practical and achievable target for primary care.

Weight loss is desirable for the health reasons explained in the previous couple of chapters but only for people who are overweight because of an excess of body fat. In other circumstances, weight loss is not always a good idea, and if not done correctly (e.g., eating insufficient protein or cutting out major macronutrients or food groups from your diet) can often be accompanied by a reduction in muscle mass and it may reduce liver and muscle glycogen stores as well which will make doing any exercise feel harder and make you feel more tired. Excessive weight loss has also been associated with chronic fatigue, irritability, and increased risk of injuries. Too much emphasis on losing weight can lead to the development of micronutrient deficiencies and eating disorders such as anorexia nervosa and bulimia nervosa, which are harmful to health. The elderly and illness-prone individuals may actually benefit from being slightly overweight rather than underweight in order to have an energy reserve when they become ill and are unable to eat properly. These are good reasons to avoid extreme dieting, but if you are a type 2 diabetic some serious dieting will be needed if you want to reverse your condition.

For those who are determined to lose some weight the first step in determining a healthy body weight goal is weighing, in a normally hydrated state, and measuring body composition as described in chapter 6. These measures can be used to determine how much body fat or weight individuals should lose to put them within an optimal range for health. An energy deficit of 500 to 1,000 kcal below estimated daily energy needs is generally recommended for effective weight loss. However, individuals with lower energy needs (women, elderly adults, and children) should minimize their total energy deficit to ensure they are getting enough nutrients for good health, and where relevant, growth, development, and reproductive functioning. As with any weight loss plan, always seek medical advice before you start if you:

- Have a history of eating disorders.

- Are taking prescribed medication.

- Are pregnant or breastfeeding.

- Have other significant medical or mental health conditions.

Don't go on a diet if you are under 18 (unless it is done under medical supervision) or if you are or are recovering from illness or surgery or are generally frail.

ABOUT FOOD CALORIES AND THE EFFECTS OF ENERGY RESTRICTION

Firstly, it is important to appreciate that some food calories are not the same as others. Predominantly carbohydrate, fat, or protein food sources are metabolized differently in the body and the energy cost of this metabolism is higher for protein than for carbohydrate or fat. In addition, ingested calories from different food sources can have very different effects on satiety, hormones, and the brain regions that control food intake – protein is known to be the most fulfilling macronutrient by far. If people increase their dietary protein intake as a percentage of their total daily energy intake (in other words they substitute some fat and carbohydrate for extra protein), they can start losing weight without counting calories. In this sense, it can be said that not all calories from food are equal. However, there is no escaping the fact that significant weight loss (i.e., more than a few kilograms) can only be achieved by substantial reductions in energy intake and improved further with increased energy expenditure with exercise.

In response to reduced energy intake, metabolic adaptation or adaptive thermogenesis occurs which results in a decrease in resting metabolic rate (RMR) which makes weight loss even harder. This phenomenon is often called "**food efficiency**" and represents the body's attempt to preserve energy; in times of famine it serves as a protective mechanism. However, it usually causes a reduction or even a plateau in weight loss and is a common source of frustration for dieters. Additionally, any lean body (muscle) mass that is lost over time will lower **resting energy expenditure** further and make exercise more efficient (because a little less energy will be expended during weight-bearing activities such as walking and running) which again makes losing weight harder to achieve. The commonly observed failure to lose more weight as diets progress over time and weight regain after stopping a diet (known as **weight cycling** or the **yo-yo effect**) is explained by these adaptations.

COMMON DIETS FOR WEIGHT LOSS AND THE ONES THAT DIABETICS SHOULD AVOID

Some diets have been designed specifically for weight loss while others have been designed with some other useful purpose in mind such as to lower and stabilize blood sugar, lower blood pressure, treat irritable bowel syndrome, etc. although they may also help to facilitate some weight loss. In this chapter, I will focus on the diets that are intended to make you lose body fat and body weight. A number of these diets have stood the test of time and are still popular because people have found that they work, and science has proved that they have some degree of success in achieving weight and/or fat loss. Some, however, are better than others either in terms of their effectiveness for weight and/or fat loss or by virtue of not having side effects or unwanted health problems associated with their use. Furthermore, some diets that may be helpful for overweight but otherwise healthy people are not as suitable for diabetics as they can worsen some aspects of an already disturbed metabolism. In this category of diets I would include many of the so-called fad diets and other diets that require an extreme modification of the usual macronutrient profile; in other words, those that are very high-fat and low-carbohydrate (e.g., Atkins, Sugar Busters) or just the opposite – very low-fat and high-carbohydrate. Although both these types of diet can be effective for weight loss, let me explain in a little more detail why some diets like these are not best suited to people with type 2 diabetes.

FASTING AND CRASH DIETING

Fasting literally means going without any food and only drinking water. Although this is the most effective form of dieting in the short-term there are significant dangers to health if it is maintained for more than even a few days due to the deficiencies of protein and micronutrients. There will also be a significant loss of lean tissue (muscle) and body water as well as fat, and you will constantly be feeling hungry, tired, and irritable, so forget it. In the diabetic state your cells are already deprived of energy in the form of glucose, and levels of blood fats are higher than normal. This situation will just be exacerbated by fasting. We all need energy for everyday tasks and without it and the essential amino acids and micronutrients that your food provides, the body tissues will be broken down and organ damage will follow. Almost all aspects of our normal physiology will become impaired. For example, immune function will become depressed and we will become more susceptible to infections; our muscles will become thinner and weaker; we will lose stamina as well as strength and our ability to think clearly, concentrate, and perform tasks that require cognitive function will worsen considerably. Although fasting and slightly less extreme crash dieting (e.g., restricting daily energy intake to less than 500 kcal) will produce significant weight loss within only a few days, much of this loss will be water because you are missing out on the water that is contained in most of the foods you eat. That means that most of the weight you lost will be regained as soon as you start eating and drinking normally again. Some forms of crash dieting require you to stick to an extremely low calorie and restricted diet (e.g., consuming only vegetable soup) which also severely limits your intake of protein and micronutrients. The other nail in the coffin for complete fasting (and crash dieting) is that it will be impossible to sustain for more than a few days, and you will probably overeat when fasting stops to compensate for what you missed during a period of abstinence from eating. For all these reasons fasting and crash dieting is definitely not recommended for anyone at all.

FAD DIETS

Every year there seems to be at least one new diet that gets promoted by the media and endorsed by some television, film, music, or fashion celebrities. These are mostly what can be called fad diets and only seem to reign in popularity for a few months until the next new fad diet comes along. Fad diets are often based on pseudoscience, myths, and ignorance but often receive much media attention. The simple fact is that many of these diets are complicated, not based on sound scientific evidence, and when tested in an appropriate controlled manner do not lead to sustained long-term weight loss. Quite frankly, most of them do not actually do what they claim to do and many pose a risk to health if sustained for more than a couple of months. There are several good reasons to avoid fad diets including:

- Some diets, especially those that require crash dieting can make you feel tired and lethargic and some can actually make you ill.

- Diets that require you to cut out certain foods altogether (e.g., meat, fish, cereal, or dairy products) could prevent you from getting enough vitamins, minerals, and other essential nutrients that your body needs to function properly.

- Some diets may be low in sugar and other carbohydrates but instead they are high in fat which can cause its own problems such as bad breath, tiredness, headaches, and **constipation**. For diabetics, these sorts of diets will worsen an already unhealthy blood lipid profile.

- Some diets claim to "detoxify" your body and that a build-up of toxins can be removed by eating certain foods and avoiding others. This is complete nonsense. They only work because your calorie intake is reduced as a result of the restrictions the diet plan places on what you can actually eat. Toxins do not normally build up in the body. Any potentially toxic substances like ammonia and **urea** are excreted in the urine well before they can accumulate to high enough levels to cause problems.

- The problem with many fad diets is that they are extreme in one form or another and while weight loss might be achieved in the short term, they are very difficult to stick to for more than a few weeks. Furthermore, diets that are unbalanced are more likely to be bad for your health, even if you do manage to stick with them!

VERY LOW-CARBOHYDRATE DIETS

Some of the best-known very low-carbohydrate diets (also known as ketogenic diets) are the **Atkins diet** and Sugar Busters that were introduced in the 1990s. These diets are based on the premise that reducing carbohydrate intake results in increased fat oxidation and are sometimes called ketogenic diets. This is because when carbohydrate is severely restricted to less than 20 g per day, the production of **ketone bodies** (acetone, acetoacetate, and β-hydroxybutyrate) will increase to supply the brain with an alternative type of fuel to glucose. Ketone bodies may suppress appetite, and some ketone bodies will be present in urine which could result in loss of some "calories" through urination. Although all of the preceding may be true, the loss of calories achieved via the excretion of ketone bodies in urine amounts to no more than 100 to 150 kcal/day. Such diets can be effective for weight loss, but they are no more effective than a well-balanced, energy-restricted diet for loss of body fat because much of the weight loss in the first few weeks is due to reduced glycogen and loss of water which will be quickly restored when the dieting stops. Although these diets may provide better satiety than high-carbohydrate diets, most of the effect can be attributed to the relatively high-protein content. For active individuals, these very low-carbohydrate or ketogenic diets are detrimental because of reduced glycogen stores which limit the ability to perform prolonged aerobic exercise due to an earlier onset of fatigue. In that sense they may limit your ability to add to your daily energy deficit by increasing your energy expenditure through exercise.

The Atkins Diet had been tested in large numbers of clinical trials and overall the evidence supports its efficacy in achieving meaningful long-term body weight loss. However, body weight loss was the only outcome measure in most of these studies and the effects of the diet on body composition (i.e., percentage body fat) were not considered. A recent comprehensive meta-analysis that considered the results of 32 controlled feeding studies involving over 500 subjects did not support the use of low-carbohydrate diets for body fat loss. In all these studies the participants had some of their dietary carbohydrate calories replaced by an equal number of calories from fat, but dietary protein content remained the same. As the proportion of dietary carbohydrate to fat changed, daily energy expenditure and body fat changes were recorded, which allowed a direct comparison of the efficacy of low-fat and low-carbohydrate diets across a wide range of study conditions. The main findings were that the average rate of body fat loss was 16 g/day (or 0.5 kg/month) greater with lower fat diets. In fact, only three out of the 32 studies examined showed a greater body fat loss with the low-carbohydrate diet, whereas the overwhelming majority showed greater body fat loss with the low-fat diet.

A major problem of very low-carbohydrate diets for people with diabetes is that they make it even more difficult for your body tissues to get glucose, and they exacerbate the already high levels of fats in the blood. When you eat a low-carbohydrate diet high in fat and protein, fatty acids are burned for energy, but they also accumulate in tissues like your muscle and liver where they are converted to triglycerides – your body's storage form of fat. When your muscle and liver begin accumulating fat, both tissues become more insulin resistant which is just what you don't want if you're diabetic! In the long-term it means that low-carbohydrate diets, high in fat and protein, can actually worsen the health of someone with type 2 diabetes, increase cancer risk, increase cholesterol, increase atherosclerosis, harden blood vessels, and increase all-cause mortality.

VERY LOW-FAT DIETS

Because fat is the most energy dense nutrient (each gram of fat contains 9 kcal compared with only 4 kcal for carbohydrate and protein) reducing the dietary fat intake can be a very effective way to reduce total daily energy intake and promote weight loss. Fat is also less satiating than either protein or carbohydrate, so we tend to eat more when consuming mostly fatty foods. Furthermore, fat is stored efficiently and requires little energy for digestion, and diet-induced thermogenesis (thermic effect of food ingestion) is lowest for fat compared with protein and carbohydrate so consuming fat results in only a very small increase in energy expenditure and fat oxidation.

Many of the very low-fat diets encourage people to consume as little fat as possible or to restrict fat intake to less than 20 g per day or less than 10% of total dietary energy intake. However, such extreme reductions in dietary fat are not recommended for healthy people or diabetics for the following reasons: (1) Replacing fat with more calories from carbohydrates results in a worsening of the blood lipid profile and increases known cardiovascular disease risk factors including the serum apoB/apoA-I ratio and triglyceride levels. (2) The high percentage of dietary energy coming from carbohydrates will further increase blood glucose levels, increasing the need for greater insulin secretion, and putting yet more stress on the pancreatic -cells that may already be starting to fail (see chapter 4 for details). (3) Eating carbohydrates in moderation seems to be optimal for health and living longer. A 2018 meta-analysis of eight studies involving a total of over 430,000 adults showed that both low-carbohydrate consumption (<40% of daily total dietary energy intake from carbohydrates) and high-carbohydrate consumption (>70% of daily total dietary energy intake from carbohydrates) conferred greater mortality risk than did moderate intake with the lowest mortality associated with carbohydrate intake of 50-55% of daily total dietary energy. (4) Fat intakes of less than 20 g/day will almost certainly not provide enough of the essential fatty acids and fat-soluble vitamins A, D, E, and K.

FOOD-COMBINING DIETS

Food-combining diets are based on a philosophy that certain foods should not be combined. Although many types of food-combining diets exist, most advise against combining protein and carbohydrate foods in a meal. It is often claimed that such combinations cause a "buildup of toxins" (which, quite frankly, is utter nonsense) with the result of this buildup being "negative side effects such as weight gain". These diets are often tempting to overweight people because they promise an easy way to rapid weight loss, and they are claimed to work for some people. However, when these diets are strictly followed, energy and fat intake are likely to be reduced compared with the normal diet, and it is this reduction in energy and fat that is the main reason for the success of the diet rather than the fact that certain foods were not combined. This is one dietary strategy I definitely do not recommend for anyone.

THE PALEO DIET

The **Paleo** (short for Paleolithic) diet is based on eating just like our ancient ancestors did. The Paleolithic era – also known as the early Stone Age – began around 2.5 million years ago and lasted until around 10,000 BC. The aim is to eat as naturally as possible, opting for grass-fed lean meats, an abundance of fruit and vegetables and other wholefoods like nuts and seeds. Some less strict versions of the diet allow some foods (e.g., low-fat dairy products and root vegetables like potatoes, carrots, and turnips) that were not necessarily available during this period. A consequence of these food choices is, of course, that the diet results in a low intake of sugar, salt, saturated fat, and zero processed foods. The diet is relatively low in carbohydrate but rich in lean protein and plant foods. These plant foods contribute the important fiber, unsaturated fats, vitamins, minerals, and phytonutrients. The diet is not low-fat but instead promotes the inclusion of natural fats from pasture-fed livestock, fish and seafood, as well as nuts, seeds, and their oils. Although people who adopt this diet are generally more concerned with healthy eating or have a digestive problem with cereals, grain, or dairy products rather than a strong desire for weight loss, the absence of such a wide range of foods like grains, dairy, processed foods, fatty foods, and sugar means the diet is more than likely to lead to some weight loss. In fact, a number of small studies have suggested that those following a Paleo diet report weight loss together with several other positive health outcomes including improved blood sugar control and a reduction in the risk factors for heart disease.

However, there are some drawbacks as the Paleo diet ignores the health benefits of consuming wholegrains as well as beans, legumes, and starchy vegetables. Numerous studies have reported a reduced incidence of heart disease in those who regularly consume three or more servings of wholegrains per day. The low glycemic index properties of beans and other legumes (which are not allowed with the Paleo diet) make them especially useful for people with blood sugar issues, and starchy vegetables are an excellent source of nutrient-dense energy. All of these foods supply essential B vitamins, which among other things help us unlock the energy in our food by acting as cofactors of enzymes involved in energy metabolism. Finally, omitting dairy may limit the intake of minerals like calcium which is essential for development and maintenance of bones as well as being needed for normal nerve and muscle function. The Paleo diet also has the problem that it is difficult to stick to, especially when socializing and eating out, because of the restriction on grains, dairy, starchy vegetables, and all processed foods. Very few cafes or restaurants have menus that allow the restrictions of the Paleo diet to be satisfied. For these reasons, although it is a healthy diet, the Paleo diet is not one I recommend for weight loss as there are better, easier to live with diets than this one.

THE ZONE DIET

The **Zone diet** was proposed in 1995 by Barry Sears in his book The Zone: A Dietary Road Map. The diet is essentially a high-protein but relatively low-carbohydrate diet. By reducing carbohydrate intake, plasma insulin responses following meals are lower. The benefits are increased fat breakdown and improved regulation of **eicosanoids**, hormone-like derivatives of fatty acids in the body that act as cell-to-cell signaling molecules. The diet is claimed to increase the "good" eicosanoids and decrease the "bad" eicosanoids which will promote blood flow and oxygen delivery to muscle tissue and stimulate fat oxidation. The diet is also claimed to reduce "diet-induced inflammation". To "enter the zone", the diet should consist of 40% carbohydrate, 30% fat and 30% protein divided into a regimen of three meals and two snacks per day. The diet is also referred to as the 40:30:30 diet. On the Zone diet you need to stick to a rather strict and restrictive regimen. You're supposed to eat a meal within an hour of waking, never let more than five hours go by without eating, and have a snack before bedtime. Worst of all, you need to stick to the 40% carbohydrate, 30% fat and 30% protein formula at every meal and snack. You can't eat mostly carbohydrate for lunch and eat lots of protein for dinner.

Although some arguments by Sears are scientifically sound, several previous studies that have manipulated the diet along these lines have been unsuccessful in stimulating the synthesis of good eicosanoids relative to bad eicosanoids. The book contains some errors in assumptions, some contradictory information, and mention of scientific studies that might support the Zone diet are limited to a few that show positive outcomes for hormonal influences on eicosanoid metabolism, while any opposing evidence is conveniently left out.

Following the consumption of a meal containing some carbohydrate, it doesn't take much to see dietary attempts to increase fat oxidation become hampered. It takes only very small rises in insulin concentration to reduce fat breakdown and oxidation significantly, and these effects persist for up to six hours after a meal. To avoid reductions in fat breakdown after a meal, the carbohydrate intake must be extremely small; much less, in fact, than the amount of carbohydrate in the Zone diet. Furthermore, from a practical standpoint, meals with the 40:30:30 carbohydrate:fat:protein ratio are quite difficult to compose, unless, of course, the dieter buys the 40:30:30 energy bars specially formulated and marketed by the author!

Although the Zone diet has been shown to achieve some degree of weight loss when applied to overweight people, such success really should be expected because the Zone diet is essentially a lower than normal energy diet that supplies 1,000 to 1,800 kcal/day. Although the theory of opening muscle blood vessels by altering eicosanoid production is correct in theory, there is very little evidence available from human studies to support any significant contribution of eicosanoids to this proposed effect. In fact, the key eicosanoid reportedly produced in the Zone diet and responsible for improved muscle oxygenation is not found in human skeletal muscle. Therefore, there is little reason to recommend this diet.

DIETS THAT WORK FOR WEIGHT LOSS AND ARE SUITABLE FOR PEOPLE WITH PREDIABETES OR TYPE 2 DIABETES

Having eliminated some diets for use by diabetics let's now examine the efficacy of some of the diets that are suitable and that have proven to have some degree of success in achieving effective loss of body fat and body weight.

LOW GLYCEMIC INDEX DIETS

Details of low glycemic index (GI) and low glycemic load (GL) foods were described in chapter 3 and will not be repeated here. Basing the carbohydrate component of your diet on the low GI or GL principle can be helpful for people who have type 2 diabetes or are at risk of developing it as it can help to control body weight by minimizing spikes in blood sugar and insulin levels. The GI and GL are not themselves diet plans but are useful tools to guide food choices. The low GI diet is a specific diet plan that uses the index as the primary or only guide for meal planning. Unlike some other plans, a GI diet doesn't necessarily specify portion sizes or the optimal number of calories, carbohydrates, or fats for weight loss or weight maintenance. Therefore, it can only be effective for weight loss if overall daily calorie intake is reduced below normal. Several of the popular commercial diets, including the Zone Diet, Sugar Busters, Slow-Carb Diet, and Blood Sugar Diet are at least partly based on the low GI principle. Most scientific studies of the low GI diet suggest that it can help achieve some loss of body fat and body weight. However, you might be able to achieve the same or even greater weight loss by eating the other diets described in this section of the chapter and/or doing more exercise.

Selecting foods based on their GI or GL value may help you manage your weight and control your blood sugar because many foods that should be included in a well-balanced, low-fat, healthy diet with minimally processed foods – wholegrain products, fruits, vegetables, and low-fat dairy products – have low GI values. Avoiding high GI foods generally means eliminating candy, chocolate, sugar-sweetened beverages, most sauces, many processed foods, and starchy vegetables like potato as well as rice, bread, and pasta from your diet. That is all well and good but to lose a significant amount of weight you need to reduce your energy intake by at least 300-500 kcal per day. For these reasons a low GI diet is not one I would recommend if your main goal is effective weight loss.

VERY LOW ENERGY DIETS

Very low energy diets (VLEDs) or very low-calorie diets are used as a therapy to achieve rapid weight loss in obese people. These diets are usually in the form of liquid meals that contain the recommended dietary allowance (daily intake) of micronutrients but provide only 400 to 800 kcal/day. These liquid meals contain a relatively large amount of protein to reduce muscle wasting and a relatively small amount of carbohydrate (less than 100 g/day). Such diets are extremely effective in reducing body weight rapidly. In the first week, the weight loss is predominantly glycogen and water. Fat and protein are lost as well during the initial phase, but those losses are a relatively small proportion of the total weight loss. After the initial rapid weight loss, the weight reduction is mainly from adipose tissue fat stores, although some loss of lean tissue also occurs. With VLEDs the restricted carbohydrate availability and increased fat oxidation result in ketosis (formation of ketone bodies, mostly in the form of acetoacetate and -hydroxybutyrate). Ketone bodies have a specific odor that is easily detectable on the breath and does not smell nice! After ketosis begins, hunger feelings may decrease somewhat as the ketone bodies can be used as a fuel by the brain, compensating for the reduced availability of blood glucose. Increased ketosis is not ideal for diabetics who may already experience this to some degree before dieting.

Because carbohydrate intake is low on VLEDs, blood glucose concentration is prevented from falling too low by synthesizing glucose from various non-carbohydrate precursors (**glycerol** from the breakdown of fat, and amino acids from the breakdown of protein). Because of the associated chronic glycogen depletion, exercise capacity is severely impaired. For this reason, such diets are not advised for those who also want to be physically active and use exercise to burn more calories in their efforts to lose weight.

Side effects of VLEDs include nausea, halitosis (bad breath), hunger (which may decrease after the initiation of ketosis), light-headedness, headaches, and low blood pressure. Dehydration is also common with such diets and **electrolyte** imbalances may occur. On VLEDs it is important to increase your daily water intake to compensate for the water you are missing by eating less food (most foods contain some water and many meats and vegetables can be 70-90% water by weight; even bread is 40% water). Dehydration is probably the main cause of light-headedness, headaches, and reduced blood pressure for people on VLEDs.

Although effective and have even been shown to reverse type 2 diabetes if maintained for long enough (see sidebar), VLEDs are hard to stick to unless you are highly motivated and determined to lose weight quickly (i.e., within weeks rather than months). People are generally advised not to try these diets without some sort of medical supervision or regular health checks, and most people will probably need strong support and encouragement from family and/or healthcare practitioners to keep going with the diet.

VLEDs are definitely not the easiest diet to sustain so are probably not the best choice for most people unless that motivation and support is there for them. Furthermore, all your eating will have to be done at home as most cafes and restaurants don't have suitable VLED meals on their menus.

INTERMITTENT FASTING DIETS

Intermittent fasting diets (IFD), of which there are several, have become popular in recent years, in part because of a lot of media coverage and backing from television and film celebrities. However, there is reasonable evidence that they can be effective, as all of them will reduce weekly energy intake to some degree. They may not be quite as beneficial for women as men, and may also be a poor choice for people who are prone to eating disorders. It is also important to bear in mind that you should aim to eat healthily as well (see chapter 3) during the normal eating phase of the diets.

The most extreme of the IFDs is the alternate day fasting diet which involves fasting every other day. This can be a complete fast or some versions of this diet allow you to consume up to 500 kcal on the fasting days. A full fast every other day is rather extreme and could lead to insufficient protein intake with negative consequences for muscle mass, so it is not recommended for older or highly physically active people. The version where you eat normally on four days of the week and consume only about 500 kcal on alternate days is sometimes referred to as the 4:3 diet. A more popular IFD is the 5:2 diet (also commonly known as the 'Fast Diet'), promoted by the British television medic Dr Michael Mosley, which involves eating normally on five days of the week, while restricting intake to 500 kcal (for women) or 600 kcal (for men) on two days of the week (usually these are separated by two to three days such as fasting on Mondays and Thursdays). On the fasting days (note this is not strictly fasting, rather just eating much less than normal on two days of the week) you could eat two small meals (250 kcal per meal for women, and 300 kcal for men). These should be high-protein meals for better satiety and to maintain muscle mass. A slightly less drastic version of the 5:2 diet with a lower risk of consuming inadequate amounts of protein is to allow up to 800 kcal on the fasting days. Of course, the most important thing on IFDs is not to compensate for the reduced calorie days by eating more than usual on the non-fasting days. On these days you should be aiming to consume no more dietary energy than you are expending (i.e., you should be in energy balance). Dr Mosley has more recently promoted a modified version of the 5:2 diet in which he recommends a healthy Mediterranean diet (see chapter 7 for details) on the non-fasting days. This is a very sensible recommendation in my opinion and is suitable for diabetics. If you want to add even more healthy variety on this IFD you could also have vegetarian meals, Japanese style meals (see chapter 7), low glycemic index meals, or high-protein and low energy density meals on the non-fasting days (see later in this chapter for the reasons why).

Another IFD involves fasting from evening dinner one day to dinner the next (i.e., skipping both breakfast and lunch for a day), amounting to a 24 hour fast, and doing this on two days of the week. You should eat a normal meal at dinner on these days and not compensate for your hunger by eating more than usual; eating slowly and having a high-protein meal will again help with satiety. Another simple IFD is to skip one meal (usually lunch) on five days of the week. The **Warrior Diet** is another type of IFD that was popularized by ex-army fitness expert Ori Hofmekler and involves eating small amounts of raw fruits and vegetables during the day, then eating one large meal in the evening. The diet also emphasizes food choices (whole, unprocessed foods) that are quite similar to the Paleo diet (described earlier in this chapter) in which you are encouraged to eat anything we could hunt or gather way back in the Paleolithic era (also known as the Stone Age) including foods like meats, fish, nuts, leafy greens, regional vegetables, and seeds, but avoiding processed foods, ready meals, pasta, bread, cereal, and candy.

Another type of IFD is what is known as **time-restricted feeding**. This is a daily eating pattern in which all your food is eaten within an 8- to 12-hour timeframe every day, with no deliberate attempt to alter nutrient quality or quantity. This usually involves abstaining from breakfast thus extending the duration of your normal overnight fast (the time when you are asleep and not eating) which gives your body more time to burn fat and do essential repairs. Outside of this time-restricted eating period, a person consumes no food items apart from drinking water or low-calorie beverages to stay well hydrated. Such beverages could also include black unsweetened coffee or green tea (without milk). Time-restricted feeding is a type of intermittent fasting because it involves skipping breakfast. It is a pattern of eating that probably is similar to what our ancient ancestors adopted: most of the daytime would be spent hunting and gathering food and most of the eating would take place after dark.

Although time-restricted eating will not work for everyone, some may find it beneficial. Some recent studies have shown that it can aid weight loss, improve sleep quality, and may lower the risk of metabolic diseases, such as type 2 diabetes. Modern humans, due to societal pressures, work schedules, and the availability of nighttime indoor illumination and entertainment, stay awake longer, which enables food consumption for longer durations of time. This extended duration itself, in addition to the caloric surplus, can be detrimental to health by reducing sleep time. A recent study using a smartphone app to monitor eating time has revealed more than 50% of adults spread their daily food and beverage intake over 15 hours or longer. Such extended eating of high-fat or high glycemic index diets is known to predispose laboratory animals to metabolic diseases.

It is probably best to start a time-restricted eating plan gradually. Try starting with a shorter fasting period and then gradually increase it over time. For example, start with a fasting period of 10:00 pm to 6:30 am Then increase this by one hour every two days to reach the desired fasting period (usually around 8:00 pm to 1:00 pm the next day – leaving a time-restricted eating period of seven hours). Studies have suggested that restricting feeding periods to less than six hours is unlikely to offer additional advantages over more extended feeding periods.

The largest evidence base for the efficacy of IFDs derives from studies that have used some of the more extreme forms, such as alternate day fasting, which according to several studies can lead to significant body weight loss amounting to 5-8 kg over a period of 15-20 weeks. With alternate day fasting the rate of weight loss averages about 0.7 kg/week (1.5 lbs/week); with other IFDs the rate of weight loss is less at about 0.35 kg/week (0.8 lbs/week). Studies comparing intermittent fasting and continuous calorie restriction show no difference in weight loss if calories are matched between groups.

REDUCED FAT DIETS

Because fat is the most energy dense nutrient (each gram of fat contains 9 kcal compared with only 4 kcal for carbohydrate and protein), reducing the dietary fat intake from 25-30% to around 10-15 % of total energy intake can be a very effective way to reduce overall daily energy intake and promote weight loss. More extreme reductions in dietary fat are not recommended for the reasons explained earlier in this chapter. A moderate reduction in dietary fat is, however, usually desirable and is best achieved by eliminating foods with high-fat content from the diet. That means cutting out fatty meats, sauces, cheese, creams, pizza, cakes, and cookies and substituting some foods or beverages with lower fat alternatives (e.g., skimmed milk, low-fat yogurt, and reduced fat coleslaw). Scientific evidence from large scale population studies suggests that reducing the percentage of fat in the diet is more effective in reducing body weight than is reducing the absolute amount of fat. However, the most important factor is always the reduction in energy intake. An important advantage of reduced fat intake is that a moderate to high-carbohydrate content can be maintained, resulting in reasonable glycogen stores and better recovery from exercise for those who also want to include exercise as part of their weight loss program. Indeed many athletes who want to lose some body fat also adopt a diet that is low in fat with a small reduction in energy intake, so that they can still replenish their carbohydrate stores to maintain their high training loads. This type of diet seems to be a sensible way of reducing weight, although weight reduction will occur relatively slowly. The magnitude of body weight and body fat losses on a reduced fat diet will largely depend on by how much daily energy intake is reduced.

HIGH-PROTEIN DIETS

For most diets, protein will provide 10 to 15% of the calories; with high-protein diets, this is increased to about 30%. Many of the most popular or fad diets recommend increased consumption of protein usually to replace calories from fat or carbohydrate. One main reason that is often given is that high-protein diets suppress the appetite, which might be a mechanism that could help to promote weight loss. Protein also has a larger thermic effect and a relatively low **coefficient of digestibility** (that is, a smaller percentage of its available energy is digested and absorbed) compared with a mixed meal of equal total calorie content. Several studies have demonstrated that increased protein content of the diet, particularly in combination with regular exercise, may improve weight loss and reduce the loss of **lean body mass** in overweight and obese individuals who are consuming a low energy diet. It is also known that less weight regain occurs after the energy-restricted period ends when protein intake is high compared with more normal dietary compositions.

A concern that some people may have is that they may have heard from some sources that high-protein diets can be damaging to kidney function. However, I can assure you that this is not true. This widely held but controversial myth was debunked in 2018 by scientists at McMaster University. The researchers examined 28 studies involving over 1,300 participants that had investigated the effects of high-protein diets on glomerular filtration rate, an index of kidney function which generally falls when kidneys become damaged or diseased. The studies involved in their meta-analysis included participants who were healthy, obese, or had type 2 diabetes, and/or high blood pressure. The high-protein diets contained either at least 20% of total caloric intake coming from protein or at least 100 g of protein per day. They found that there is simply no evidence linking a high-protein diet to kidney disease in healthy individuals or those who are at risk of kidney disease due to conditions such as obesity, hypertension, or even type 2 diabetes.

On a high-protein (30% protein, 50% carbohydrate, 20% fat) diet, satiety is increased compared with a normal weight-maintaining diet (10-15% protein, 50-55% carbohydrate, 30-35% fat) of equal calorie content. In one study, when subjects were on an ad libitum (eat as desired) high-protein diet for 12 weeks, their mean spontaneous daily energy intake decreased by 441 kcal and they lost, on average, 4.9 kg (11 lbs) body weight and had a mean decrease in fat mass of 3.7 kg (8 lbs). Of course, increasing the proportion of protein in the diet also permits a simultaneous reduction in the proportion of fat which is good because extra calories from fat (and carbohydrate) are more fattening than calories in the form of protein.

Another effect of protein that can facilitate weight loss is its relatively high thermogenic effect (i.e., the increase in resting metabolic rate that occurs after feeding). The **metabolizable energy** (that is the energy available from a nutrient after it has been digested and absorbed) of dietary protein is 4 kcal/g. Protein, however, is particularly thermogenic, and the **net metabolizable energy** is actually only 3.1 kcal/g (that is the available energy after taking into account the energy lost as heat in its metabolism), making it lower than either carbohydrate or fat (4.0 kcal/g and 8.1 kcal/g, respectively). Reported values for diet-induced thermogenesis for separate nutrients are 0 to 3% for fat, 5 to 10% for carbohydrate, and 20 to 30% for protein. Thus, a high-protein diet induces a greater thermic response in healthy subjects compared with a high-fat or high-carbohydrate diet. This conclusion implies even higher fat oxidation on a high-protein diet. The relatively strong thermic effect of protein may be mediated by the high energy costs of protein synthesis following the absorption of amino acids from digested protein after a meal. Protein from meats (e.g., pork, beef, chicken) generally produces higher diet-induced thermogenesis than protein derived from plants (e.g., soy).

A third possible mechanism by which a high-protein intake may aid weight loss is by maintaining muscle mass during periods of dietary energy restriction. A high-protein intake helps to prevent some of the muscle mass loss that is otherwise inevitable with energy restriction. This means that a larger muscle mass can be maintained, and because muscle is the most active tissue metabolically, the resting metabolic rate can be better maintained, thus helping weight loss. In one study, 31 overweight or obese postmenopausal women were put on a reduced calorie diet of 1,400 kcal/day (with 15%, 65%, and 30% calories from protein, carbohydrate, and fat, respectively) and randomized to receive either 25 g of a whey protein or carbohydrate (maltodextrin) supplement twice a day for the 6-month study period. The group receiving the additional protein lost 4% percent more body weight than the carbohydrate supplement group and preserved more of their muscle mass. In another intervention study, young, overweight, recreationally active men were placed on an intense 4-week diet and exercise program that included circuit training and sprints to help build muscle. Their diet contained 40% less energy each day than necessary for weight maintenance. Half of the men were randomly selected to receive a higher-protein diet (2.4 g/kg body weight, 35% protein, 50% carbohydrate, and 15% fat) and the others were placed on a lower-protein diet (1.2 g/kg body weight, 15% protein, 50% carbohydrate, and 35% fat). Both groups lost body weight, with no significant difference between groups. However, men in the higher-protein group gained 1.2 kg (2.6 lbs) of muscle and lost 4.8 kg (10.6 lbs) of body fat, while men in the lower-protein group gained only 0.1 kg (0.2 lbs) of muscle and lost 27% less fat. Both groups similarly improved measures of strength, **power**, and fitness.

Some of the more important reasons for selecting a high-protein diet are summarized in the following sidebar.

Why dietary protein is helpful in weight loss and maintenance

Protein may be an effective and healthy means of supporting weight loss and maintenance for several reasons:

- Eating protein makes you feel fuller for longer as protein has a greater effect on satiety than carbohydrate or fat does.

- Ingested protein has less net metabolizable energy available than carbohydrate or fat does as its nitrogen component cannot be oxidized and it has a higher thermogenic effect.

- A high-protein intake helps to maintain muscle mass during periods of dietary energy restriction thereby preserving metabolically active tissue.

- High-protein diets are associated with less severe hunger pangs because the levels of ghrelin, the hormone that stimulates appetite are lower.

- The amino acids obtained from the digestion of ingested protein can be used to support glucose synthesis in situations of low-carbohydrate availability.

- High-protein diets are associated with lower plasma triglyceride concentrations.

For these reasons a high-protein diet is one that I highly recommend for safe and effective weight loss. It can be even more effective if the carbohydrate foods you consume are low glycemic index and you trim the fat off cuts of meat and avoid other high-fat foods.

LOW ENERGY DENSITY DIETS

The energy density of the diet can play an important role in weight maintenance. A small quantity of food rich in fat has very high energy content. Visual cues that may prevent a large intake of energy on a high-carbohydrate diet, which is commonly of high bulk and volume, may be absent on a high-fat diet. Several studies have shown that subjects tend to eat a similar weight of food regardless of the macronutrient composition. Because a 500 g meal consisting mainly of carbohydrate will contain significantly less energy than a 500 g high-fat meal, lower energy intake will automatically result.

Studies in the 1990s showed that when subjects received a diet that contained 20%, 40%, or 60% fat and could eat ad libitum (i.e., they were free to choose as much as desired), the weight of the food that they consumed was the same (see figure 8.1). Because of differences in energy density, however, the total amount of energy consumed with the higher-fat diets was greater and therefore weight gain was greater. This result happened in both controlled laboratory conditions and free-living conditions. When the fat content of the diet was altered but the energy density was kept the same, the subjects still consumed the same weight of food, indicating that the energy density of the meals is a major determinant of energy intake.

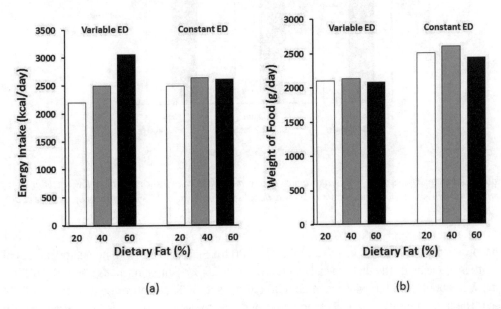

Figure 8.1 Ad libitum energy intake (a) and weight of food consumed (b) in subjects who consume diets that have 20, 40, and 60% of their energy as fat. In one of these projects the energy density (ED) between diets was different (variable ED). In the other study, the energy density was the same despite differences in composition (constant ED). Data from Stubbs et al. (1995) and Stubbs et al. (1996).

Several large scale longitudinal and cross-sectional studies involving thousands of participants have clearly shown that an increase in energy density results in an increase in energy intake, whereas a decrease in the energy density of the diet results in a decrease in intake as illustrated in figure 8.2. These studies demonstrate the important role of the energy density of the diet and suggest that manipulation of energy density is a good tool in weight management. What these studies also indicate is that normal-weight people consume diets with a lower energy density than obese people and that people who have a high fruit and vegetable intake have the lowest dietary energy density values and the lowest prevalence of obesity. This is not surprising as fruits and vegetables generally have high water and fiber content which provides bulk but less energy than most other food sources. Only subtle changes to the diet are needed to alter its energy density. For example, the energy density of many popular foods such as pies, pizzas, sandwiches, and stews can be decreased by reducing the fat content and adding vegetables and/or fruits – and without noticeably affecting **palatability** or portion size. In fact, the portion size will generally be larger for a low energy density meal, and the changes to food selection can lead to healthier eating patterns consistent with the 2015-2020 Dietary Guidelines for Americans as explained in chapters 3 and 7.

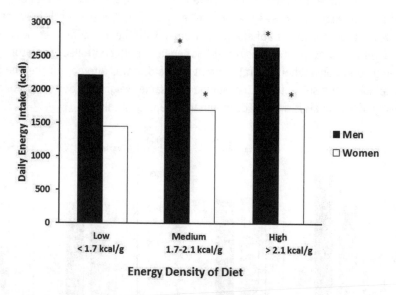

Figure 8.2 Energy intakes of men (closed columns) and women (open columns) consuming a low, medium, or high energy-dense diet. Data comes from a cross-sectional study involving 7,356 participants by Ledikwe et al. (2006).

The low energy density diet provides a total of 1,300 to1,500 kcal/day with an energy density of less than 1.5 kcal/g. The diet typically contains about 25-30% protein (that's about 90-105 g/day) with about 20% fat (which is around 30 g/day) and 50% carbohydrate (less than 180 g/day). The main principle of a low energy density diet is to avoid fatty foods (or use reduced fat versions of foods like cheese and milk), use only lean meat (trim off any visible fat and remove skin from poultry) and fish, and include lots of fruit and non-starchy vegetables such as asparagus, broccoli, cauliflower, green beans, spinach, or salad leaves with tomatoes, onion, celery, etc.

Gourds which are fleshy, typically large fruits, with a hard skin (the edible plant structure of a mature ovary of a flowering plant; a selection are illustrated in photo 8.1.), including aubergine (eggplant), squash, marrow, melon, and zucchini (courgette), are a particularly good choice as all have an energy density less than 0.5 kcal/g. Many people might consider them to be vegetables, but the term "vegetable" is not a scientific name – any part of a plant consumed by humans as food as part of a meal is called a vegetable. In fact, many fruits and most vegetables have an energy density less than 1.0 kcal/g (e.g., tomatoes, salad leaves and spinach are 0.2 kcal/g; apples, oranges, and carrots are 0.4 kcal/g; and beans are about 0.9 kcal/g). The energy density of some common foods is illustrated in figure 8.3. Using the principles of energy density, it is possible to achieve a lower calorie intake which will help towards weight loss, while allowing generous, voluminous portions of food that provide an overall balanced healthy diet that is high in protein, fiber, micronutrients, and phytonutrients. Foods that have a low energy density also usually have a low glycemic index which is another bonus for diabetics. Another significant advantage of consuming a low energy density diet is that because the majority of the ingredients contain relatively few calories per gram, you can eat that much more of those food items. This helps to avoid the hunger pangs that are many a diet's downfall. For these reasons a low energy density diet with high protein is my number one choice for safe and effective weight loss for people with type 2 diabetes.

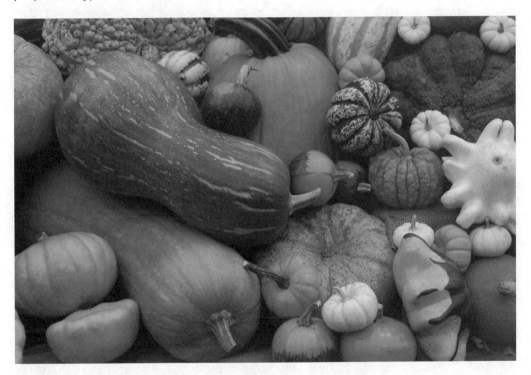

Photo 8.1: A selection of gourds, all of which have a low energy density

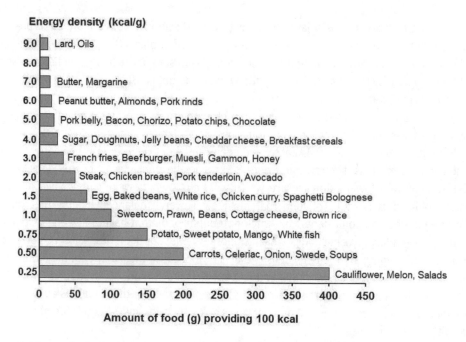

Figure 8.3 Energy density (kcal/g) of some common foods and the amount of food (in grams) that provides 100 kcal.

COMPARISONS OF THE DIFFERENT DIETS FOR WEIGHT LOSS IN PEOPLE WITH TYPE 2 DIABETES

Many scientists still support the view that weight changes are not primarily determined by varying proportions of carbohydrate and fat in the diet, but instead by the number of calories ingested. I certainly agree that overall daily calorie intake in comparison with daily energy expenditure is the most important factor when it comes to weight and fat loss. Diet-induced changes in energy expenditure, which metabolic pathways are used, and other considerations are quite modest when compared with the importance of actual calorie intake. Table 8.1 provides a summary of expected body fat tissue losses on different diets.

When it comes to choosing which is the best diet for yourself you need to take into account not only the efficacy of the diet for body weight and fat loss but also how likely you are going to be able to stick to the diet for 10 weeks or more, how healthy (or unhealthy) the diet is, and how safe it is. Table 8.2 shows my own personal ratings and overall rankings for the eight diets that were listed in the previous table. Of course you will have increased sensation of hunger on just about any diet but how much hungrier you feel is influenced by the degree of energy restriction and the diet's macronutrient composition. You will not be as hungry if the diet is high in protein (because protein intake promotes satiety) or has a low energy density (because these diets contain a relatively high weight and volume of food due to their high water and fiber content). Some ways by which you can abate your hunger when dieting are listed in the sidebar.

Table 8.1 A summary of the efficacy of different diets for body fat tissue loss in overweight adults with prediabetes or type 2 diabetes

Diet	What it involves	Weekly energy deficit	Weekly body fat tissue loss
Very low energy	800 kcal/day liquid meals high in protein	8,400 kcal	1.0 kg (2.2 lbs)
Alternate day fast	Fast completely every other day	7,000 kcal	0.8 kg (1.8 lbs)
4:3	Only 500 kcal on 3 days a week	4,500 kcal	0.5 kg (1.1 lbs)
5:2	Only 500 kcal on 2 days a week	3,000 kcal	0.35 kg (0.8 lbs)
Skip lunch	No 500-kcal lunch, 5 days a week	2,500 kcal	0.3 kg (0.6 lbs)
Reduced fat	1,500 kcal/day with 10-15% fat	3,500 kcal	0.4 kg (0.9 lbs)
High protein	1,500 kcal/day with 30% protein	4,200 kcal	0.5 kg (1.1 lbs)
Low energy density	1,400 kcal/day with 25-30% protein	4,900 kcal	0.6 kg (1.3 lbs)

Assumes (1) normal energy intake is 2,000 kcal/day with 15% coming from protein, (2) some diets will reduce appetite compared with normal due to higher protein or lower energy density, (3) body fat tissue losses are average weekly loss over a 10-week period on each diet, and (4) approximately 0.46 kg of body fat tissue is lost for each 3,500 kcal energy intake deficit in the first five weeks, and 0.34 kg is lost for each 3,500 kcal energy intake deficit thereafter (accounting for metabolic adaptation to energy restriction). Note that body weight losses with be higher than the losses of body fat tissue shown here as some diets will also cause some additional loss of body water, glycogen, and lean tissue (see main text for details).

Table 8.2 My own personal star ratings and overall rankings of the different diets after considering how effective they are for body fat loss together with taking into account how easy they are to stick to, their health effects, and their safety

Diet	Efficacy for body fat loss	How easy to stick to	Health and safety	Overall rating (and rank)
Very low energy	☆☆☆☆☆	☆	☆	☆☆ (8)
Alternate day fast	☆☆☆☆	☆☆	☆☆	☆☆ (7)
4:3	☆☆☆	☆☆☆	☆☆☆	☆☆☆ (4=)
5:2	☆☆	☆☆☆☆	☆☆☆☆	☆☆☆☆ (3)
Skip lunch	☆	☆☆☆☆	☆☆☆☆	☆☆☆ (4=)
Reduced fat	☆☆	☆☆☆	☆☆☆☆	☆☆ (6)
High protein	☆☆☆	☆☆☆☆	☆☆☆☆	☆☆☆☆☆ (2)
Low energy density	☆☆☆	☆☆☆☆	☆☆☆☆☆	☆☆☆☆☆ (1)

☆ = lowest rating; ☆☆☆☆☆ = highest rating

How to abate your hunger when dieting

There are several things you can do to make you feel fuller and more satisfied when eating a meal without eating more calories. These are useful things to know when you are dieting. The strategies listed below will help to abate your hunger when dieting to lose weight, making it more likely you will stick to your diet for longer.

- *Drinking water before eating:* Drinking a glass or two of water or a low-calorie beverage before eating a meal is a good idea as it makes the stomach feel fuller quicker.

- *Foods and beverages that increase the volume in the stomach but with low energy density:* Eating foods with a high water and/or fiber content but low-fat and sugar content (e.g., beansprouts, tomato, melon, salad leaves, celery, zucchini/courgette, green beans, broccoli, asparagus, pickled vegetables) also add to the bulk volume of a meal which is one of the things that signals satiety.

- *Eating meals with high-protein content:* Because protein has a much stronger effect on satiety than fat and carbohydrate do, meals with high-protein content (e.g., from meat, fish, and beans) are satisfying even when relatively low in calories.

- *Eating the high-protein and lower energy food items on your plate first:* Because you may start to feel full before you start consuming the higher energy food items containing carbohydrate and/or fat.

- *Eating your food slowly:* Because this will allow more time for nutrients to be digested and absorbed and the satiety signals to kick in, meaning that you may eat smaller portions or no longer want a dessert after your main meal.

- *Sprinkling dried mixed herbs and a pinch of ground pepper and salt or a splash of vinegar or lemon juice over your food:* Because this adds to the flavor and satisfies your desire for tasty foods without adding hardly any calories and much salt at all.

EXERCISE FOR WEIGHT LOSS

As an alternative to dieting, exercise is another way to create a negative energy balance. In obese people (BMI of 30 kg/m² or more), the effectiveness of exercise programs to achieve weight loss has been questioned because of problems related to a lack of motivation to do physical activity, non-compliance with exercise programs lasting more than a few weeks, and impaired ability (e.g., poor fitness, flexibility, or stamina) to perform some forms of exercise, particularly weight-bearing activities like jogging and step aerobics. In moderately overweight people (BMI of 25-29 kg/m²) with a real desire to lose weight, these factors are less likely to be a problem. Most people can include exercise sessions with the specific aim of increasing energy expenditure, and they can exercise at an intensity high enough or for a duration long enough to cause a significant increase in the amount of energy expended. Working people may have difficulty finding time to exercise, so for them higher intensity with relatively short duration would be the exercise of choice, at least on working days. For those lucky enough to have time on their hands such as retired folk like myself, long walks (e.g., 5 miles or 8 km taking about two hours) are a great way to exercise while enjoying the local scenery and still being able to engage in conversation.

Using exercise to induce weight loss generally results in loss of body fat while lean tissue is preserved. If some short (10-15 minute) resistance exercise sessions are included in the weight loss program and dietary protein intake is adequate muscle mass may even be increased which also tends to increase the resting metabolic rate. Moderate to high-intensity aerobic exercise can also increase the resting metabolic rate for several hours after exercise although this is not a significant factor in weight loss, despite some claims to the contrary by so-called fitness experts. In this chapter the efficacy of different forms of exercise for weight loss will be explained. Let's begin by examining which types of exercise are best for fat loss.

AEROBIC EXERCISE

Aerobic exercise (also known as cardio) is physical exercise of low to high-intensity that depends primarily on the aerobic (oxygen requiring) energy-generating process. During aerobic exercise oxygen is used to oxidize stored fat or carbohydrate to provide energy in the form of **adenosine triphosphate (ATP)** for muscle contraction. Generally, light- to moderate-intensity activities that are sufficiently supported by **aerobic metabolism** can be performed for extended periods of time and will predominantly use fat as the main fuel. High exercise intensities that approach the **aerobic capacity** (or maximal oxygen uptake) of the individual also activate **anaerobic** (non-oxygen requiring) ATP production and cause **lactic acid** accumulation which contributes to fatigue. High-intensity exercise (that is exercise at more than 70% of aerobic capacity) will predominantly use carbohydrate as the main fuel. Exercise at an intensity of 80-100% of a person's aerobic capacity can only be sustained for a matter of minutes, especially if you are unfit. So what intensity of exercise is best for fat burning and weight loss?

Some scientists argue that the optimal exercise intensity for weight and fat loss is related to fat oxidation and should be the intensity with the highest fat oxidation rate. Fat oxidation increases as exercise increases from low to moderate intensity, even though the percentage contribution of fat may decrease (see figure 8.4). Increased fat oxidation is a direct result of increased energy expenditure when going from light-intensity to moderate-intensity exercise. Compared with rest, light-intensity activities may increase the metabolic rate (i.e., energy expenditure) three- to fivefold (table 8.3). At moderate exercise intensities the metabolic rate may be six to nine times the value at rest. High-intensity activities generally increase the metabolic rate more than 10 times the resting value (and up to about 20 times in elite endurance athletes). However, at high exercise intensities, fat oxidation is inhibited, and both the relative rate and the absolute rate of fat oxidation decrease to negligible values. Also, at such high intensities of exercise (sometimes called **anaerobic exercise**) the activity cannot be sustained as fatigue develops within a few minutes. In other words, high-intensity exercise is really no good for fat burning.

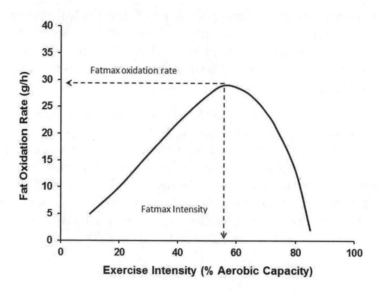

Figure 8.4 Fat oxidation rate as a function of exercise intensity. In this example the maximum rate of fat oxidation is about 29 g/hour and occurs at a relative exercise intensity of about 55% of aerobic capacity (maximum oxygen uptake).

Table 8.3 The rate of energy expenditure during various activities

Activity	Rate of energy expenditure (kcal/min)	Examples
Resting	1	Sleeping, reclining, sitting in relaxed pose
Very light activities	2-3	Standing activities including most household chores, and some active sitting activities such as driving, card playing, typing
Light activities	4-6	Walking (3 to 5 km/h), baseball, bowling, horseback riding, golf, gardening
Moderate activities	7-9	Cycling at 10-15 km/h, hiking, jogging, badminton, basketball, soccer, swimming, tennis, volleyball
Strenuous activities	10-13	Cycling at 20 km/h, running at 10-13 km/h, cross-country skiing (8 to 10 km/h)
Very strenuous activities	>13	Cycling at 35 km/h, running at >14 km/h, cross-country skiing at >12 km/h

The maximal rate of fat oxidation (typically around 0.4-1.0 g/min or 25-60 g/hour depending on an individual's aerobic capacity) generally occurs between 50% and 65% of aerobic capacity (maximum oxygen uptake) and has been referred to as the "**Fatmax**" intensity. In relatively unfit people, Fatmax tends to occur at lower relative intensity (50-55% of aerobic capacity or maximal oxygen uptake) than in athletic individuals (60-65% of aerobic capacity) because fitter people are better adapted to burning fat as a fuel for exercise. If you are unfit or perform exercise only occasionally it is likely that your maximum rate of fat oxidation is around 0.5 g/min or 30 g/hour and will occur at about 55% of your aerobic capacity. At this moderate intensity of exercise in a middle-aged relatively sedentary or recreationally active person, the heart rate will be about 140-150 beats/min, and wearing a heart rate monitor will therefore enable you to know that you are exercising at the desired intensity. Whether regular exercise at the Fatmax intensity is more effective than exercise at other intensities for body weight and fat loss remains to be determined. However, one of the advantages of moderate-intensity exercise is that it can be sustained for a long time (hours) and will feel easier when it is performed regularly.

The rate of fat oxidation during moderate-intensity aerobic exercise increases as exercise duration increases (see figure 8.5) as it takes some time for fatty acids to accumulate in the blood (from the breakdown of fat stores in adipose tissue) so that the working muscles have a ready supply of fat fuel to burn. Thus, the longer you exercise, the more fat you burn.

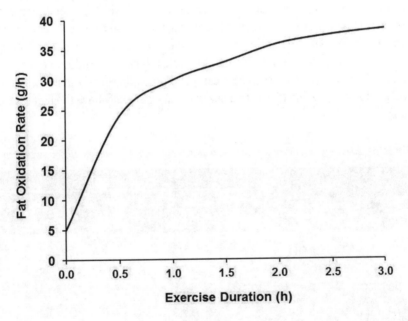

Figure 8.5 Fat oxidation rate as a function of exercise duration. In this example the exercise intensity is fixed at 55% of aerobic capacity (maximum oxygen uptake). You can see that after 30 minutes of exercise the fat oxidation rate is 24 g/hour but after 2 hours of exercise it has increased to 36 g/hour.

There can be no doubt that aerobic exercise is best for burning fat and losing weight but there are several different modes of aerobic exercise that can be performed including walking, running, aerobics, cycling, and swimming as well as sports such as tennis, soccer, and rugby which involve a variety of movements but are predominantly aerobic activities. Some physical activities obviously expend more energy than others, as shown in table 8.4. The amount of energy expended per minute is related to the intensity of the exercise, but the total amount of energy expended is more closely related to the duration of the activity or the total distance covered. For weight-bearing activities the energy expended is higher the greater the body weight of the person. But even within the same activity there can be considerable differences in the energy expenditure dependent on the level at which it is performed. Tennis, for example, has relatively low energy expenditure if played recreationally, and because each player has to move less when playing doubles the energy cost is lower than for singles. At this level of play, it could be classified as a light to moderate activity, although at occasional times during a game the activity can sometimes be extremely intense, requiring high rates of energy expenditure, but only in short bursts lasting no more than a few seconds. However, the majority of the time in recreational tennis, and even in moderate level club play, involves longer periods of low-intensity activity like moving side to side, walking, or just standing, and even some sitting (at change of ends). This is the reason why the average energy expenditure for tennis is relatively low. The advantage, of course, is that this game can be enjoyed by many people right into old age. In contrast, tennis played at a high level has shorter periods of rest, and the average exercise intensity is much higher. The players are fitter and more skillful meaning that rallies can be prolonged and a lot more energy is expended. A five-set match in men's grand slam events can often last over four hours and total energy expenditure may exceed 2,500 kcal. Games like soccer, rugby, and American football also involve intermittent activity but match duration is fixed by the rules of the sport, so the average amount of energy expended (e.g., typically 1,600 kcal for professional soccer) does not vary much from game to game. Continuous sports such as cycling and running, which usually include little or no recovery during the activity and can last for several hours, generally have the highest total energy expenditures.

Table 8.4 The estimated energy cost of various sporting activities in kcal/min according to body weight in kg (or lbs)

Activity	Body weight				
	50 kg (110 lbs)	60 kg (132 lbs)	70 kg (154 lbs)	80 kg (176 lbs)	90 kg (198 lbs)
Aerobics	7.0	8.3	10.0	11.3	12.8
Badminton	5.0	5.7	6.7	8.3	9.3
Ballroom dancing	2.8	3.3	3.8	4.3	4.8
Basketball	7.2	8.8	10.0	11.5	13.0
Canoeing Easy	2.3	2.8	3.3	3.8	4.3
Hard	5.5	6.5	7.5	8.5	9.8
Circuit training	5.5	6.5	7.5	8.5	10.0
Baseball/Cricket (batting)	4.3	5.3	6.0	7.0	8.0
Cycling 10 km/h	3.3	4.0	4.5	5.3	6.0
15 km/h	5.3	5.7	6.7	8.3	9.5
25 km/h	8.8	10.5	12.3	14.0	15.8
Football/Soccer	7.0	8.3	9.8	11.0	12.5
Golf	4.5	5.5	6.3	7.0	8.0

Activity		Body weight				
		50 kg (110 lbs)	60 kg (132 lbs)	70 kg (154 lbs)	80 kg (176 lbs)	90 kg (198 lbs)
Gymnastics		3.5	4.0	4.8	5.5	6.3
Hockey		4.5	5.0	6.0	7.3	8.3
Judo		10.3	12.3	14.3	16.3	18.3
Running	11 km/h	10.0	12.3	14.3	16.3	18.3
	12 km/h	11.0	13.0	15.3	17.5	19.5
	13.5 km/h	12.0	13.8	16.3	18.8	21.3
	15 km/h	13.5	16.3	19.0	21.8	24.5
Skiing	Cross-country	8.8	10.5	12.3	14.0	15.8
	Downhill (easy)	4.5	5.5	6.3	7.3	8.3
	Downhill (hard)	7.3	8.8	10.0	12.3	13.8
Squash		11.0	13.3	15.5	17.8	19.8
Swimming						
	Freestyle	8.3	10.0	11.5	13.0	14.8
	Backstroke	9.0	10.8	12.3	14.0	15.8
	Breaststroke	8.5	10.3	11.8	13.5	15.3
Table tennis		3.5	4.3	4.8	5.8	6.5
Tennis	Social	3.8	4.3	5.0	5.8	6.5
	Competitive	9.3	11.0	12.5	14.5	16.3
Volleyball		2.5	3.0	3.6	4.3	4.8
Walking	4 km/h	3.9	4.7	6.0	6.9	7.5
	5 km/h	4.6	5.6	6.7	7.8	8.6
	6 km/h	5.3	6.5	7.5	8.8	9.8

The mode of exercise also affects maximal rates of fat oxidation. For example, it is known that fat oxidation is significantly higher during uphill walking and running compared with cycling at the same relative exercise intensity or heart rate. Although no long-term studies have been conducted to compare different types of exercise and their effectiveness in achieving or maintaining weight loss, there have been numerous studies that have examined the volume of exercise or weekly amounts of energy expended in relation to weight loss. More on this a little later in the chapter but before that let's consider the case for two other popular forms of exercise, namely resistance exercise and **high-intensity interval exercise**.

RESISTANCE EXERCISE

Comparisons of resistance training with endurance training have demonstrated some favorable effects on body composition but resistance training is not so effective in facilitating body-fat loss. However, resistance training certainly seems more effective in preserving or increasing lean muscle mass. In turn, the amount of metabolically active tissue also increases, and the increase is suggested as one of the mechanisms by which exercise helps to maintain lower body weight after weight loss that has been achieved mostly through dietary energy restriction. The exercise preserves (or even increases) muscle mass, resulting in a smaller reduction (or even an increase) in the resting metabolic rate. The disadvantage of resistance exercise, however, is that it cannot be sustained for long periods and is intermittent rather than continuous as the muscles are worked hard and need time for recovery between sets of contraction repetitions. Thus, actual fat loss with resistance exercise is likely to be considerably less than with continuous, moderate-intensity aerobic activities such as brisk walking, jogging, cycling, and swimming.

Few studies have compared the effectiveness of various types of exercise. Current evidence, however, indicates that resistance training is at least as effective as aerobic exercise in reducing body fat for the same (but relatively short) duration of actual exercise. The duration of the exercise is, of course, an important factor which largely determines the total amount of energy expended. People who can spend more time exercising at relatively high exercise intensity have a greater opportunity to achieve a negative energy balance and thus lose body fat and body weight. However, this is limited by fatigue, and in reality it is easier to expend more energy in more moderate aerobic activities (e.g., walking, running, cycling, or swimming) that can be sustained for an hour or more.

Combining resistance training with aerobic training has been shown to be superior for body weight and fat loss and to result in greater lean body mass when compared with aerobic exercise alone in several randomized controlled trials. Furthermore, most studies combining resistance training with dietary energy restriction report better maintenance or even increased lean body mass compared to dieting alone. The take home message is that resistance exercise helps to preserve muscle mass during periods of dieting but does not, in itself, assist much with fat loss.

By the way, don't worry that increasing your muscle mass with resistance exercise will cause you to lose less weight overall. The crucial thing for your health is to lose your excess body fat and this will be lost at least as effectively if not more by adding some resistance exercise to your weekly activities. In later years you will benefit from having a little extra muscle as we all lose some as part of the aging process anyway.

HIGH-INTENSITY INTERVAL EXERCISE

Most exercise protocols designed to induce fat loss have focused on regular participation in relatively prolonged aerobic exercise such as walking and jogging at a low to moderate intensity. For most people, in the absence of dietary energy restriction, these kinds of protocols have led to rather slow and small losses of body fat and/or weight. This should not be surprising, as even exercising at the intensity that elicits maximal fat oxidation (i.e., about 55% of aerobic capacity for a people with below average fitness) only results in a rate of fat oxidation of about 0.5 g/min, or 30 g/hour (i.e., one ounce per hour). Some scientists and fitness gurus have claimed that high-intensity interval exercise (HIIE) has the potential to be an economical and effective exercise protocol for reducing body fat in overweight individuals. But can it really be as effective as some are claiming? Let's stop to consider what HIIE actually involves.

HIIE protocols typically involve repeated bouts of brief anaerobic exercise such as sprinting at an all-out intensity (or at least at exercise intensities that exceed 90% of aerobic capacity) immediately followed by low-intensity exercise or rest. The length of both the sprint and recovery periods has varied from six seconds to four minutes. A commonly used protocol has been the Wingate test, which consists of 30 seconds of all-out sprint cycling on a cycle ergometer with a hard resistance that is performed four to six times with each bout separated by two to four minutes of recovery. This protocol amounts to three to four minutes of actual exercise per session with each session being typically performed three to seven times a week. This form of training is commonly called **high-intensity interval training** (HIIT). Other less demanding HIIE protocols have also been utilized with either shorter sprints or somewhat lower exercise intensities (but still close to 100% of aerobic capacity) but with shorter recovery periods. Thus, one of the characteristics of HIIT is that it involves markedly lower training volume making it a time-efficient strategy to accrue training adaptations, fitness improvements, and possible health benefits compared with traditional aerobic exercise programs. These benefits have been shown to include increased aerobic and anaerobic fitness, lowering of insulin resistance, and increased muscle capacity for fat oxidation. While this is good from the fitness and health perspective, there is limited evidence that HIIT results in significant body fat and weight loss even when performed for weeks or months.

Studies that have carried out relatively short HIIT interventions (e.g., three to six weeks) in young adults with normal body mass and BMI have reported negligible weight loss. Research examining the effects of longer term HIIT on body weight and fat loss in slightly overweight people has produced evidence to suggest that it can result in only rather modest reductions in body fat. Unfortunately, this type of exercise is usually distressing for those who are not used to it (photo 8.2). Heart rate and blood pressure are elevated and the hyperventilation it causes makes people who are unaccustomed to this form of exercise feel faint and sick which does not provide much motivation to stick with it. People who have existing hypertension (which is often the case for people with type 2 diabetes) and women who are pregnant should avoid any form of HIIE.

The mechanisms underlying the small degree of body fat reduction induced by HIIT appear to include elevated fat oxidation in the post-exercise period and suppressed appetite. However, the actual energy cost of HIIE is rather low; despite the intensity of the exercise being high, the duration is so short that the actual amount of energy expended in each HIIE session usually does not exceed 100 kcal. Even taking into account a prolonged post-exercise elevation of resting metabolic rate (which could be as much as a 10% increase over the first 12 hours after the HIIE session) this only adds on another 100 kcal at most, making the overall daily energy cost of a HIIE session to be no more than 200 kcal. If performed five times per week this amounts to a 1,000-kcal energy deficit. To put this into perspective, this amount of energy loss could be achieved with a single 10-mile (16-km) walk or run. Therefore, as previously mentioned, the moderately overweight person who seriously wants to lose body weight relatively quickly (i.e., in a matter of weeks or months) would be best advised to do aerobic exercise at moderate intensity for longer durations together with at least some degree of dietary energy restriction.

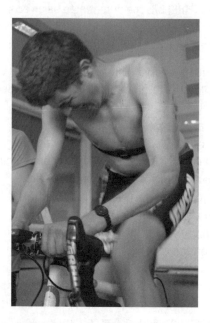

Photo 8.2: Performing a HIIE session can be distressing, even for individuals who are used to exercising

So what sort of exercise is best for losing body fat?

Taken as a whole, the evidence suggests that for maximum fat burning during exercise itself, you should exercise aerobically at an intensity close to that which elicits your maximal fat oxidation rate. Depending on your fitness, this will be around 55-65% of your aerobic capacity (or 60-80% of your maximum heart rate which can be estimated as 220 minus your age in years). As for the duration and frequency of exercise sessions, the most important factor is your total energy expenditure over any given period of time. So for example, six dynamic exercise (e.g., cycling or running) training sessions per week of one hour duration at 75% of your maximal heart rate would be equivalent to three sessions of two hours duration at the same relative exercise intensity. The goal is to increase your total volume of exercise (within reasonable limits) so that you will burn more fat. Fewer but longer sessions may be more advantageous as fat oxidation becomes an increasingly important fuel as the duration of exercise increases. An additional benefit of structuring sessions this way is that it allows longer periods of recovery in between each bout of exercise and/or some of that recovery time could be used to do HIIE sessions which should increase your aerobic capacity, further increasing your muscles' ability to burn fat. If you are undecided about whether to run or cycle it is worth knowing that rates of fat oxidation have been shown to be slightly higher for a given rate of oxygen uptake during running compared with cycling.

Furthermore, any fat loss program should ideally include some resistance training because this increases muscle mass and lean body mass, which is desirable as lean tissue is metabolically far more active than adipose tissue. Increasing your muscle mass by including some resistance training means that your resting metabolic rate can be increased to a small degree, helping you to achieve your negative energy balance more easily. Two or three short sessions (10-15 minutes) of resistance training per week comprising of several different exercises designed to work all the major muscle groups (one to two sets of 10-15 repetitions per exercise with enough weight set so that the repetitions can only just be completed is best) should produce good results in those who are not experienced resistance trainers.

HOW MUCH EXERCISE IS NEEDED TO ACHIEVE SIGNIFICANT BODY WEIGHT AND FAT LOSS?

A negative energy balance generated by regular exercise will result in weight loss and the larger the negative energy balance, the greater the weight loss. Extreme amounts of physical activity performed by military personnel, endurance athletes, and mountaineers offer the potential for substantial weight loss; however, it is difficult for most individuals to achieve and sustain these high levels of physical activity.

A limited number of studies that have examined moderate levels of physical activity as the only intervention in sedentary overweight or obese individuals have reported about 2-3 kg decreases in body weight after 12 weeks. Therefore, most individuals who require substantial weight loss may need additional interventions (i.e., dietary energy restriction) to meet their weight loss needs. Better controlled studies that supervised and verified the volumes of exercise performed have generally found larger losses of body mass in overweight individuals, but as expected, the magnitude of the weight loss depended on the weekly volume (duration) of physical activity. Several studies that targeted 90-150 min/week of physical activity for 12 weeks found only small changes in body weight (0.5-1.5 kg) but increasing this to 150-225 min/week increased weight loss to 2-3 kg and further increasing the exercise dose to 225-350 min/week (incurring a 500-700 kcal/day energy deficit) has generally resulted in body weight losses of 5.0-7.5 kg. Thus, as expected, a dose response effect is apparent for the impact of physical activity on weight loss. The bad news for the ladies is that exercise seems to be a little less effective for weight and fat loss than it is for men. The reasons for this are explained in the following sidebar.

Gender differences in weight loss with exercise

Numerous studies of weight loss after aerobic exercise training have shown that weight loss, although modest, was generally greater for males. These findings confirm earlier research in males concerning exercise-training effects on body mass and body composition and extend them both to females and to a broader range of exercise types including running, cycling, circuit training, and aerobics. These gender differences appear to be related to differences in body-fat distribution. Women store more fat in the buttocks and thighs, whereas men store more fat in the visceral (abdominal) area. Fat located in the upper body and abdominal regions (central fat) is more metabolically active and therefore has higher rates of fat breakdown in response to sympathetic nervous stimulation which occurs during exercise. This means that during exercise, fat is preferentially mobilized from these regions. In addition, fat storage after eating may be higher in subcutaneous adipose tissue in women than in men. All these differences may play a role in the variation in net regional fat storage between men and women and women's greater resistance to weight loss with exercise.

As the energy expenditure of various activities has been measured in laboratory studies, it is possible to estimate the amount of body fat tissue loss when regularly performing such activities for one hour per day, five days per week as illustrated in table 8.5.

Table 8.5 Weekly amounts of energy deficit and expected body fat tissue loss for a 70 kg person with different exercise protocols when exercising for one hour per day, five days per week

Activity	Daily energy deficit kcal	Weekly energy deficit kcal	Weekly body fat tissue loss kg (lbs)
Aerobics	522	2,610	0.35 (0.8)
Badminton	480	2,400	0.32 (0.7)
Circuit training	450	2,250	0.30 (0.65)
Cycling 15 km/h	400	2,000	0.26 (0.6)
Running 11 km/h	860	4,300	0.57 (1.25)
Walking 4 km/h	275	1,375	0.18 (0.4)
Swimming	720	3,600	0.47 (1.0)

Table 8.6 shows the amount of exercise needed to incur a 500-kcal daily energy deficit and the amount of exercise needed to lose 0.46 kg (1 lb) of body fat tissue (equivalent to 3,500 kcal) per week when exercising five days per week.

Table 8.6 Daily duration of exercise needed to (A) expend 500 kcal and (B) lose 0.46 kg (1 lb) of body fat tissue (equivalent to 3,500 kcal) per week when exercising five days per week for a 70 kg person

Activity	(A) minutes	(B) minutes
Aerobics	56	79
Badminton	61	86
Circuit training	66	92
Cycling 15 km/h	76	106
Running 11 km/h	34	48
Walking 4 km/h	109	153
Swimming	42	59

Remember that doing exercise, especially with family or friends, can be fun. Some examples of enjoyable physical activities are shown in photos 8.3 to 8.6. You can tell from these pictures that the participants are not overexerting themselves as they all look happy!

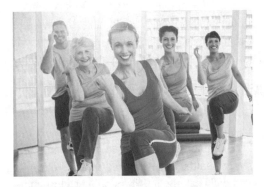

Photo 8.3: A simple aerobics class which is good for cardiorespiratory fitness, flexibility, and fun

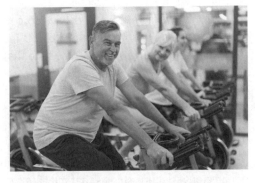

Photo 8.4: A stationary cycling (spinning) class which is a non-weight-bearing aerobic exercise which is great for overweight people

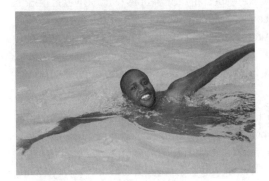

Photo 8.5: Swimming is another form of non-weight-bearing aerobic exercise which is great for overweight people and will improve cardiorespiratory fitness and flexibility

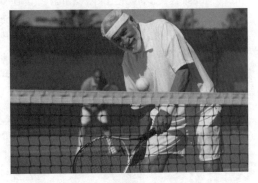

Photo 8.6: Games like doubles tennis involve intermittent physical activity but can burn significant amounts of fat when played for a couple of hours

WHY COMBINING DIETING AND EXERCISE IS BEST FOR BOTH WEIGHT LOSS AND HEALTH

It is often said that dieting is more effective for weight loss than doing more exercise. Indeed, the scientific evidence suggests that this is the case in most circumstances, even after taking into account the adaptive reduction in metabolic rate that occurs after a few weeks of reduced energy intake. Of course, many authors of diet books hammer this point home and often one can be left wondering is it worth doing any more exercise at all? There are several reasons why dieting is more effective than exercise for losing weight and the main ones are probably as follows:

- People who are not used to doing exercise are concerned that they will find the experience painful and unpleasant; some do and so they don't keep up the exercise regimen for long.

- They don't want to have to strip off or go to a gym where they may be surrounded by other people who are much slimmer than them as it is likely to make them feel embarrassed about their body.

- Doing exercise requires a significant time investment. For example, to incur a 500-kcal energy deficit by walking you would have to cover about 5 miles which would take the average person around two hours. In reality it is much easier to lose weight by cutting back on what we eat, and it can also save some time that is normally spent in preparing and eating food.

- It is simply much easier to skip a meal like lunch to achieve a 500-kcal energy deficit that it is to burn it off through exercise.

What the diet books generally don't tell you is that combining both dieting and exercising more is actually the best strategy for weight loss and for your health. This is backed up by the results of numerous scientific studies that indicate for a given daily calorie deficit, people will lose more body weight by a combination of dieting and exercise than with dieting alone. Not only is more weight lost but virtually all of it is achieved by a reduction in body fat. With dieting alone, some muscle mass is usually also lost which is undesirable, especially for people over 50 years of age when age-related loss of muscle (sarcopenia) becomes a significant concern. If the energy deficit achieved via reduced energy intake through dieting is supplemented by the energy burned with exercise, then the dieting can be less severe which reduces the impact on metabolic rate and makes it less likely that protein or micronutrient intakes will be insufficient to support optimal health.

Significant weight loss (i.e., more than a few kilograms) can only be achieved by substantial reductions in dietary energy intake and be improved further with increased energy expenditure with exercise. Generally, a combination of dieting and exercise is the most effective way to lower body weight and to maintain it at a lower level after weight reduction; it is nearly always more successful for weight loss than dieting or exercise alone. There are several potential reasons for this and there are also some other very good reasons for doing more exercise as follows:

- If you are looking to generate a 1,000 kcal/day energy deficit it is easier to do this by a combination of dieting (e.g., lower your energy intake by 500 kcal/day) and exercise (burn 500 kcal/day) than it would be to achieve this by dieting alone.

- Compared with moderate energy deficits resulting from exercise alone, acute dietary energy restriction results in rapid changes in appetite and food cravings during the day that often result in compensatory eating, which may initially limit potential success in weight loss efforts. In contrast, a similar energy deficit created by exercise does not induce any significant change in appetite, thereby allowing the attainment of a short-term negative energy balance.

- Exercise training helps to preserve muscle mass which can be lost to some degree with an energy deficit that is brought about by dietary energy restriction alone. Furthermore, including some resistance exercise can result in an increase in muscle mass even when energy balance is negative (provided that dietary protein intake is adequate) which increases the amount of metabolically active tissue, producing a small increase in the resting metabolic rate.

- Exercise training, especially aerobic exercise, results in a shift from carbohydrate to fat metabolism and the oxidative capacity of the muscle is improved due to the production of more mitochondria and blood capillaries. These effects allow an increase in the supply of blood-borne fuels and oxygen to the muscle as well as an increase in the capacity to take up oxygen and oxidize fat. Studies have consistently observed a decreased reliance on carbohydrate as a fuel and an increased capacity to oxidize fat in response to as little as four weeks of exercise training. This increased ability to oxidize fat may help to reduce fat mass even more in a situation of energy restriction.

- Regular exercise will preferentially reduce visceral (belly) fat, particularly in men, which is good because an excess of visceral fat is the worst kind to have when it comes to your health.

- Exercise has lots of additional health benefits including helping to maintain muscle and bone mass, improving fitness, flexibility, cardiovascular function, and immune function, as well as increasing insulin sensitivity, a particular bonus for diabetics. Furthermore, exercise reduces the risk of health complications in overweight and type 2 diabetic people such as coronary heart disease, stroke, kidney disease, dementia, and some cancers.

The take home message is that combining some additional but regular exercise with dietary energy restriction is likely to be the most effective strategy for body fat and weight loss. In the next chapter I will explain how you can put together a combined diet and exercise program that can be personalized to your own preferences and will be guaranteed to provide effective weight loss.

Key Points

- A person who has been diagnosed with type 2 diabetes will have to lose a significant amount of weight (at least several kilograms and probably for most people maybe as much as 10-20 kg) to get their diabetes into remission.

- Calories from different macronutrients or food items can have markedly different effects on hunger, hormones, resting energy expenditure, and the brain regions that control food intake. However, the most effective means of losing weight by dieting is to reduce total energy intake by at least 300 kcal/day.

- Substantial weight loss (i.e., more than a few kilograms) can only be achieved by more substantial reductions in energy intake (i.e., eating at least 500 kcal/day less than normal) and improved further with increased energy expenditure through doing more exercise.

- The resting metabolic rate decreases in response to weight loss. This effect, referred to as food efficiency, makes losing weight more difficult.

- Diets that have proven to be effective in achieving moderate weight loss and are suitable for people with type 2 diabetes include very low energy diets, intermittent fasting diets, reduced fat diets, high-protein diets, and low energy density diets.

- A low energy density diet provides about 1,400 kcal/day with an energy density of less than 1.5 kcal/g. The main principle of a low energy density diet is to avoid fatty foods (or use reduced fat versions of foods like cheese and milk), use only lean meat (trim off any visible fat and remove skin from poultry) and fish, and include lots of fruit and non-starchy but bulky, high-fiber vegetables such as spinach, broccoli, cauliflower, green beans, or salad leaves with tomatoes, onion, celery, etc.

- Several strategies can be used to help to abate hunger when dieting to lose weight. These include drinking water before eating a meal; eating foods with a high water and/or fiber content but low-fat and sugar content; eating meals with high-protein content; eating the high-protein and lower energy food items first; eating food slowly; and sprinkling a small amount of dried mixed herbs, ground pepper, vinegar, or lemon juice over your food.

- Exercise can help to create a negative energy balance, maintain muscle mass, and compensate for the reductions in RMR seen after weight loss.

- Resistance exercise and high-intensity interval exercise are not as effective for fat burning and weight loss as continuous aerobic exercise which can be sustained for much longer duration.

- For maximum fat burning during exercise itself, you should exercise aerobically at an intensity close to that which elicits your maximal fat oxidation rate. Depending on your fitness, this will be around 50-60% of your aerobic capacity (or 60-75% of your maximum heart rate).

- The mode, duration, and intensity of exercise influence the amount of energy expended and the amount of fat that is burnt. The most effective way to create a 500-kcal energy deficit is to exercise aerobically at low to moderate intensity for a continuous period of one to two hours.

- Compared with moderate energy deficits resulting from exercise alone, acute dietary energy restriction results in rapid changes in appetite that result in compensatory eating, which may initially limit potential success in weight loss efforts.

- Generally, adding exercise to a weight loss program results in weight loss that is fat loss (rather than lean tissue loss) and a combination of dieting and exercise is the most effective way to lower body weight and to maintain it at a lower level after weight reduction; it is nearly always more successful for weight loss than dieting or exercise alone.

Chapter 9

How to Personalize Your Weight Loss Plan to Beat Type 2 Diabetes

Objectives

After studying this chapter, you should:

- Know how to combine dieting and exercise for effective loss of body fat and body weight.

- Realize that you do not have to stick to just one method of dieting, and that using multiple methods will help keep up your motivation to achieve your weight loss goals.

- Know how much exercise you need to do to burn 600 kilocalories per day.

- Understand how to modify your diet and exercise habits to maintain your weight loss after finishing your weight loss plan.

- Understand how you will know if you have beaten type 2 diabetes.

In this chapter I will describe a personalized weight loss plan which I guarantee will be effective for body weight and fat loss. What's more is that it is a plan that is much easier to stick to than those that use a single diet strategy. My plan involves using multiple diets (a different one every week) and you can choose your own preferred type(s) of physical activity to further promote fat burning, minimize loss of lean tissue, and help to maintain your resting metabolic rate. Keeping to my weight loss plan should see the average overweight person lose about one kilogram (2.2 lbs) per week, and most of this will be body fat.

THE COMBINATION 1,000GPW (GRAMS OF FAT PER WEEK) WEIGHT LOSS PLAN FOR DIABETICS

This is my idea of an effective weight loss plan for people with prediabetes or type 2 diabetes. It is based on an adaptation of the 1,000GPW weight loss plan for non-diabetic people that I described in my previous book Eat, Move, Sleep, Repeat published by Meyer and Meyer in 2020. The "1,000GPW" means the aim is to lose, on average, **1,000 G**rams of fat **P**er **W**eek which will mean losing the same or slightly greater amount of body weight. Your initial goal is to adhere to the 1,000GPW weight loss plan for 10 weeks. By the end you should have lost about 10 kg (22 lbs) of body fat tissue and 11-12 kg (24-26 lbs) of body weight. The originality of the plan lies in how I suggest this is achieved. It is not done by dieting alone but by combining dieting with more exercise. But that is not all: the really clever and novel aspect of the plan is that you do not stick to just one diet for 10 weeks; in fact, you change the diet each week.

To lose one kilogram of body fat tissue per week, you will need a weekly total energy deficit of about 8,400 kcal or 1,200 kcal per day. I have chosen this size of energy deficit to match the one in the 2018 UK study that used an 800 kcal/day VLED to achieve it as this is the only study to date to provide proof of principle that type 2 diabetes can be put into remission by losing sufficient weight by dieting. So a reasonable aim is to reduce your dietary energy intake by 600 kcal per day and burn off an additional 600 kcal per day with exercise. For the vast majority of overweight people, their daily resting energy requirement to maintain energy balance and be weight stable will be about 1,800 to 2,200 kcal; my weight loss plan with its 1,200 kcal per day energy deficit should put anyone into substantial negative energy balance and therefore be highly effective for weight loss. As we are all different and genetics play a role in how much weight we lose by dieting or exercise, not everyone will lose exactly one kilogram per week. For some it will be a bit less and for others a little more. You will also probably find that you lose more weight per week in the first five weeks than you will after that, but don't worry as that is only to be expected as your body adapts to the daily energy deficit. One advantage of combining exercise with dieting and selecting diets with a high-protein content is that this food efficiency adaptation is not as great as it would be if you were attempting weight loss by dieting alone.

DECIDE YOUR TARGET WEIGHT AND HOW MUCH WEIGHT YOU NEED TO LOSE

The first thing you need to do is to decide what target weight you are aiming for and – depending on your current body weight – how much weight you are trying to lose. You can decide this yourself by referring to the body weight for height chart (figure 6.1) or in consultation with your healthcare professional.

WHY STICK TO JUST ONE WEIGHT LOSS DIET WHEN YOU CAN PICK AND MIX FROM SEVERAL DIETS THAT ARE EFFECTIVE AND SAFE?

You can personalize the dietary energy restriction part of the weight loss plan as there is no need to stick to the same diet every week for 10 weeks to achieve your goal. Of course, virtually all the books and articles you will have read before will almost certainly have promoted one particular diet because the author has had this one idea and wants to sell it (and their book!) to you. Forget it. You will soon get bored with eating the same foods and probably give up. Instead give yourself some variety. The previous chapter described several different diets that can be used to achieve the 600-kcal energy deficit that you are aiming for here. Table 9.1 illustrates exactly what you have to do to achieve this with the different diets.

So why not choose a different diet each week? You can choose the diets that suit you best according to your personal preferences and to fit in with what you are doing that week. This is a very simple approach and you won't get bored; every week will be different to the previous one. You can follow the suggested sequence in table 9.1 which ensures you will be having different foods each week, or you can come up with your own sequence. To achieve the desired weekly dietary energy deficit on some diets (the 4:3 and very low energy diet) you won't need to diet every day of the week as indicated by the frequency needed column in table 9.1. On the other days you can eat normally, but don't overcompensate by eating more than usual. Whenever possible on the normal eating days adhere to the principles of healthy eating that I described in chapter 7. You could try out the Mediterranean or Japanese diet or go vegetarian on these days to add further healthy variety to your program.

In this plan your average daily dietary energy deficit is 600 kcal (which is 4,200 kcal/week). The plan uses the strategy of varying the diet each week but there is some variation in the energy deficit from week to week as it ranges between 3,500 and 4,800 kcal/week.

Table 9.1 What you need to do to achieve an average of 600 kcal/day (4,200 kcal/week) energy deficit with different diets in overweight adults, and which weeks to apply the diet

Diet	What it involves	Frequency needed and weekly energy deficit	Week number of your 10-week plan
4:3	Only 500 kcal on 3 days/week	3 days per week 4,500 kcal	Weeks 1 and 6
Reduced fat	1,500 kcal/day with 10% fat (that's about 20 g fat)	7 days per week 3,500 kcal	Weeks 2 and 7
Very low energy	800 kcal/day with 35% protein (that's about 70 g protein)	4 days per week 4,800 kcal	Weeks 3 and 8
High-protein	1,400 kcal/day with 30% protein (that's about 105 g protein)	7 days per week 4,200 kcal	Weeks 4 and 9
Skip lunch	No 500-kcal lunch (so no more than 1,500 kcal/day)	7 days per week 3,500 kcal	Week 5
Low energy density	1,400 kcal/day with 25% protein (that's about 90 g protein)	7 days per week 4,200 kcal	Week 10

Assumes that you normally consume 2,000 kcal/day to achieve energy balance.

As indicated in the footnote to table 9.1, the figures are based on the assumption that your daily energy intake is normally 2,000 kcal. This amount of food energy is the number of calories you need to achieve energy balance if your resting daily energy expenditure is 2,000 kcal/day. You can calculate your own personal resting daily energy expenditure as described in the sidebar if you wish and adjust the energy intakes shown in Table 9.1 accordingly to achieve the desired 600 kcal/day energy deficit. For example, if your resting daily energy expenditure works out to 2,100 kcal per day you can add an extra 100 kcal to the energy intakes indicated in the second column of table 9.1.

How to estimate your personal resting daily energy expenditure

To most accurately calculate your resting metabolic rate (RMR), a scientist would take measurements of oxygen uptake and carbon dioxide production after a 12-hour overnight fast with eight hours of sleep. However, a rough estimation of the RMR can be obtained using the **Mifflin-St. Jeor equation** which was introduced in 1990. This equation is currently considered to be the best for estimating RMR.

Mifflin St. Jeor Equation:

For men: RMR (kcal/day) = 10 x weight (kg) + 6.25 x height (cm) − 5 x age (years) + 5

For women: RMR (kcal/day) = 10 x weight (kg) + 6.25 x height (cm) − 5 x age (years) − 161

The RMR will be about 5-10% higher for a man than a woman of the same age and body weight since body composition (ratios of lean muscle, bone, and fat) differ between men and women. The heavier you are, the more energy you need to sustain the larger muscle mass and larger organs, which is why heavier and taller individuals have a higher RMR. The other important factor is age as your RMR decreases as you get older because muscle mass declines by 5-10% each decade after the age of 30, unless that is, you participate in regular resistance training to prevent this (and believe me it is preventable). Nowadays many apps on mobile devices can be used to calculate RMR. After calculating your own RMR add an extra 10% to it to account for diet-induced thermogenesis (the increase in RMR that occurs following ingestion of a meal which represents the energy expended in the digestion, absorption, and storage of the nutrients in the meal). Now to this value add another 100 kcal to cover the energy expended in essential daily physical activities such as getting dressed, moving around the house, keeping an upright posture when seated or standing, and doing a few household chores. This value will now be a reasonable estimate of your personal resting daily energy expenditure.

Here is an example calculation for a 50-year-old female, who is 172 cm tall and weighs 90 kg. The appropriate equation is:

For women: RMR (kcal/day) = 10 x weight (kg) + 6.25 x height (cm) − 5 x age (years) − 161

(continued)

Inputting her weight, height, and age gives:

RMR (kcal/day) = 10 x 90 (kg) + 6.25 x 172 (cm) – 5 x 50 (years) – 161

= 900 + 1,075 – 250 – 161

= 1975 – 411

= 1,564

To this value we add 10% (which is 156 kcal/day) to account for the diet-induced thermogenesis component of daily energy expenditure, so that means her value increases to 1,720 kcal/day. Now we need to add 100 kcal for essential physical activities, bringing her daily energy expenditure 1,820 kcal/day.

The sequence of diets over the 10 weeks I have suggested in table 9.1 does have its advantages: Starting with the 4:3 intermittent fast diet in week one will get you off to a good start, and the reduced carbohydrate availability should speed up your exercise training adaptations by promoting the molecular signals that lead to increases in the numbers of mitochondria which increases your ability to oxidize fat. You follow this in week two with a switch to a reduced fat diet which means you get to eat more carbohydrate which is what you will have been missing most in week one. Next up in week three is the very low energy diet (but for only four days of the week). Week four brings the high-protein diet followed by week five where you just eliminate lunch every day. For the next four weeks you can simply repeat this sequence of diets except in week 10 you have the low energy density diet. The final chapter that follows provides some meal ideas for the various diets listed in table 9.1.

I have devised the 1,000GPW Weight Loss Plan because it will be suitable for most people with prediabetes or type 2 diabetes, is safe, and provides a good outcome in a reasonable amount of time. The multiple diets and the variety of the dieting strategy each week largely eliminates increases in appetite and cravings for particular foods compared with a weight loss plan that uses a single diet, but it is just as, if not more, effective for weight loss.

THE EXERCISE PART OF THE WEIGHT LOSS PLAN

Now for the exercise part of the weight loss plan that aims to burn 600 kcal per day. This part of the plan can also be personalized to match your preferred type(s) of physical activity. The best choice of exercise is going to be one that you want to do and that you will enjoy. There is no point in choosing to run for 30 minutes if you don't really like running and will put off going or make excuses for not going. If the thought of doing one activity continuously is too much to handle then why not split it up? Do one activity for half that amount of time and burn 300 kcal and then change activity, or later in the day do a different activity until you have worked off another 300 kcal. That way you will have some variety and will be training different muscle groups.

Selecting Your Choice of Exercises to Burn Fat

Selecting which exercises you want to do and determining the duration and frequency of the sessions in a day is about personalizing your plan to suit you. The exercises I have suggested in Table 9.2 are all predominantly aerobic forms of exercise, the best way to burn fat, but it is also a good idea to include some additional resistance exercise (say three 10-15 minute sessions per week) in order to help maintain or even increase muscle mass in the face of the energy deficit. This resistance training can either be done separately and in addition to your fat burning aerobic exercise sessions, or it can be included as part of these sessions. For example, you could include some resistance exercise as part of a circuit training session in the gym or by holding bar weights in your hands while taking part in an aerobics class as illustrated in photo 9.1. The weight of the bars that you feel comfortable with will depend on the strength of your upper arms; for most people a weight of between 2 kg and 5 kg would be suitable.

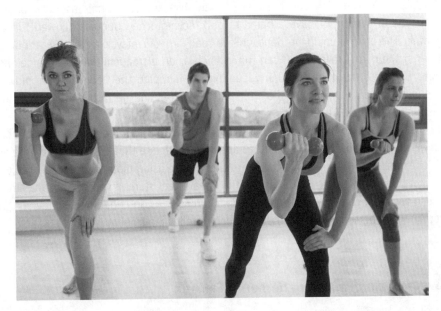

Photo 9.1: Doing some resistance exercise by holding 2-5 kg bar weights while taking part in an aerobics class

The calories you burn in the activities listed in table 9.2 below are all approximate and based on a person weighing 70 kg (154 lbs). The number of calories you burn will depend on your body weight and how much effort you are putting into it. If you are heavier then you will burn more calories, if you are laid back and taking the activity easy you will burn less calories than if you push yourself harder and work at a higher intensity.

Table 9.2 Duration of exercise needed to expend 600 kcal for a 70 kg person

Activity	Exercise time (minutes)
Aerobics	68
Badminton	73
Circuit training	80
Cycling 15 km/h (10 mph)	92
Running 8 km/h (5 mph)	50
10 km/h (6 mph)	40
Walking 4 km/h (2.5 mph)	131
Walking 5 km/h (3.1 mph)	105
Swimming	51

There are, of course, some fairly equivalent (in terms of calorie burn) alternatives to the activities listed in table 9.2. You could do dancing instead of aerobics, soccer or tennis instead of badminton, rowing instead of cycling, or have a game of golf (no motorized buggies allowed!) instead of a long walk. The cycling could be done on the road on your bicycle or on a stationery cycle ergometer in the gym; similarly you can run outside or on a treadmill indoors. Remember that everything you do burns calories, even vacuuming or mopping the floor, dusting, mowing the lawn, cleaning the car, walking up the stairs, and just standing up rather than sitting or lying down uses more calories. Although these activities alone do not burn many calories it all helps so next time you need to do housework or chores think of them as additional ways to burn calories. You can also take advantage of the opportunities to do exercise that arise when you are out and about. For example, you can walk to the shops rather than using motorized transport or take the stairs rather than the elevator in the mall or the department store. If you want to maximize your fat burning then you can exercise at your Fatmax intensity as described in the previous chapter. To determine your personal Fatmax intensity see the following sidebar.

How can I determine my personal Fatmax intensity?

For maximum fat burning during exercise you should exercise aerobically at an intensity close to that which elicits your maximal fat oxidation rate. For a person of low to average fitness this will be about 55 to 60% of your aerobic capacity. Actually, measuring your aerobic capacity (or maximum oxygen uptake) requires specialist laboratory equipment and performing an incremental exercise test to exhaustion, so an alternative is to use a method that only requires the measurement of your heart rate using a simple and inexpensive heart rate monitor. Firstly, you can easily calculate your maximum heart rate which can be estimated as 220 minus your age in years. So for a 50 year-old person, this would be 220 − 50 = 170 beats/min. Secondly, by wearing a monitor or counting your pulse at the wrist, measure your resting heart rate. Start the measurement after lying down and relaxing for 10 minutes. For a person of low to average fitness (and a non-smoker) this will be about 70 to 80 beats/min. Thirdly, calculate your **heart rate reserve** which is simply your maximum heart rate minus your resting heart rate. In our example, this would be 170 − 75 = 95 beats/min. Your Fatmax intensity (let's imagine you are pretty unfit and it's 55% of your aerobic capacity) will be achieved when exercising at a heart rate equal to your resting heart rate plus 55% of your heart rate reserve. In our example this would be 75 + (95 x 55 ÷ 100) = 75 + 52 = 122 beats/min. So when you go out for a run or cycle whilst wearing your heart rate monitor, start off slowly and gradually increase your pace until your heart rate reaches your personal target value and try to keep it at this value ± 5 beats/min for the duration of your workout.

If possible, stick to the exercise part of the plan every day of the week. Don't worry if circumstances mean that you have to miss out on exercise on one or two days of the week; it will not have a significant impact on your weight loss over 10 weeks and you may be able to make up for it by exercising a little more than usual on the day after your off-exercise day.

The amount of body fat and weight you will lose will vary slightly from one week to the next but this is not a concern. Keep in mind that you will achieve the overall goal of the plan after the 10 weeks is up. Sticking to the plan means you should expect to lose, on average, about 1,000 g or 1 kg (2.2 lbs) of body fat tissue per week. Keep that up for 10 weeks and you will have lost 10 kg (22 lbs) of body fat tissue, which should equate to an 11-12 kg (24-26 lbs) drop in body weight.

It is a good idea to record what you do in terms of physical activity and what you eat on a daily basis using a simple weekly food and activity chart. Organizations, such as the UK National Health Service, often offer free downloads on their websites. You don't necessarily have to use premade templates or include so much detail but it does no harm to celebrate what you are achieving by noting in a diary what you have eaten and what amount and type of exercise you have done each week. This may help to further strengthen your resolve to continue with your weight loss plan.

What If I Don't Want to Go to the Gym?

Quite a number of the aerobic activities I have suggested are often done in a gym or leisure center, but these can be expensive and not everyone has one available near where they live. Some people, particularly if they are overweight, may feel too embarrassed to go to the gym, although it can be a great way to socialize and make new friends if you make the effort to go. However, if it is not possible or you just don't want to go to a gym you can choose other activities that you can do at home or in your local park or neighborhood. Suitable exercises include jogging, cycling, and walking. You could also consider buying a cycle ergometer that you set up in a spare room in your house or apartment. I have one in my garage. You can get ones with a simple adjustable pedal resistance and a battery-operated display. A new one will cost around $200-300 (£160-240). You can get secondhand ones on Ebay for about $50-100 (£40-80). These are a great investment and give you the opportunity to carry on with your daily exercise when the weather outside is bad. Because your body weight is supported by the seat of the cycle you don't put as much stress on your joints as you do with jogging. Some people might find cycling for an hour or so on their own a bit boring but there is nothing to stop you listening to music or the radio while you cycle. You can even watch television or set up two cycle ergometers in the same room and cycle together with your partner. Finally, if none of these suggestions are to your liking, why not just walk? Walking is a great way to burn fat if you can find enough time to fit it into your daily routine. I like playing doubles tennis, but I won't do that more than once or twice per week. But walking, well I try to do that every day for at least one hour and preferably two. It's easy to keep a track of how many calories you burn by keeping a small pedometer in your pocket. These devices measure how many steps you take and most will display the distance you have covered if you input your usual stride length. From this you can calculate quite accurately how much energy you expended on your walk. How to do this is explained in the following sidebar.

How to estimate your energy expenditure for walking by using a pedometer

Simple inexpensive pedometers that record steps taken and distance covered for walking are available and usually just require the user to input their normal stride length which can be determined by measuring the distance covered (using a normal tape measure) when walking a given number (e.g., 20) of strides. The device can then reasonably estimate the distance covered over a long walk (say 6 miles or 10 km). If you have one of the more expensive devices that incorporates a Global Positioning System (GPS) function (just like the satnav in your car) the distance covered on a walk or run can be even more accurately determined without having to know your stride length. There is a relatively simple relationship between the distance covered (either walking or running) and the amount of energy expended. A person expends one kcal per km distance covered per kg body weight, so the following equation can be used to estimate the energy expended when completing any known distance on foot (and it's the same for a man or a woman):

Amount of energy expended (kcal) = Distance covered (km) x body weight (kg)

Thus, a person weighing 70 kg (154 lbs or 11 stone) would expend 700 kcal if they covered a distance of 10 km (6 miles). As a rough approximation you can say about 110 kcal per mile (or 70 kcal per km). This is for covering distance over relatively flat terrain. The amount of energy expended would be about 10-20% higher if walking mostly uphill (photo 9.2).

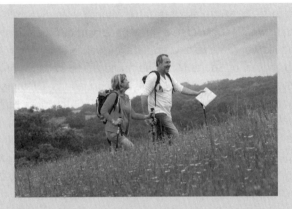

Photo 9.2: Walking is great for fat burning at about 110 kilocalories per mile on the flat and about 10-20% more when walking uphill

Note though that it is the distance covered, not the pace at which it is covered, nor the time taken to complete the distance that determines the amount of energy expended.

You can do the same calculation for jogging but when you are running, the stride length will, of course, be longer than it is for walking so you will have to measure this as you did for walking but while running at your usual pace. For a 70 kg runner, the amount of energy expended when completing a marathon race (26.2 miles or 42.2 km) is 42.2 x 70 kcal which is 2,954 kcal.

Just Going for a Brisk Walk Is a Great Way to Burn Fat and Lose Weight

As explained in the sidebar you will expend about 110 kcal for each mile you complete so to reach the target of burning 600 kcal per day by exercising you will need to cover 5.5 miles (8.7 km). If you do that distance at a leisurely stroll it could take you three hours but at a normal average pace it should take only just over two hours. If you walk briskly it could take only just over an hour and three quarters. If you split that up into three shorter walks during the day (e.g., one in the early morning, one around midday and the other in the afternoon or evening) that would be only three 35- to 40-minute brisk walks per day. There are some advantages to walking at a "brisk pace" and it is often mentioned that it is very good for getting the health benefits of exercise and is better than walking at a slow pace. While this is certainly true, what does a "brisk pace" actually mean? Obviously the actual distance covered in a certain amount of time (say one hour) depends on a person's stride length and the stride rate or cadence (steps per minute) so the actual speed for brisk walking will be different for a tall person with long strides than for a shorter person with smaller strides when their stride rate is the same. The US Centers for Disease Control and Prevention advice indicates that brisk walking is movement that calls for heavy breathing, so although you may be able to roughly approximate a brisk pace by asking "Am I getting a little breathless?" or "Am I moving faster than a leisurely stroll?", how do you really know if you're walking at what's considered a "brisk pace" without the use of scientific equipment to measure something like your rate of oxygen uptake? Well, a new review of research published in 2018 in the British Journal of Sports Medicine found that a cadence of about 100 steps per minute indicated a moderately intense brisk walk for most adults. Of course, you don't need to be at exactly 100 – some people might be at 95, others 105 – but close to 100 steps per minute constitutes a brisk walk, the research suggests, regardless of age, fitness, or athletic ability. So if this is what you want to achieve, the next time you're on a walk, take 20 seconds to mentally count how many steps you take, and then multiply that number by three to get your step count per minute. Obviously to be walking at 100 steps per minute you need to be completing about 33 steps every 20 seconds.

WHAT IF I WANT TO LOSE MORE WEIGHT THAN THIS?

I appreciate that the 1,000GPW weight loss plan may not be suitable for everyone's goals. If you want to lose more than 10 kg (22 lbs) of body fat then you could just continue with the plan for another 5-10 weeks or as long as it takes to reach your target weight. The longer you stick with the plan, the fitter you will get because your body adapts to exercise training. The function of your muscles, heart, and lungs all improve, your muscles increase their ability to oxidize fat, and your aerobic capacity also increases. As you get fitter any exercise you do starts to feel easier and you may feel that you can increase the intensity of the exercise you were doing or keep it going for longer without feeling tired. So if you want to speed up your weight loss after the first 10 weeks you can do so by doing more exercise to get your daily exercise energy expenditure up to around 700-800 kcal per day. This would be a better option than trying to reduce your dietary energy intake more.

WEIGHT MAINTENANCE FOLLOWING SUCCESSFUL WEIGHT LOSS

Having put in the hard work in achieving successful weight loss it would be a shame to put the weight back on in the months that follow. So be aware of the pitfalls. Remember that losing body weight usually becomes increasingly difficult as weight loss progresses because the body responds to weight loss by becoming more efficient, which is usually referred to as "food efficiency". With the 1,000GPW weight loss plan that combines dieting and exercise it should not be an important issue but it is still likely that some fall in your resting metabolic rate will have developed, so when resuming your normal pattern of food intake it is best to employ some of the strategies you have learnt such as continuing to exclude high-fat processed foods and sugar-sweetened beverages in favor of low-fat or low calorie equivalents, and generally aim to maintain a low energy density diet with 15-25% protein and lots of fruit and vegetables. In other words, make sure that your altered eating habits stay altered, at least to some degree.

Often, the considerable effort applied to achieve weight loss is exceeded by the effort required to maintain the new lower body weight. After the weight is lost, if you are not careful, it can be regained in a relatively short period. This effect is usually referred to as the yo-yo effect. Studies in animals have documented this pattern of weight cycling. After a period of food restriction and weight reduction, animals tend to regain the weight quickly if they are allowed free access to food. Several **prospective cohort studies** have shown that weight fluctuation (gain–loss or loss–gain) or weight variability is associated with increased mortality, independent of the direction of weight change. When taking limited account of preexisting disease, however, studies show little evidence of negative side effects of weight cycling. Thus, from your own health perspective, the risks from overweight and obesity far exceed the potential risks of weight cycling. But try to avoid it anyway by not succumbing to cravings to eat more or going back to your old bad habits. Remember that it is always far easier to put weight on than it is to lose it.

Finally, to maintain the long-term health benefits of exercise you need to keep exercising. What you did activity-wise 5, 10, or 20 years ago will not protect you in later life if regular exercise is not maintained. If you do some exercise it means you can afford some indulgences such as a nice glass of wine with dinner or some ice cream with your fruit for dessert without risking a return to a positive energy balance and cumulative weight gain. Always remember that doing exercise is good for your health in so many ways. It makes no sense whatsoever to avoid it.

HOW WILL I KNOW IF I HAVE BEATEN TYPE 2 DIABETES?

Let's say you have reached your target weight which means it should now be somewhere in the "healthy weight" range according to the chart in figure 6.1. When you have lost the excess fat that was causing you to be overweight the mechanisms that caused your diabetes will have been put into reverse gear meaning that your blood lipid profile should have improved (lower serum total cholesterol and triglycerides, lower LDL/HDL and apoB/apoA-I ratios) and your blood sugar levels should have started to stabilize and return to the normal range. The normalization of blood glucose may take a little longer as your pancreatic β-cells will need time to recover particularly if you have had type 2 diabetes for a number of years. Allow at least a few months and then request a blood test from your healthcare practitioner. You blood test should show the expected improvements in your blood lipid profile, but the critical measurement that determines if you are still classed as diabetic or not is your blood glycated hemoglobin (HbA1c) level. If this has fallen to less than 6.5% (48 mmol/mol) you are probably no longer diabetic. If it is between 5.7 and 6.4% (42-47 mmol/mol) – which is quite likely – you are back to being prediabetic and you can think of it as being in remission from your type 2 diabetes. The important thing is to keep it that way or, better still, by continuing with sensible healthy eating and keeping up your exercise regimen, bring your blood HbA1c further down to less than 5.7% (42 mmol/mol). Then you can truly claim to have beaten your type 2 diabetes.

But again, let's be honest: People are different and some of us have genes that increase our risk of having or retaining type 2 diabetes. Not everyone who reaches their weight target will drop below the critical HbA1c level of 6.5% (48 mmol/mol). However, I would expect that everyone who achieved their desired weight loss will have lowered their HbA1c level to some degree and shown some improvements in their blood lipid profile. Such people can also comfort themselves in the knowledge that they will have almost certainly decreased their risk of the serious health consequences that would otherwise ensue had they not made the effort to lose their excess body fat.

But always remember that your type 2 diabetes will come back if you revert to your bad habits of eating too much, drinking too much alcohol, and not doing much exercise. Having worked so hard to get where you are now it would be a real shame to become diabetic all over again.

Key Points

- It is essential to decide on your weight loss goals right at the start. These goals should be carefully thought out and be realistically achievable. Goals also have to be defined with a time schedule in mind. How much weight must be lost and how soon?

- The 1,000GPW weight loss plan generates a 1,200 kcal per day energy deficit using a combination of diet and exercise which should result in a loss of about 10 kg (22 lbs) of body fat in 10 weeks.

- You can personalize the plan by making your own selection of the diets to use and in the order that you do them, changing the diet week by week. You can also personalize the exercise part of the weight loss plan to suit the activities that you are capable of and like to do – in the gym, at home, or outdoors.

- Weight maintenance following weight loss requires that you continue to employ some of the strategies you have learnt such as continuing to exclude high-fat processed foods and sugar-sweetened beverages in favor of low-fat or low calorie equivalents, and generally aim to maintain a low energy density diet with 15-25% protein and lots of non-starchy fruit and vegetables.

- By remaining physically active and sticking with sensible healthy eating and drinking you will reap the benefits of a healthier life as you get older, as well as assisting with your weight maintenance.

Chapter 10

Meal Ideas for Diets for People Who Are Trying to Manage or Beat Type 2 Diabetes

Objectives

After studying this chapter, you should:

- Be able to plan suitable low glycemic index meals for managing blood sugar levels.

- Be able to plan suitable meals for the very low energy diet and "fasting days" on the 4:3 diet.

- Be able to plan suitable meals for the Mediterranean, Japanese, and vegetarian diets.

- Be able to plan suitable meals for the reduced fat diet.

- Be able to plan suitable meals for the high-protein diet.

- Be able to plan suitable meals for the low energy density diet.

- Appreciate that you can vary many of the meal plans to some degree to suit your personal food and taste preferences.

- Appreciate the value of adding low energy density foods and natural flavoring to your meals when dieting.

- Know what to drink and what to avoid drinking when dieting.

If you are planning to follow any of the weight loss diets suitable for people with type 2 diabetes described in chapter 8 or my multi-diet 1,000GPW weight loss plan described in chapter 9, then you need to know some example meal plans for breakfasts, lunches, and evening dinners for these diets. This chapter provides some example meal plans but you can vary them to some degree to suit your personal food and taste preferences, substituting like for like for the meats, green vegetables, legumes, breads, and pasta items that are mentioned below. For example, it is perfectly fine to use turkey instead of chicken; lean pork or non-oily fish like cod instead of beef;

asparagus, spring greens, leeks, cabbage, or green beans instead of spinach; sweet potato, corn, or rice instead of potato; peas or butter beans instead of red beans or baked beans; and penne pasta, macaroni, linguine, or noodles instead of spaghetti. Just stick to the guideline amounts in grams and the calorie (kcal) amounts will not be very different. The meal plans described in this chapter give the amounts per meal for just one person. If you are preparing meals for two people simply double the amounts.

I have not attempted to provide full recipes with cooking times and temperatures here. Just bear in mind that generally steaming is preferable to boiling for most vegetables that need cooking because more of the essential nutrients are retained and that grilling is preferable to frying for most meats as no oil needs to be added. When you do fry food such as steak, use a non-stick frying pan and only enough extra virgin olive oil (no more than two teaspoons which is 80 kcal and 9 g of fat) to thinly coat the bottom the pan, and if you are only cooking for one person use a small diameter pan. Alternatively, brush each side of your steak with one half teaspoon of extra virgin olive oil before placing it in a hot non-stick frying pan. Better still, use an extra virgin olive oil spray to just thinly coat your meat or the pan surface. Many of these sprays are an emulsion – a mixture of oil and water – and are claimed to give you just one calorie (kcal) per spray, but you will probably find that you need six to ten sprays to provide enough oil to fry your meat or use in a stir-fry. Even so, that is a big saving on calories compared with using teaspoon quantities of olive oil or any other oil for that matter. Do check the label, though, as some of these sprays use different vegetable oils such as sunflower and rapeseed which are not as good for you as extra virgin olive oil. Extra virgin is the highest quality and most expensive olive oil classification. It should have no defects and a flavor of fresh olives. It must be produced entirely by mechanical means from cold pressed olives without the use of any added processed oils, solvents, and under temperatures that will not degrade the oil.

For all meal plans described in this chapter I give you the ingredients with their weight or volume and the energy (kcal) content of the individual ingredients or the whole meal. For some meal plans I give you the energy content (kcal) of all the individual items to give you an idea of the energy value of various foods. Otherwise, I just give you the approximate energy content (rounded up to the nearest 10 kcal) of the whole meals Note that some meal plans specify dry uncooked weights for rice and pasta items while others give the cooked weight. Take care to check which it is as the energy content of boiled rice or pasta is about 130 kcal per 100 g but that of uncooked dry rice or pasta is nearly three times that value at 370 kcal per 100 g.

It is also worth remembering that some tasty vegetables such as sauerkraut, beansprouts, and pickled silver-skin onions, red cabbage, and beetroot can be used as an accompaniment to most lunches or dinners on all the diets provided that they are agreeable to your stomach. Onion, for example, can be a problematic food for some people. Many find their stomachs are sensitive to onions, and they find that unpleasant tummy upset symptoms reduce when they remove them from their diets. So if things are new to you, try them in small amounts first. The advantage of these tasty vegetables is that they have a low energy density and contain very little carbohydrate (except fiber) and very few calories (typically only 5-15 kcal in a 50 g serving) but provide flavor, fiber, and bulk which will make your food on the plate look more substantial and make you feel fuller and more satisfied. The fiber is also good for your gut and will help to keep your bowel movements regular. These foods, along with other vegetables such as spinach, kale, and cabbage are particularly useful on the very low energy diet, "fasting" days on the 4:3 intermittent fasting diet, and the high-protein diet where the usual filling carbohydrate staples like potatoes, rice, pasta, and bread are restricted or absent altogether. They are also an absolutely essential part of the low energy density diet.

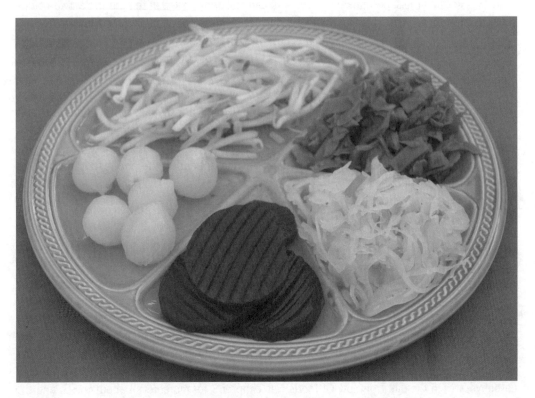

Photo 10.1: A selection of 50 g portions of low-calorie accompaniments to main meals.

If, like me, you enjoy casseroles, curries, and tagines as hot, healthy, and tasty meals don't use liquid ready-made liquid sauces as these are usually high in calories and added sugar. The dry powdered sauce mixes usually have lower fat, sugar, and energy content (typically only about 50-60 kcal per tablespoon which is all you need for one person, but remember to check the nutrition facts label to be sure), or better still make your own sauce by using dry curry powder (one tablespoon of medium or high strength is usually enough) or paprika powder, with some garlic granules, dried ginger, chili bits, or mixed herbs to add flavor. Mix these with a half a tin of chopped tomatoes (only 50 kcal) and two tablespoons of low-fat yogurt (or 100 g spinach – only 22 kcal) to thicken. You can also enhance the flavor of many other foods that you eat by adding a teaspoon of dried mixed herbs, dried chili bits, ground garlic, ginger powder, turmeric, or paprika powder to your cooking of stews, soups, and roast meat dishes. These can provide a huge boost to flavor but only add five calories per teaspoon at most.

Another important point is to be careful with what you choose to drink. For all the diets described in this chapter, you don't want to add extra calories from hot or cold beverages. That means cutting out altogether any sugar-sweetened beverages such as energy drinks, sports drinks, flavored soft drinks, and cordials and avoiding milkshakes and creamy or milky hot drinks like latte coffee and cocoa. Obviously, water is fine but there is an excellent selection of artificially sweetened fruit flavored soft drinks, mixers, and cordials. Look for the "low calorie", "diet", or "light" versions on the supermarket shelves. You can still drink coffee or tea but use a zero-calorie artificial sweetener instead of sugar, and a dash of skimmed or semi-skimmed milk instead of whole milk or cream. For all the meal plans described in this chapter that require the addition of milk, I have suggested using semi-skimmed milk (48 kcal per 100 mL), but you can use skimmed milk (35 kcal per 100 mL) if you prefer. There is little point having whole milk if you are looking to lose weight as it contains 18 kcal more per 100 mL than semi-skimmed. Other alternatives, including ones that are suitable for vegetarians and vegans, are soymilk (35 kcal per 100 mL), rice milk (53 kcal per 100 mL), or unsweetened almond milk (only 17 kcal per 100 mL). Finally, you should not drink any alcoholic beverages like wine, beer, or spirits on most of the diets although you could allow yourself just one glass of wine or beer on the non-fasting days of the 4:3 intermittent fasting diet.

MEALS FOR THE LOW GLYCEMIC INDEX DIET FOR MANAGING BLOOD SUGAR LEVELS

The low glycemic index (GI) diet is a bit of a misnomer as the GI is a value that is only related to carbohydrate containing foods; it does not consider other things such as the total energy content or the amount of protein and fat. So really a low GI diet is just one that generally seeks to avoid the intake of high GI foods, limit the intake of medium GI foods, and get most of your carbohydrates in the diet from low GI foods. See chapter 3 for more detail about the GI and the glycemic load (GL). One way to introduce lower GI foods into your diet is to substitute them for some of the foods you're eating now. For example:

- Replace ordinary pasta with wholewheat pasta.

- Replace white processed bread with 100% wholegrain bread or wholemeal bread as these contain more micronutrients than processed bread.

- Replace sugar-sweetened beverages with low calorie versions.

- Eat breakfast cereals based on oats, barley, and bran or occasionally have a boiled or poached egg or two slices of grilled bacon with some sliced avocado instead.

- Have baked sweet potatoes instead of baked white potatoes.

- Instead of drinking fruit juice eat whole fruits with relatively low-carbohydrate content such as melon, grapes, and blueberries.

- Snack on soybeans, nuts, celery, or miniature tomatoes instead of candy, chips, and pretzels. Or use hummus as a spread on rye crispbread or as a dip for sticks of celery or carrot.

The GI shouldn't be the only thing you consider when making choices about what to eat. The fact a food has a low GI doesn't mean it's particularly healthy, or that you should eat a lot of it. The food's energy, vitamin, and mineral content are still important. For example, potato chips have a lower GI than oatmeal and about the same as green peas, but oatmeal and green peas contain more nutrients. Portion sizes matter, too. The more carbohydrate you eat – no matter what kind of carbohydrate it is – the more it will affect your blood sugar. That's what the GL tells you. The GL helps you to account for both the quantity and the quality of your carbohydrates at the same time. As a simple guide: a GL less than 10 is low; more than 20 is high.

For a diet with a lower GL you should eat:

- More wholegrains, legumes, vegetables that contain little or no starch, nuts, melon, and other foods with a low GI (these were listed in chapter 3).

- Limit foods with a high GL, like potatoes and white rice, to no more than two or three servings per week, and eat these with some low GL vegetables like asparagus, broccoli, cauliflower, green beans, or spinach.

- As little as possible sugary foods, including candy, cookies, cakes, and sugar-sweetened beverages.

You can still eat some foods with a high GI, but have them less often, in smaller portions, and offset with nutritious, low GI foods when you do. Remember that the low GI diet doesn't cover everything you eat or should eat for a healthy diet. Some relatively high GI foods, such as sweet potato, are still healthy for you, and some low GI foods, like nuts, can pack a lot of calories if you eat too many. Although the GI and GL can guide your choice of carbohydrate foods, you'll have to monitor how much protein and fat you're getting, as well.

Also bear in mind that a low GI or GL diet is not designed for weight loss, and there are other diets that are far more effective for weight loss if this is your main goal. If you are at risk for diabetes or have prediabetes, type 2 diabetes, or the metabolic syndrome, then incorporating the GI principle into your meal planning may help you keep your blood glucose levels in check. The American Diabetes Association recommends traditional carbohydrate counting for blood sugar control with the GI being used to help "fine tune" meal planning. Some example meals that incorporate the low GI (or GL) principle are listed below, and to help with weight maintenance I have indicated their approximate calorie content:

LOW GL BREAKFASTS (250-400 KCAL)

Two egg omelet with one tablespoon of extra virgin olive oil, 30 g grated cheese, and one whole sliced red pepper (390 kcal).

100 g smoked salmon with half a sliced ripe avocado and 50 g cottage cheese, sprinkled with black pepper. Serve with one slice of wholegrain bread (400 kcal).

Three thick slices of grilled lean bacon, one poached egg, one grilled tomato sprinkled with oregano, and 50 g sauerkraut (310 kcal).

Porridge oats (50 g) made with 130 mL skimmed milk and topped with a tablespoon of honey and 20 raisins (320 kcal).

One 80 g fried pork or beef sausage, one fried egg, one fried tomato (using two teaspoons of extra virgin olive oil for pan frying), and 50 g sauerkraut (400 kcal).

Three slices of Parma ham or boiled ham, two poached eggs, and one tomato (310 kcal).

One-half cup of oatmeal and one-half cup of plain Greek yogurt with 10 chopped pecan nut halves (330 kcal).

Two scrambled eggs made with 50 mL semi-skimmed milk and two teaspoons of margarine with four steamed chopped asparagus spears and one slice of lean bacon. Serve with one slice of toasted wholegrain bread (330 kcal).

Two poached eggs with 80 g sliced mushrooms fried in two teaspoons of extra virgin olive oil and 30 g spinach leaves seasoned with ground black pepper and a pinch of salt (270 kcal).

LOW GL LUNCHES (300-400 KCAL)

Goat's cheese salad made with 80 g salad leaves, five olives, five cherry tomatoes, half a small sliced ripe avocado, 50 g cubed cucumber, and 50 g crumbled goat's cheese. Drizzled with juice from half a lemon or lime. Serve with one piece of rye bread or cracker (400 kcal).

100 g roast chicken breast served over 40 g mixed salad leaves, half a chopped red pepper, six cucumber slices, and 100 g new potatoes. Topped with 30 g grated cheese (400 kcal).

Two celery stalks each filled with 30 g cottage cheese and wrapped in 25g of thin sliced roast chicken, ham, or beef, and served with 30 g beansprouts and two slices of wholegrain bread (330 kcal).

Greek salad including five olives, two large vine tomatoes cut into wedges, half a chopped red onion, 50 g cubed peeled cucumber, and 30 g feta cheese cut into chunks, 50 g baby spinach leaves, and half a small sliced ripe avocado. Drizzled with one teaspoon of extra virgin olive oil and sprinkled with dried oregano (400 kcal).

One small tin of salmon served over 50 g baby spinach leaves, five cherry tomatoes, one quarter of thinly sliced cucumber. Drizzled with one teaspoon of extra virgin olive oil. Serve with two slices of wholegrain bread (350 kcal).

One small tin of tuna or mackerel in brine, drained, served over 50 g spinach leaves, 30 g crumbled feta cheese, and half a chopped red pepper (300 kcal).

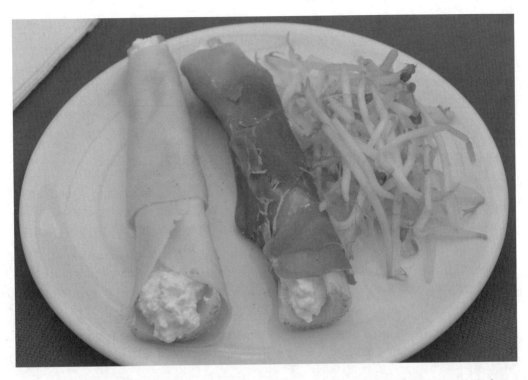

Photo 10.2: Two celery stalks filled with 30 g cottage cheese. One is wrapped in a thin slice (25 g piece) of roast chicken and the other with Parma ham and served with 30 g beansprouts.

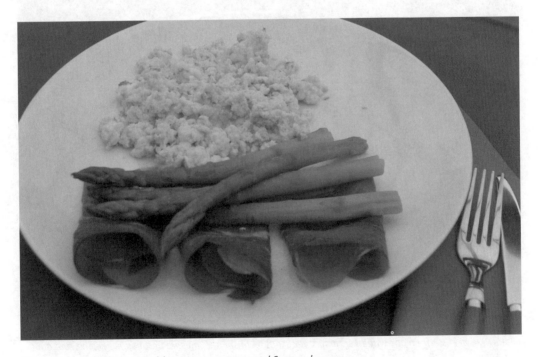

Photo 10.3: Scrambled eggs with asparagus spears and Serrano ham.

One small tin of salmon with half a small chopped avocado, served over a two-thirds of a cupful of boiled brown rice or wholewheat pasta (390 kcal).

Two scrambled eggs cooked with 50 mL semi-skimmed milk and two teaspoons of margarine, served with five steamed asparagus spears, three slices of Serrano (or Parma) ham, and a slice of wholegrain bread (390 kcal).

LOW GL DINNERS (700-900 KCAL, INCLUDING DESSERT)

The following main courses can be followed with a 220-kcal dessert consisting of one cup of chopped melon, watermelon, or mango with 10 grapes or 20 blueberries, two tablespoons of low-fat yogurt, and a sprinkling of two crushed walnuts or six crushed almonds.

200 g pork tenderloin served with 100 g broccoli and 100 g cauliflower mashed with one teaspoon of butter. Topped with 30 g grated cheddar cheese. Serve with two-thirds of a cup of boiled brown rice (660 kcal).

Lamb tagine casserole made with 140 g lean diced cubes of lamb, tagine powdered sauce mix, two whole dried figs, 100 g sliced carrots, half a can of chopped tomatoes, 50 g button mushrooms, and half a sliced aubergine (eggplant). Serve with one cup of boiled couscous (680 kcal).

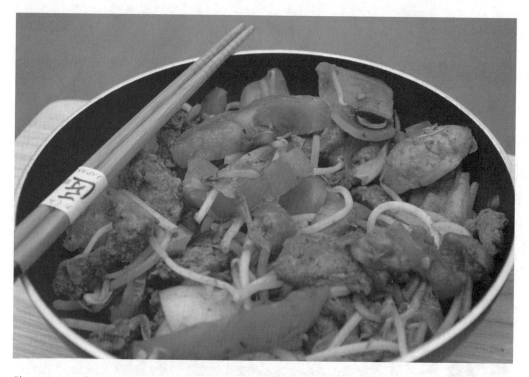

Photo 10.4: Beef stir-fry made with beef rump steak strips, beansprouts, mushrooms, pepper, onions, and dark soya sauce.

Three oven-baked pork sausages with one teaspoon of extra virgin olive oil and served with 80 g green beans and 100 g chopped steamed leek or cauliflower, with topping of one tablespoon of cream cheese. Serve with one large oven baked sweet potato (540 kcal).

One-half roast chicken breast wrapped in two slices Parma ham. Served with one oven baked potato, 80 g sliced zucchini, 100 g chopped leeks or celeriac, mashed with one teaspoon of butter (600 kcal).

Beef stir-fry made with 200 g beef rump steak strips, 100 g beansprouts, five sliced mushrooms, half a sliced red or green pepper, and one medium chopped onion or 30 g water chestnuts. Stir-fried with two teaspoons of extra virgin olive oil and two tablespoons of dark soya sauce. Serve with one cup of boiled whole-wheat pasta (650 kcal).

130 g salmon, topped with one teaspoon of butter and one teaspoon of chopped parsley, and baked in foil. Served with half a sliced medium avocado, 100 g steamed cauliflower, and 80 g sautéed kale cooked in one tablespoon of extra virgin olive oil with one finely chopped slice of lean bacon (540 kcal).

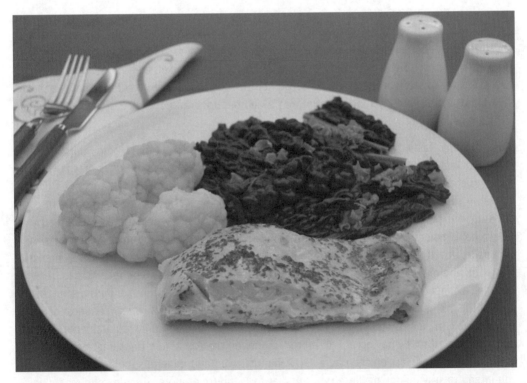

Photo 10.5: Oven baked salmon with butter and parsley, served with steamed cauliflower and sautéed kale cooked in extra virgin olive oil with bacon bits.

MEALS FOR DAYS ON THE VERY LOW ENERGY DIET AND "FASTING DAYS" ON THE INTERMITTENT FASTING 4:3 DIET

On a very low energy diet it is common practice to take nutrition in the form of liquid, high-protein meals, supplemented with vitamins and minerals. Such supplements are only really necessary if this type of diet is being kept up for more than two to three weeks. Liquid meals usually have to be purchased from specialist manufacturers and are usually in the form of a soup or a milk-based beverage (with or without added egg) in the form of a shake or smoothie. Milk-based shakes are available as powders that are reconstituted with water and come in a variety of flavors including, banana, strawberry, chocolate, cookie, toffee, and vanilla. Each 50 g serving of a shake or smoothie provides about 200 kcal, 6-8 g fat, 15-20 g carbohydrate, 15-20 g protein, about 5 g fiber, and 1 g salt, together with vitamins and minerals. Consuming three or four of the 50 g servings will usually provide sufficient micronutrients and protein to meet recommended daily intakes. It is usually recommended to consume these four times per day, at regular intervals, three to four hours apart.

However, in the 1,000 GPW weight loss plan, the very low energy diet is only employed on four days every five weeks, so normal foods like soups and low-calorie meals can be consumed on the VLED days, just as they can for the 4:3 intermittent semi-fasting diet. Half a can (200 g) of soup (normal soup that you find on grocery store or supermarket shelves) generally provides 100-130 kcal, so three of these can be consumed per day together with some mixed leaf salad, sauerkraut, beansprouts, shredded carrot, or pickled beetroot, and one slice of wholemeal bread (70 kcal) per serving.

Meals for the "fasting days" on the 4:3 intermittent fasting diet should amount to no more than 500 kcal/day (for women) and 600 kcal/day (for men), whereas for days on the very low energy diet the calorie intake should not exceed 800 kcal/day. Simply pick and mix from the meal and snack options shown below or read food labels and use the same principles to come up with your own meal ideas. In order not to add extra calories from drinks consumed with meals, have mineral water, low calorie (diet) versions of fruit juices/cordials, tonic water, cola, lemonade, etc. If you cannot do without your tea or coffee with every meal, use skimmed or semi-skimmed milk rather than whole milk and artificial low-calorie sweeteners instead of sugar. Avoid all alcohol on these low-calorie intake days. The very low energy intake on the semi-fasting days of the 4:3 intermittent fasting diet is limited to 500-600 kcal/day and will almost certainly not provide sufficient protein and micronutrients to meet minimum daily requirements. This can be compensated for by having a high-protein dinner on the day before the semi-fasting day and a high-protein breakfast on the day after. A multivitamin and mineral supplement is advised if you intend to stay on one of these types of diet for a month or more. Some example breakfasts, lunches, dinners, and snacks are as follows:

BREAKFASTS CONTAINING ABOUT 125 KCAL

Spinach or tomato omelet

One medium egg: 78 kcal

Just enough low-calorie olive oil spray to coat a small frying pan: 10 kcal

60 g fresh spinach or two tomatoes: 15 kcal

Add a pinch of ground pepper and a sprinkling of herbs (e.g., chives, oregano, parsley, sage, or a mixture) to the omelet for more flavor.

Cup of tea or coffee with 20 mL semi-skimmed milk: 12 kcal

Total kcal = 115

Blueberries, cranberries, raisins, or sultanas with Greek yogurt and almonds or walnuts

One tablespoon of blueberries/cranberries/raisins/sultanas: 42 kcal

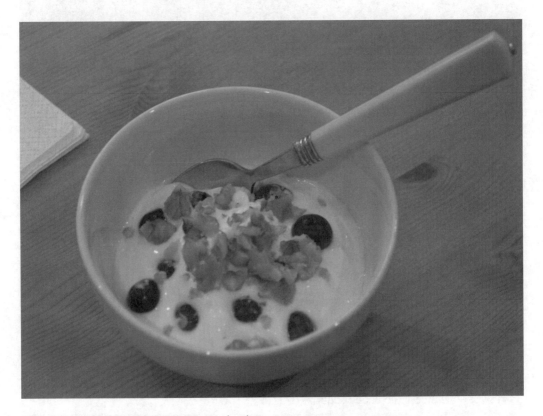

Photo 10.6: Blueberries with Greek yogurt and walnuts.

Three tablespoons of fat-free Greek yogurt: 24 kcal

Four whole almonds or two walnuts with skin crushed: 28 kcal

Cup of tea or coffee with 20 mL semi-skimmed milk: 12 kcal

Total kcal = 106

BREAKFASTS CONTAINING ABOUT 250 KCAL

Grapefruit half and a blueberry or cherry muesli

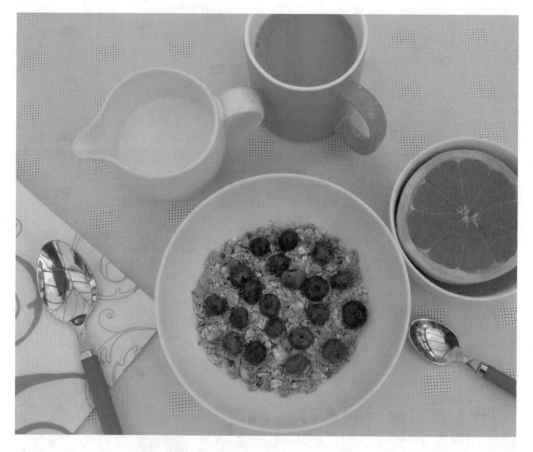

Photo 10.7: Grapefruit half and a blueberry muesli.

Half a pink grapefruit: 55 kcal

35 g swiss style muesli (no added sugar): 110 kcal

75 mL semi-skimmed milk: 36 kcal

20 blueberries or four pitted chopped red cherries: 16 kcal

150 mL glass of low-calorie cranberry juice: 10 kcal

Cup of tea or coffee with 20 mL semi-skimmed milk: 12 kcal

     Total kcal = 239

Orange or Grapefruit and all bran cereal with sliced banana

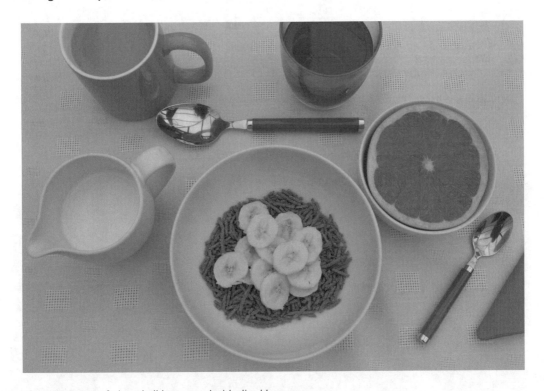

Photo 10.8: Grapefruit and all bran cereal with sliced banana.

Half a large orange or a small pink grapefruit: 45 kcal

35 g all bran cereal (no added sugar): 102 kcal

75 mL semi-skimmed milk: 36 kcal

Half a small banana, chopped into 10 thin slices: 44 kcal

Cup of tea or coffee with 20 mL semi-skimmed milk: 12 kcal

     Total kcal = 239

LUNCHES CONTAINING ABOUT 125 KCAL

Soups

Hot soups are also a suitable alternative for some meals. Half a can of soup (amounting to 200 g) such as pea and ham, lentil and bacon, chicken and vegetable, mulligatawny, minestrone, tomato, or mushroom normally contains about 100-130 kcal, 3-5 g fat, 10-20 g carbohydrate, 5-10 g protein, about 3-5 g fiber, and 1 g salt. The soups that contain a mixture of meat and vegetable tend to be the most nutritious.

Salads (without salad cream, mayonnaise, or coleslaw)

Lettuce/Rocket/Watercress/Spinach/Mixed (60 g): 15 kcal

Celery (two stalks, 100 g): 20 kcal

Tomato (one medium size, 120 g): 22 kcal

Thin sliced ham/chicken/turkey (two slices, diced, 50 g): 60 kcal

Juice from half a squeezed lime or lemon: 5 kcal

>   Total kcal = 122

Hummus and ham with celery

Celery (two stalks, 100 g): 20 kcal

Hummus (40 g): 60 kcal

Thin sliced ham (or chicken/turkey/beef; two slices, 50 g): 60 kcal

>   Total kcal = 140

LUNCHES CONTAINING ABOUT 250 KCAL

Tasty substantial soups with bread

As stated previously, hot soups are an excellent option, but you can also have some bread and a little extra protein can be added in the form of small pieces of sliced cold meats (about 25 g) to help ensure that daily protein requirements are met. Use wholegrain or wholemeal bread as these contain more micronutrients than processed bread. You can add up to 100 mL water to increase the volume of the soup, and adding a small amount (e.g., one teaspoon) of red or green pesto will help to thicken it and add extra flavor.

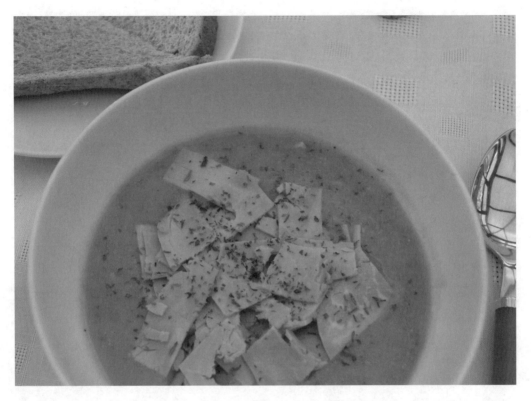

Photo 10.9: Pea and ham soup with added ham, green pesto, and mixed herbs.

Soup such as pea and ham, chicken and mushroom, lentil and bacon, or beef and tomato (200 g): 125 kcal

Thin sliced cooked ham/chicken/turkey/beef (one slice, diced, 25 g): 30 kcal

One teaspoon of red or green pesto: 20 kcal

Add sprinkle of mixed herbs or chili bits to add flavor

Wholemeal bread (one slice, 30 g): 70 kcal

> Total kcal = 245

Salads (without salad cream, mayonnaise, or coleslaw; add ground pepper, herbs, lemon juice to flavor) with bread

Mixed leaf salad with spring onion, green olives, and diced roast ham with a slice of toasted wholemeal bread

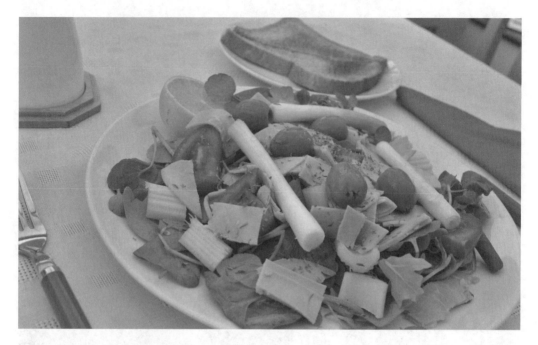

Photo 10.10: Mixed leaf salad with spring onion, green olives and diced roast ham with a slice of toasted wholemeal bread.

Lettuce/Rocket/Watercress/Spinach/Mixed (60 g): 15 kcal

Celery (two stalks, 100 g): 20 kcal

Tomato (one medium size, 120 g): 22 kcal

Five spring onions (small size, 10 cm long, 60 g): 25 kcal

Five pitted green olives: 25 kcal

Thin sliced ham/chicken/turkey (two slices, diced, 50 g): 60 kcal

Juice from half a squeezed lime or lemon: 5 kcal

Toasted wholemeal bread (one slice, 30 g): 70 kcal

     Total kcal = 242

DINNERS CONTAINING ABOUT 250 KCAL

Chicken with new potatoes and spinach

100 g lean skinless chicken breast or lean beefsteak (grilled): 135 kcal

60 g steamed spinach: 15 kcal

Celery (two stalks, chopped and steamed): 20 kcal

100 g steamed new potatoes: 75 kcal

Two slices of pickled beetroot: 5 kcal

Total kcal = 250

Bacon, mushroom, broccoli, celery, and tomato stir fry

Two rashers of lean bacon: 150 kcal

80 g sliced mushrooms: 20 kcal

50 g broccoli florets: 15 kcal

5 cherry tomatoes: 20 kcal

Celery (two stalks, chopped): 20 kcal

Total kcal = 225

Oven-baked cod loin with lemon and parsley accompanied by tenderstem broccoli, mangetout, and new potatoes

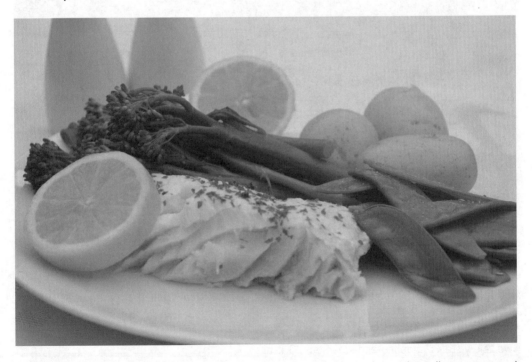

Photo 10.11: Oven-baked cod loin with lemon and parsley accompanied by tenderstem broccoli, mangetout, and new potatoes.

100 g cod fillet or cod loin (oven baked with lemon and parsley): 125 kcal

130 g steamed tenderstem broccoli: 35 kcal

60 g steamed mangetout (snow peas): 15 kcal

100 g steamed new potatoes: 75 kcal

      Total kcal = 250

DINNERS CONTAINING ABOUT 400 KCAL

Chicken breast, new potatoes, and vegetables with chopped mango for dessert

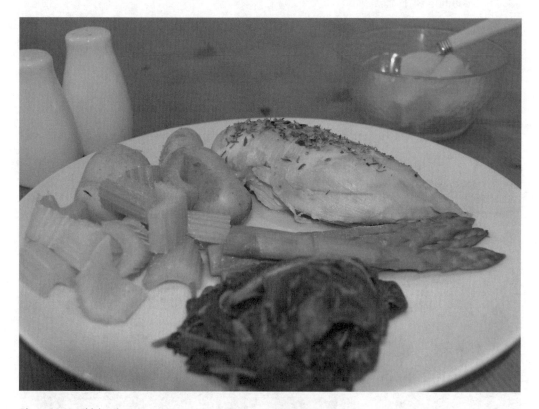

Photo 10.12: Chicken breast and vegetables with chopped mango for dessert.

150 g lean skinless chicken breast, lean beef steak, or lamb steak (grilled or pan-fried): 200 kcal

60 g steamed spinach: 15 kcal

Two celery stalks, chopped and steamed: 20 kcal

Five asparagus spears (medium size, 15 cm long, steamed): 15 kcal

BEATING TYPE

100 g steamed new potatoes: 75 kcal

80 g chopped mango: 73 kcal

      Total kcal = 398

Chicken and bacon casserole

150 g skinless, boneless chicken breast or thighs chopped into 6 pieces: 200 kcal

50 g lean bacon, chopped: 35 kcal

80 g tomato puree: 30 kcal

80 g small onions or shallots, whole and peeled: 30 kcal

60 g mushrooms, sliced: 15 kcal

120 g carrots, cut into chunks: 50 kcal

One stalk of celery, cut into chunks: 10 kcal

Sprinkle of mixed herbs (oregano, thyme, parsley, black peppercorns): 5 kcal

300 mL (10fl oz) water, plus one chicken stock cube: 20 kcal

Serve with 50 g sauerkraut: 5 kcal

      Total kcal = 400

Chicken saag curry

150 g skinless, boneless chicken breast or thighs chopped into 6 pieces: 200 kcal

One tablespoon of medium strength curry powder: 20 kcal

80 g tomato puree: 30 kcal

80 g onions peeled: 30 kcal

60 g mushrooms, sliced: 15 kcal

One red pepper (100 g), cut into chunks: 40 kcal

One stalk of celery, cut into chunks: 10 kcal

60 g spinach: 15 kcal

300 mL (10fl oz) water, plus one chicken stock cube: 20 kcal

Serve with 100 g fresh beansprouts: 30 kcal

      Total kcal = 410

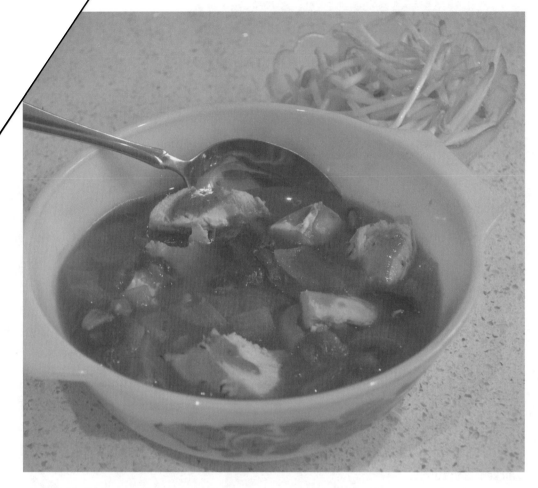

Photo 10.13: Chicken saag (with added spinach) curry served with beansprouts.

Beef steak with beetroot salad and corn on the cob

150 g grilled lean beef steak (e.g., sirloin or rump with fat removed): 280 kcal

10 cm length of corn on the cob: 80 kcal

50 g mixed salad leaves: 10 kcal

Five cherry tomatoes: 15 kcal

50 g finely chopped pickled beetroot: 30 kcal

      Total kcal: 415

For further meal ideas see: https://www.goodtoknow.co.uk/recipes/538311/5-2-diet-meal-plans-what-to-eat-for-500 caloric fast days

MEALS FOR "NONFASTING DAYS" ON THE INTERMITTENT FASTING 4:3 DIET

On the non-fasting days do not resort to eating unhealthy foods. A great idea is to have meals from the Mediterranean or Japanese diets on these days. Alternatively, try the occasional vegetarian meal or revert to a low glycemic index meal plan. Some example meal plans for the Mediterranean, Japanese, and vegetarian diets are as follows:

MEALS FOR THE MEDITERRANEAN DIET

Only meals suitable for lunches or dinners are shown below. For breakfast, choose fruit with an oat or wheat-based cereal with semi-skimmed milk, or an egg-based meal (e.g., scrambled or poached egg with toasted wholegrain bread or an omelet).

Beef stifado stew with onions and tomato served with salad leaves (400 kcal)

150 g of lean beef cubed, 80 grams of shallots, one medium chopped onion, one medium tomato cut into wedges, clove of garlic, vegetable stock cube, tablespoon of extra virgin olive oil, one tablespoon of red wine vinegar, one tablespoon of tomato puree, one bay leaf, teaspoon of dried rosemary, pinch of nutmeg, salt and black pepper. Serve with 50 g mixed salad leaves and a slice of wholegrain crusty bread.

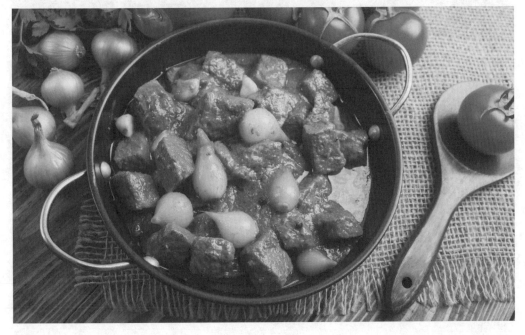

Photo 10.14: Beef stifado stew with onions and tomatoes.

Brown rice paella with peas, chicken, and seafood (500 kcal)

50 g chopped chicken thigh or breast, 50 g peeled prawns with one tablespoon of extra virgin olive oil, 50 g garden peas, one chopped red pepper, one chopped medium onion, and one vegetable stock cube with 100 mL water and 50 g (uncooked weight) brown rice. Sprinkle with parsley.

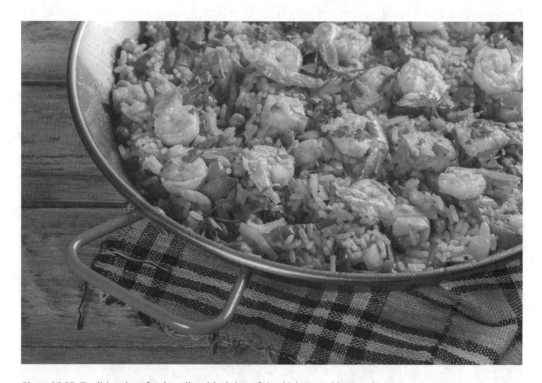

Photo 10.15: Traditional seafood paella with shrimp, fish, chicken, and brown rice.

Greek salad with tomato, cucumber, onion, feta cheese, olives, and lemon juice with a slice of wholegrain crusty bread (400 kcal)

Five olives, two large vine tomatoes cut into wedges, half a chopped red onion, 50 g cubed peeled cucumber, and 30 g feta cheese cut into chunks. Drizzled with one teaspoon of extra virgin olive oil, juice from half a lemon, and sprinkled with dried oregano. Serve with one slice of crusty wholegrain bread.

Grilled sardines, tomato, onion, and salad greens with wholegrain bread (250 kcal)

Same as for the Greek salad above but replace the feta cheese with 100 g of grilled sardines (or one small can of sardines in brine; you can use canned tuna or mackerel as an alternative to sardines).

Omelet with mixed vegetables and olives (340 kcal)

Two medium eggs cooked with one tablespoon of extra virgin olive oil, 60 g fresh spinach, two chopped tomatoes, four sliced mushrooms, one chopped red or green pepper, five pitted olives. Add a pinch of ground pepper and a sprinkling of herbs (e.g., chives, oregano, parsley, sage, or a mixture) to add flavor.

Grilled lamb, pork or chicken on a skewer with tomato, zucchini, onion, and peppers (400 kcal)

150 g of large cubes of lamb, pork, or chicken on two 25 cm (10 inch) skewers alternated with tomato, zucchini, onion, aubergine (eggplant), red, green, or yellow pepper.

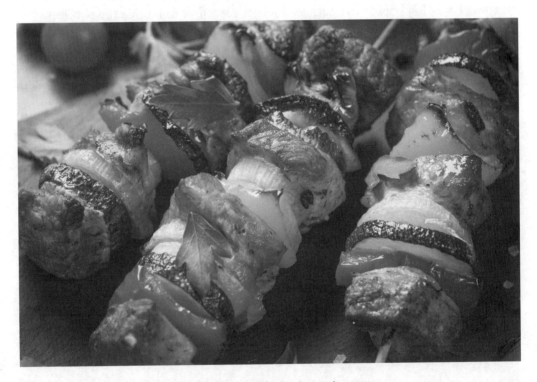

Photo 10.16: Grilled pork on skewers with tomato, zucchini, onion, and peppers.

Lean lamb mince with onion, diced aubergine (eggplant) and mashed sweet potato (500 kcal)

150 g of lean lamb mince, two medium chopped onions, two medium tomatoes cut into wedges, half an aubergine (eggplant) cut into chunks, one meat stock cube, one tablespoon of tomato puree. Serve with one large oven baked sweet potato, mashed.

Lean beef or lamb casserole with onions, tomato, aubergine (eggplant), and figs (400 kcal)

150 g of lean beef or lamb cut into cubes, 80 grams of shallots, one medium chopped onion, two medium tomatoes cut into wedges, half an aubergine (eggplant) cut into chunks, one tablespoon of extra virgin olive oil, one tablespoon of red wine vinegar, one tablespoon of tomato puree, one bay leaf, one dried fig.

MEALS FOR THE JAPANESE DIET

Only meals suitable for lunches or dinners are shown next. For dessert, just have a cup of chopped fruit such as apple, pear, peach, or melon which will contain about 100 kcal. For a 300-kcal breakfast, have 50 g smoked fish (such as mackerel, salmon, or eel) with a cup of boiled white rice. The Japanese prefer to use a short-grain glutinous white rice called "Koshihikari" which has short, round, opaque grains. It becomes quite sticky when cooked which gives it a firmer and chewier texture than other types of rice. But for the dishes described here, you can use any standard short-grain or medium-grain white rice. For some dishes you can have brown rice which comes from the same grains as white rice. The only difference is that brown rice has an outer layer of bran and the rice germ left on, and these layers give brown rice a delicious nutty flavor as well as an extra helping of vitamins and fiber. An alternative meal for a 200-kcal breakfast is to have fruit and an oat- or wheat-based cereal with semi-skimmed milk, or an egg-based meal (e.g., two poached eggs with toasted wholegrain bread or a two egg omelet with 50 g chopped mushrooms cooked together using a low-calorie olive oil spray in a small frying pan).

Miso chicken and rice soup (230 kcal)

400 mL Dashi stock, one tablespoon of miso paste, 100 g tofu (or pan-fried cubes of pork or chicken), two tablespoons of dry wakame, four sliced green shallots and 10 g (uncooked weight) white rice.

Spicy soup with seafood, prawns, vegetables, lime, parsley, and hot pepper (200 kcal)

50 g peeled prawns, 50 g small clams, 30 g chopped celery, 30 g water chestnuts or mushroom, one sliced lime, 20 g watercress, a little parsley, hot pepper powder or chili bits.

Salmon and avocado rice (500 kcal)

150 g oven baked salmon, broken up and mixed with chopped pieces of half an avocado and 100 g boiled short- or medium-grain white rice. Drizzle with one tablespoon of light reduced-salt soy sauce.

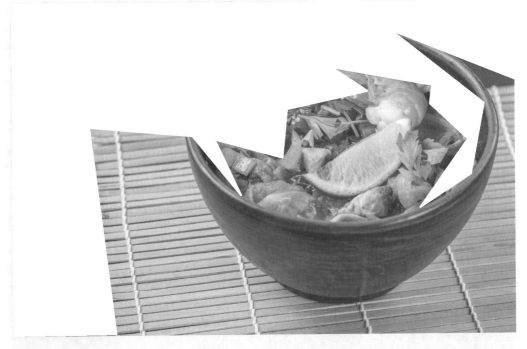

Photo 10.17: Japanese spicy soup with seafood, prawns, vegetables, lime, parsley, and hot pepper or chili.

Teriyaki noodle broth (200 kcal)

300 mL hot vegetable stock, one teaspoon of grated fresh root ginger, one tablespoon of teriyaki marinade or light reduced-salt soy sauce, pinch of Chinese five-spice powder, 70 g fresh stir-fry vegetables, 25 g mushrooms, 50 g skinless roast chicken chopped into small pieces, 30 g (uncooked weight) fine egg or rice noodles.

Soba noodle and edamame (soybean) salad with grilled tofu (350 kcal)

40 g soba noodles, 80 g fresh or frozen podded edamame (soy) beans, two shredded spring onions, 80 g beansprouts, one quarter of a cucumber, peeled and sliced, 70 g tofu, one teaspoon of olive oil, pinch of chopped fresh or dried coriander leaves. Topped with a dressing made from one tablespoon of mirin or sweet white wine, one teaspoon of tamari, one tablespoon of orange juice, pinch of chili bits.

Miso marinated salmon or chicken (300 kcal)

Two teaspoons of miso paste, one tablespoon of light reduced-salt soy sauce, one teaspoon of sesame oil, pinch of dried chili bits, ginger powder, and garlic granules, 150 g skinless chicken breast fillet or salmon fillet, one sliced carrot, two spring onions. Served with 20 g lettuce leaves.

...ng (300 kcal)

...quarters, 30g watercress, 200 g frozen shelled edamame (soy) ...into long matchsticks, 140 g radish thinly sliced and covered ...r using one tablespoon of rice wine vinegar, one tablespoon of ...a chopped small onion, one tablespoon of chopped sushi ginger, ...ée, one tablespoon of olive oil.

Chicken... with white rice (650 kcal)

175 g sliced rump... k or chicken breast, one tablespoon of Japanese soy sauce, one tablespoon of sake, two tablespoons of mirin (or a sweet white wine), one teaspoon of caster sugar or honey, one teaspoon of grated ginger, one garlic clove, crushed, one tablespoon of olive oil, one teaspoon of ground black pepper, one finely chopped small green chili. Serve with 100 g boiled white rice and 80 g broccoli or 40 g watercress.

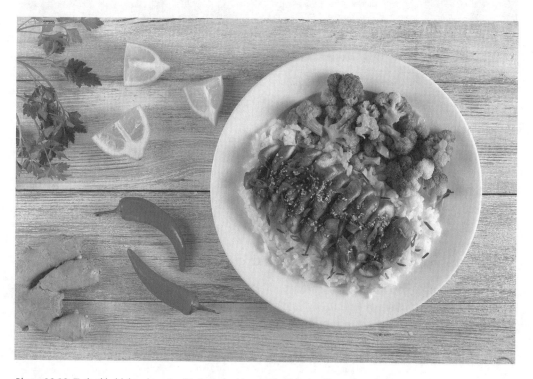

Photo 10.18: Teriyaki chicken breast with boiled white rice and broccoli.

Stir fry with chicken, mushrooms, broccoli, and peppers (300 kcal)

150 g chopped chicken breast, 50 g mushrooms, 80 g broccoli, and one chopped red/green/yellow pepper.

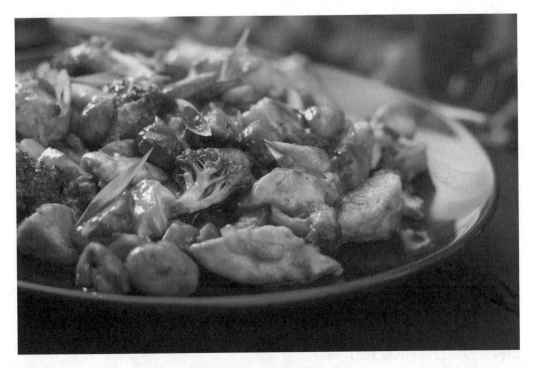

Photo 10.19: Stir fry with chicken, mushrooms, broccoli, and peppers.

Miso brown rice and chicken salad (250 kcal)

60 g boiled brown basmati rice, 150 g skinless chicken breast, 70 g sprouting broccoli, two diced spring onions, one teaspoon of toasted sesame seeds. Topped with a dressing made of one teaspoon of miso paste, one tablespoon of rice vinegar, one tablespoon of mirin or sweet white wine, and one teaspoon of grated ginger.

Japanese-style brown rice (350 kcal)

70 g boiled brown basmati rice, 50 g frozen soya beans, one teaspoon of light reduced-salt soy sauce, one teaspoon of extra virgin olive oil, one teaspoon of finely grated ginger, pinch of garlic granules, two diced spring onions.

DESSERTS FOR THE JAPANESE OR MEDITERRANEAN DIETS (ALL LESS THAN 200 KCAL)

Cup of mixed chopped fruits (e.g., apple, grapes, persimmon, nectarine, melon, cherries) with Greek yogurt and walnuts.

120 g chopped watermelon with a dozen grapes.

120 g slice of Honeydew or Piel de Sapo (frog skin) melon sprinkled with ginger powder.

Peeled orange segments (from one medium-sized orange) with 20 blueberries.

One dark chocolate coated 50 g piece of vanilla ice cream (choc-ice).

One 50 g piece of chocolate ice cream sprinkled with one tablespoon of unsweetened shredded coconut.

MEALS FOR THE VEGETARIAN DIET

Some of the following vegetarian meals include dairy products (e.g., semi-skimmed milk, cheese, yogurt) or eggs, so are not suitable for vegans. Meals that contain no animal products that are suitable for vegans are indicated by a "(V)". Skimmed milk can be used instead of semi-skimmed milk or plant-based alternatives such as almond milk, soymilk, or rice milk can also be used if preferred and plant-based syrup sweeteners can replace honey.

Breakfasts (200-400 kcal)

Porridge oats (30 g) made with 100 mL semi-skimmed milk, and topped with a tablespoon of honey and 20 raisins (260 kcal).

One cup of blueberries, cranberries, raisins, or sultanas with one cup of low-fat Greek yogurt and a quarter of a cup of crushed almonds, pecans, or walnuts (400 kcal).

Two whole-wheat biscuits (such as Shredded Wheat, Weetabix, or Oatibix) with 100 mL semi-skimmed milk and 10 medium-sized strawberries (220 kcal).

Fruit smoothie – one large ripe banana, 300 mL cranberry juice (no added sugar version), and 100 g frozen mixed red berries blended together and served with an English muffin toasted and spread with jam or marmite (V), (350 kcal).

Half a pink grapefruit or orange followed by 50 g swiss style muesli (no added sugar) with 100 mL semi-skimmed milk and 20 blueberries or four pitted chopped red cherries. An alternative cereal is 35 g all bran cereal (no added sugar) with 75 mL semi-skimmed milk and half a banana, chopped into 12 thin slices (270 kcal).

Two scrambled eggs made with 50 mL skimmed milk and two teaspoons of margarine with four steamed asparagus spears and half a small avocado, sliced. Serve with one slice of rye crispbread (400 kcal).

Two egg omelet with one tablespoon of extra virgin olive oil, 30 g grated cheese, and one whole sliced red pepper. Add a pinch of ground pepper and a sprinkling of herbs (e.g., chives, oregano, parsley, sage, or a mixture) to the omelet for more flavor (390 kcal).

Two egg omelet with one tablespoon of extra virgin olive oil, 60 g fresh spinach, and two tomatoes. Add a pinch of ground pepper and a sprinkling of herbs (e.g., chives, oregano, parsley, sage, or a mixture) to the omelet for more flavor. Serve with one slice of rye crisp bread (360 kcal).

One large mashed banana on two thick slices of toasted wholemeal bread (V), (260 kcal).

Lunches (300-400 kcal)

Goat's cheese salad made with 80 g salad leaves, five olives, five cherry tomatoes, half a sliced ripe avocado, 50 g cubed cucumber, and 50 g crumbled goat's cheese. Drizzled with juice from half a lemon. Serve with one piece of rye bread or cracker (400 kcal).

Greek salad including five olives, two large vine tomatoes cut into wedges, half a chopped red onion, 50 g cubed peeled cucumber, 30 g feta cheese cut into chunks, 50 g baby spinach leaves and half a sliced small ripe avocado). Drizzled with one teaspoon of extra virgin olive oil and sprinkled with dried oregano (400 kcal).

One large baked potato served with 30 g cottage cheese and 30 g sauerkraut, and a 30 g mixed leaf side salad with juice from half a squeezed lemon or lime (350 kcal).

Half a can (200 g) of baked beans on two slices of toasted wholemeal bread (V), (300 kcal).

Macaroni cheese made with 30 g low-fat cheddar, one cup of boiled macaroni pasta, and 150 ml semi-skimmed milk. Served with 50 g chopped steamed asparagus and 50 g broccoli (380 kcal).

Sandwich made with two thick slices of wholemeal bread with one teaspoon of margarine, 40 g hummus, and plenty of vegetables like lettuce, cucumbers, watercress, and tomatoes (V), (300 kcal).

Vegetable soups are also a suitable alternative for some meals. Half a can of a vegetarian soup (200 g) such as lentil, tomato and red pepper, mixed vegetable, minestrone, butternut squash, tomato, or mushroom normally contains about 100-130 kcal, 3-5 g fat, 10-20 g carbohydrate, 4-8 g protein, about 3-5 g fiber and 1 g salt. To provide extra protein and calories, add half a cup of cooked mixed beans and serve with one crusty wholegrain bread roll. You can add up to 100 mL water to increase the volume of the soup and adding a small amount (e.g., one teaspoon) of red or green pesto will help to thicken it and add extra flavor (V).

Dinners (600-800 kcal, including dessert)

The following main courses can be followed with a 200-kcal dessert consisting of one cup of chopped apple, pear, persimmon, melon, or watermelon with 10 grapes, cherries, or blueberries (V), two tablespoons of low-fat yogurt, a sprinkling of two crushed walnuts or six almonds.

Brown rice paella with mixed beans, peas, onion, and tofu

100 g tofu, 100 g canned mixed beans, 50 g garden peas, one chopped red pepper, one chopped medium onion and 100 g (uncooked weight) brown rice cooked in a frying pan with one tablespoon of extra virgin olive oil and one vegetable stock cube dissolved in 150 mL water. Sprinkle with parsley (V), (600 kcal)

Omelet with mixed vegetables and olives

Three medium eggs with one tablespoon of extra virgin olive oil, 60 g fresh spinach, two chopped tomatoes, one chopped onion, five chopped mushrooms, one chopped red or green pepper, and five pitted olives. Add a sprinkling of ground black pepper and herbs (e.g., chives, oregano, parsley, sage, or a mixture) to add flavor (470 kcal).

Cottage pie

Made with Quorn (150 g), 50 g peas, 50 g carrots, two tomatoes, one vegetable stock cube, two teaspoons of marmite, 150 mL water. Place 200 g mashed potato on top and oven bake. Serve with 50 g red cabbage (V), (470 kcal).

Mixed vegetable rice risotto

Made with 15 g margarine, one finely chopped garlic clove, half a cup of dry Arborio rice, one vegetable stock cube dissolved in 150 mL boiling water, 50 g canned chickpeas, drained and rinsed, 100 g mixed fresh vegetables, such as asparagus, diced red pepper, baby corn, onion, aubergine (eggplant), button mushroom slices, broccoli, courgette (zucchini), mangetout (snow peas), pinch of salt and black pepper, one tablespoon of chopped fresh herbs, such as parsley or thyme (V). Non-vegans can add one tablespoon of grated hard Italian cheese (550 kcal).

Spaghetti Bolognese

Made with 200 g Quorn, 200 g Bolognese sauce, 60 g cannellini beans, half a can of chopped tomatoes, garlic, and 75 g boiled whole-wheat spaghetti (V), (650 kcal).

Spicy Linguini Carbonara

Made with 100 g Quorn, 100 g Carbonara sauce (contains egg and milk), 60 g cannellini beans, 60 g chopped shallots, 30 g grated cheddar cheese, garlic, chili, and 100 g boiled linguini pasta. After cooking sprinkle on one tablespoon of grated hard Italian cheese (660 kcal).

Thai vegetable curry

Made with one red pepper, half of a finely chopped red onion, 100 g butternut squash or aubergine (eggplant), one tablespoon of Thai red curry paste, one vegetable stock cube dissolved in 150 mL boiling water, one tablespoon of sushi ginger, 30 g spinach, 30 g tomato puree, juice of one lime, coriander leaves to garnish. Serve with 100 g boiled medium-grain white rice and one small naan bread (V), (550 kcal).

MEALS FOR THE REDUCED FAT DIET

The reduced fat diet typically provides a total of 1,500 kcal/day with about 10% fat or no more than 20 g/day fat. From the listed meals below choose one breakfast, one lunch, and one dinner per day.

BREAKFASTS (250-350 KCAL)

Two whole-wheat biscuits (such as Shredded Wheat, Weetabix, or Oatibix) with 100 mL semi-skimmed milk and 10 medium-sized strawberries (250 kcal).

Porridge oats (30 g) made with 100 mL semi-skimmed milk and topped with a tablespoon of honey and 20 raisins (260 kcal).

Fruit smoothie – one large ripe banana, 300 mL cranberry juice (no added sugar version), and 100 frozen mixed red berries blended together and served with an English muffin, toasted and spread with a "light" spread or marmite (350 kcal).

Lean bacon sandwich – two slices of lean back bacon, trimmed of all fat and grilled or microwaved. Served between two slices of wholemeal bread or in a toasted bun with one finely chopped tomato (260 kcal).

Kedgeree made from 100 g poached smoked haddock, 100 g boiled brown rice ,and one tablespoon of curry paste or red pesto, topped with one sliced hardboiled egg (320 kcal).

Muesli (50 g) comprising rolled oats, wheat flakes, and a variety of dried fruits (e.g., cranberries, raisins, sultanas) served with low-fat yogurt and topped with a large strawberry (280 kcal).

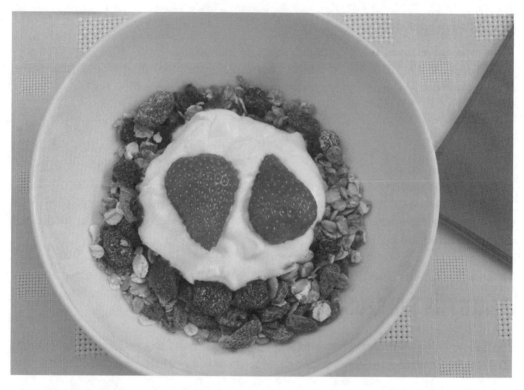

Photo 10.20: Muesli comprising rolled oats, wheat flakes, dried raisins, and sultanas, served with low-fat yogurt and topped with strawberry.

LUNCHES (300-400 KCAL)

One baked potato served with 30 g cottage cheese and 30 g sauerkraut, and a 30 g mixed leaf side salad with juice from half of a squeezed lemon or lime (340 kcal).

Chunky vegetable soup (300 mL) and a crusty wholegrain bread roll (340 kcal).

Sandwich consisting of two slices of wholemeal bread with 40 g lean ham, 30 g grated cheddar cheese, and watercress, or 40 g tinned tuna, 30 g grated cheddar cheese, and sliced cucumber (340 kcal).

Half a can of baked beans on two slices of toasted wholemeal bread (300 kcal).

Tagliatelle pasta (100 g) with one cup of tomato sauce and 40 g finely chopped roast ham or chicken pieces (300 kcal).

Mixed salad leaves with 100 g penne pasta, half a cup of tomato sauce, and 100 g roast chicken pieces (390 kcal).

DINNERS (600-800 KCAL)

Poached or grilled white fish (180 g) served with 200 g new potatoes and 50 g peas (340 kcal).

Cottage pie made with Quorn or very lean minced beef (150 g), 100 g mashed potato, 50 g peas, 50 g carrots, two tomatoes, one vegetable stock cube, two teaspoons of marmite, 150 mL water. Place 200 g mashed potato on top and oven bake. Serve with 50 g red cabbage (470 kcal).

Stir-fried 150 g pork tenderloin with chopped onion, one green pepper, 30 g mushrooms, and 100 g (uncooked weight) egg noodles (710 kcal).

Burger made with lean mince (150 g) and on finely chopped onion with one tablespoon of chili sauce and 20 g sauerkraut. Served on a wholemeal bread cob (710 kcal).

Mixed vegetable and fish rice risotto made with 15 g half fat butter, 100 g diced cod loin one finely chopped garlic clove, half a cup of dry Arborio rice, one vegetable stock cube dissolved in 150 mL boiling water, 50 g canned chickpeas, drained and rinsed, 100 g mixed fresh vegetables, such as asparagus, diced red pepper, baby corn, onion, aubergine (eggplant), button mushroom slices, broccoli, courgette (zucchini), mangetout (snow peas), pinch of salt and black pepper, one tablespoon of chopped fresh herbs, such as parsley or thyme, 10 g hard Italian cheese (590 kcal).

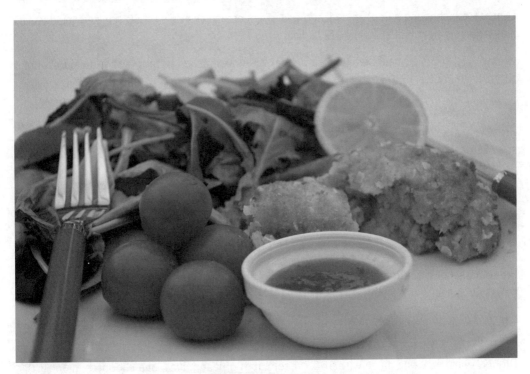

Photo 10.21: Cod and prawn Thai-style fishcake with mixed leaf salad, cherry tomatoes, and sweet chili sauce.

Chicken saag curry (see earlier recipe) with 50 g beansprouts and 120 g boiled brown or white rice (550 kcal).

Oven-baked cod and prawn Thai-style fishcake (buy ready-made one, 250 g size, from supermarket cold cabinet) served with 50 g mixed leaf salad, five cherry tomatoes, and a sweet chili sauce (460 kcal).

DAILY MEAL PLANS FOR THE HIGH-PROTEIN DIET

The high-protein diet typically provides a total of 1,400 to 1,500 kcal/day with 30-35% protein or 100-130 g/day protein. The sample daily meal plans below, each provide about 110 grams of protein per day and no more than 1,500 kcal. However, you can adjust the portions to meet your needs or add a 200-kcal dessert such as 40 g cheese with three cream crackers, a cup of Greek yogurt containing 10 crushed strawberries, or a 60 g slice of sponge cake.

Breakfast: Three eggs, one slice wholegrain toast with one tablespoon of almond butter, and a medium pear (500 kcal).

Lunch: Fresh chopped half of an avocado and 30 g cottage cheese with 30 g mixed salad leaves and segments from half an orange (220 kcal).

Dinner: 170 g grilled beef steak or lamb steak, one oven baked potato, and a grilled chopped zucchini (courgette) (530 kcal).

Breakfast: One cup of low-fat yogurt, one tablespoon of shredded dessicated coconut, and five strawberries (210 kcal).

Lunch: 120 g canned salmon, mixed greens, one tablespoon of extra virgin olive oil and vinegar, and an apple (400 kcal).

Dinner: 170 g grilled chicken with quinoa and Brussels sprouts (550 kcal).

Breakfast: Half a cup of oatmeal and half a cup of low-fat yogurt with six chopped pecan nut halves (300 kcal).

Lunch: 120 g grilled chicken mixed with half a chopped ripe avocado and red bell pepper, and a peach (470 kcal).

Dinner: Chili con carne made with 100 g beef cubes or lean mince, one chopped onion, 100 g red kidney beans, half a can of chopped tomatoes, and one tablespoon of chili powder. Served with 120 g boiled white or brown rice (620 kcal).

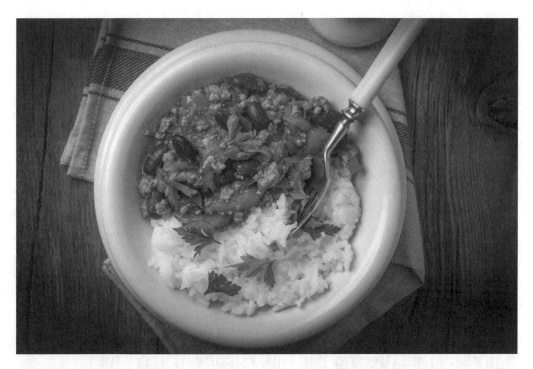

Photo 10.22: Chili con carne made with lean minced beef, accompanied by boiled white rice.

Breakfast: Spanish omelet made with three eggs, one tablespoon of extra virgin olive oil, 30 g cottage cheese, one chopped chili pepper, five pitted black olives, and a tablespoon of salsa (400 kcal).

Lunch: Two celery stalks each filled with 30 g cottage cheese and wrapped in thin sliced 25 g piece of roast chicken, ham, or beef with two slices of wholegrain bread (330 kcal).

Dinner: 180 g halibut, 100 g boiled lentils, 100 g steamed broccoli, and 100 g steamed new potatoes (430 kcal).

Breakfast: One cup of cottage cheese with a quarter of a cup of chopped walnuts, diced apples, and cinnamon (390 kcal).

Lunch: 120 g canned salmon mixed with one tablespoon of low-fat yogurt on sprouted grain bread, and carrot sticks (290 kcal).

Dinner: 170 g grilled chicken breast (skin removed) wrapped in two slices Parma ham. Served with one oven baked potato, 80 g sliced zucchini, 100 g chopped leeks or celeriac, mashed with one teaspoon of butter (740 kcal).

Breakfast: Omelet made with three eggs, one tablespoon of extra virgin olive oil, 30 g cottage cheese, and half a cup of diced boiled potatoes, and one chopped onion (480 kcal).

Lunch: 75 g thin sliced ham with tomato and mixed salad leaves, and an apple (230 kcal).

Dinner: 150 g king prawn fajitas with grilled onions and bell peppers, guacamole, one cup of black beans on a corn tortilla (520 kcal).

Breakfast: Two scrambled eggs made with 50 mL semi-skimmed milk and two teaspoons of margarine and one chopped green pepper and one diced 25 g slice of cooked ham. Serve with one slice of toasted wholegrain bread (380 kcal).

Lunch: One cup of plain Greek yogurt mixed with a quarter of a cup of chopped mixed nuts and one cup of diced pineapple (400 kcal).

Dinner: 200 g grilled salmon, 200 g boiled new potatoes, and 50 g sautéed spinach with a teaspoon of butter (500 kcal).

DAILY MEAL PLANS FOR THE LOW ENERGY DENSITY DIET

The low energy density diet provides a total of 1,300 to 1,500 kcal/day with an energy density of less than 1.5 kcal/g. The diet contains 25-30% protein with low-fat (less than 30 g/day) and limited carbohydrate (less than 130 g/day). Here are some low energy density meals that you might like to try. You could also try adapting your own favorite dishes to reduce their energy density too. The main principle is to avoid fatty foods or use reduced fat versions of foods like cheese and milk, use only lean meat and fish, and include lots of fruit and non-starchy vegetables. Most vegetables have an energy density less than 1.0 kcal/g (e.g., salad leaves and spinach are only 0.2 kcal/g, carrots and most gourds are 0.4 kcal/g, and beans are about 0.9 kcal/g). Using the principles of energy density you can achieve a lower calorie intake which will help towards weight loss, whilst allowing you to continue to enjoy generous portions of food and get an overall balanced diet. Essentially you are reducing the number of calories in a meal and increasing the size of it by weight (total grams of food on your plate) and volume by lowering the amount of fat while increasing the amount of water and fiber rich ingredients.

BREAKFASTS WITH LOW ENERGY DENSITY AND FEWER THAN 250 KCAL

Half a pink grapefruit followed by 35 g swiss style muesli (no added sugar) with 75 mL semi-skimmed milk and 20 blueberries or six seedless green grapes (220 kcal).

Half a large orange followed by 35 g all bran cereal (no added sugar) with 75 mL semi-skimmed milk and six seedless red grapes (230 kcal).

Cup of seedless grapes followed by two Weetabix with 75 mL semi-skimmed milk.

300 mL (11 fl oz) fruit smoothie made with fruit, nonfat yogurt, and crushed ice (280 kcal).

LUNCHES WITH LOW ENERGY DENSITY AND FEWER THAN 250 KCAL

Half a can of soup (200 g) such as pea and ham, lentil and bacon, chicken and vegetable, mulligatawny, minestrone, tomato, or mushroom. Add small pieces (about 40 g) of sliced cold meats (e.g., ham, turkey, chicken, or beef) to help ensure that daily protein requirements are met. Serve with one slice of wholegrain or wholemeal bread (300 kcal).

Macaroni cheese made with 30 g low-fat cheddar, one cup of boiled macaroni pasta, and 150 ml semi-skimmed milk. Served with 50 g chopped steamed asparagus and 50 g broccoli (380 kcal).

Half a small tin of chopped tuna in pitta bread, stuffed with mixed salad leaves and chopped tomato (300 kcal).

Sandwich made with two thick slices of wholemeal bread with one teaspoon of margarine, 40 g hummus or lean sliced meat, and plenty of vegetables like lettuce, cucumbers, onion, and tomatoes (300 kcal).

Green salad made with 20 g mixed salad leaves (e.g., lettuce, rocket, spinach, watercress), two celery stalks, two tomatoes, five spring onions, five pitted green olives, and drizzled with juice from half a squeezed lime or lemon. Served with two diced 25 g slices of cold meat (e.g., ham, chicken, turkey, or beef) and one slice of wholemeal bread (260 kcal).

Greek salad made with five olives, two large vine tomatoes cut into wedges, half a chopped red onion, 50 g cubed peeled cucumber, 10 g watercress, 30 g feta cheese cut into chunks and half a small sliced ripe avocado. Drizzled with one teaspoon of extra virgin olive oil and sprinkled with dried oregano (400 kcal).

DINNERS WITH LOW ENERGY DENSITY AND FEWER THAN 800 KCAL

Spaghetti Bolognese made with 200 g lean mince, 200 g reduced calorie Bolognese sauce, 60 g cannellini beans, half a can of chopped tomatoes, garlic, and 75 g wholewheat spaghetti (650 kcal).

200 g grilled lean meat (e.g., beefsteak, chicken breast, pork tenderloin) with your choice of three of the following steamed vegetables: 100 g cauliflower, broccoli, aubergine (eggplant), mangetout, zucchini (courgette), spinach, cabbage, or kale. Serve with 120 g boiled penne pasta or boiled brown rice (500 kcal).

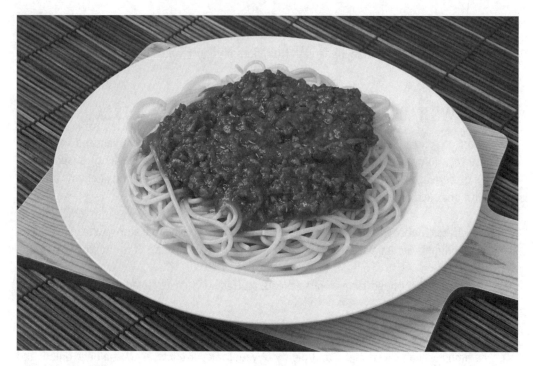

Photo 10.23: Spaghetti Bolognese.

Chili con carne made with 100 g beef cubes or lean mince, one chopped onion, 100 g red kidney beans, half a can of chopped tomatoes, and one tablespoon of chili powder. Served with 120 g boiled white or brown rice (620 kcal).

180 g oven baked cod fillet or cod loin with lemon and parsley, accompanied by 60 g steamed mangetout, 130 g steamed tenderstem broccoli, and 100 g steamed cauliflower (270 kcal).

Chicken saag curry (see recipe described earlier in this chapter) served with 50 g beansprouts and 120 g boiled brown rice (550 kcal).

Two whole, oven-baked red peppers, deseeded and stuffed with 100 g lean minced beef or lamb, one chopped onion, and two chopped tomatoes. Served with 150 g steamed sliced zucchini (courgette) and a wedge of crusty wholegrain bread (420 kcal).

Oven baked casserole with 150 g cubed lean lamb, beef, pork, or chicken breast accompanied by 100 g sliced aubergine (eggplant), one diced onion, 50 g sliced mushrooms, 50 g carrot, meat stock cube dissolved in 150 mL water, and one tablespoon of paprika (420 kcal).

For 100 kcal desserts have one cup of chopped fruit (e.g., apple, grapes, orange, persimmon, plums, melon, or mango) or a cup containing a mixture of two or three different fruits topped with a tablespoon of low-fat yogurt.

Key Points

- Low GI or GL diets are not designed for weight loss and there are other diets that are far more effective for this purpose. If you are at risk for diabetes or have prediabetes, type 2 diabetes, or the metabolic syndrome, then incorporating the GI principle into your meal planning may help you keep your blood glucose levels in check.

- Very low energy diets with specially formulated liquid meals are designed to provide about 800 kcal/day with sufficient protein and micronutrients to meet minimum daily requirements. Soups with added chopped meat or meals with relatively low fat and carbohydrate content are suitable alternatives if such diets are only used intermittently for a few days per week.

- The energy intake on the semi-fasting days of the 4:3 intermittent fasting diet is limited to 500-600 kcal/day and will almost certainly not provide sufficient protein and micronutrients to meet minimum daily requirements. This can be compensated for by having a high-protein dinner on the day before the semi-fasting day and a high-protein breakfast on the day after. A multivitamin and mineral supplement is advised if the intention is to stay on this type of diet for more than one month.

- Other diets that supply a total of about 1,500 kcal/day, are high in either fat or carbohydrate but supply at least 15% of calories as protein, should provide sufficient protein and micronutrients to meet minimum daily requirements.

- For the low energy density diet you reduce the number of calories in a meal and increase the size of it by weight (total grams of food on your plate) and volume by lowering the amount of fat in a meal and by increasing the amount of water and fiber rich ingredients like fruit and non-starchy vegetables. An advantage of low energy density foods is that the fewer calories a food contains, the more of it you can eat. This helps keep you from the hunger pangs that are many a diet's downfall.

- When dieting you should avoid drinking any sugar-sweetened beverages, milkshakes, creamy or milky hot drinks, and alcohol. Stick to water, artificially sweetened "low calorie", "diet", or "light" versions of fruit flavored soft drinks, mixers, and cordials. You can still drink coffee or tea, but use a zero calorie artificial sweetener instead of sugar, and skimmed or semi-skimmed milk instead of whole milk or cream.

My Final Message to You

Being diagnosed with type 2 diabetes can come as a shock. It certainly was to me. I didn't think I was unfit or particularly overweight at that time. I have a fairly slight build with rather skinny arms and legs. Yes, I had a bit of belly fat, but nowhere near as much as some, and I just put that down to drinking a little too much alcohol. Being an academic can actually be quite a stressful job at times – standing in front of over 200 students to give a lecture, organizing research and trying to secure funding to keep it going, writing papers, review articles, and books, marking exams, travelling to conferences, giving talks about your research to an audience of critical scientists, sometimes having heated debates with your fellow scientists, as well as the tedium of marking seemingly endless coursework assignments and exam papers (often within tight deadlines) and attending long meetings. There is always pressure to publish and bring in money. Well I had been for my annual health check at my local doctor's clinic – something I had been doing since I was diagnosed with high blood pressure several years previously – and a week later got a letter asking me to revisit the clinic to discuss my results. It was then that I was told that tests on my blood had revealed that I had developed type 2 diabetes; in other words, my HbA1c level had gone above 48 mmol/mol or 6.5%. I was advised to change my diet, do more exercise, and lose some weight; otherwise I would soon have to go on some medication to help control my blood sugar level. I realized then that I was actually about 10 kg or 15% above my ideal healthy body weight and discovered that it is possible to cure type 2 diabetes without the need for medication, and that is what I set out to do.

I succeeded, and what's more, it took me less than six months to get my type 2 diabetes into remission. Just by becoming more physically active, dieting to lose my excess weight, and then sticking to a healthier low energy density diet and cutting down my wine and beer consumption. Five years ago, when I was first diagnosed with type 2 diabetes, my body weight was close to 80 kg with a BMI of 27.0 kg/m². My current weight is 67 kg and my BMI is 22.7. My diabetes is in remission, and I intend to keep it that way.

My mission to get rid of my type 2 diabetes by self-help succeeded, and yours can, too. I hope that my book will help you. But you must act now. Do something about it. Follow the guidelines I have given in this book. Beat your type 2 diabetes. Good luck.

Glossary

absorption—The transport of nutrients from the intestine into the blood or lymph system.

acanthosis nigricans—A condition in which areas of darkened skin start to appear in the folds and creases of the body — usually in the armpits, groin and neck. The condition occurs in some people with type 2 diabetes and may be a sign of insulin resistance as it is caused by high levels of insulin in the blood which stimulate the growth of cells in the outer layer of the skin.

ad libitum—As much as desired (e.g., in regard to eating, how much a person eats when given free access to food).

adenosine triphosphate (ATP)—A high-energy compound that is the immediate source for muscular contraction and other energy-requiring processes in the cell.

adipocyte—An adipose tissue cell whose main function is to store triaglyceride (fat).

adipokine—Chemical messenger molecule secreted from adipose (white fat) tissue.

adiponectin— A hormone-like protein which is produced by adipose tissue and is involved in regulating blood glucose levels as well as fatty acid breakdown. The actions of adiponectin increase insulin sensitivity by increasing fatty acid oxidation and inhibiting liver glucose production. These actions lower circulating fatty acid and glucose levels, respectively.

adipose tissue—White fatty tissue that stores triglyceride.

aerobic—Occurring in the presence of free oxygen.

aerobic capacity—The highest rate of oxygen consumption by the body that can be determined in an incremental exercise test to exhaustion. Also known as maximal oxygen uptake.

aerobic exercise—Dynamic physical activity at an intensity below that which elicits the maximum oxygen uptake (aerobic capacity) that can be sustained for long periods. Also known as cardio or endurance exercise.

aerobic metabolism—The resynthesis of ATP using the energy generated from the oxidation of predominantly fat and/or carbohydrate.

albumin—The most abundant protein found in human plasma. Its presence in urine is abnormal and is an indicator of kidney inflammation or disease.

alcohol—A colorless liquid that has depressant and intoxicating effects. Ethyl alcohol or ethanol (C_2H_5OH) is the alcohol found in wines, spirits, and beers.

Alzheimer's disease—A progressive mental deterioration that can occur in middle or old age, due to generalized degeneration of the brain. It is the commonest cause of premature senility.

amino acid—The chief structural molecule of protein, consisting of an amino group (NH_2) and a carboxylic acid group (CO_2H), plus another so-called R-group (an organic side chain) that determines the properties of the amino acid. Twenty different amino acids can be used to make proteins.

anaerobic—Occurring in the absence of free oxygen.

anaerobic exercise—Very high-intensity physical activity that does not require the use of oxygen as it relies on muscle ATP and phosphocreatine as fuel (e.g., all out sprinting). This type of exercise can only be sustained for a matter of seconds. Anaerobic exercise may also sometimes be used to describe exercise in which anaerobic metabolism provides the major portion of the energy needed (e.g., exercising at a high intensity that can be sustained for only a few minutes).

anorexia nervosa—An eating disorder characterized by abnormally small food intake and refusal to maintain a normal body weight (according to what is expected for gender, age, and height), a distorted view of body image, an intense fear of being fat or overweight and gaining weight or "feeling fat" when clearly the person is below normal weight, and the absence of at least three successive menstrual cycles in women (amenorrhea).

antioxidant—Molecules that can prevent or limit the actions of free radicals, usually by removing their unpaired electron and converting them into something far less reactive.

apoB/apoA-I ratio—The ratio of two apolipoproteins in the blood (i.e., the serum apolipoprotein B concentration divided by the apolipoprotein A-I concentration) which represents the balance of pro-atherogenic and anti-atherogenic lipoproteins. It is known to be superior to any of the cholesterol ratios in predicting risk of coronary heart disease.

apolipoprotein—Proteins that bind fats (lipids) to form a complex of triglycerides, cholesterol, and protein called lipoproteins that are used to transport fats through the lymphatic and circulatory systems.

appetite—A desire for food for the purpose of enjoyment that is developed through previous experience. Controlled in humans by an appetite center in the hypothalamus.

arteriosclerosis—Hardening of the arteries. See also atherosclerosis.

arthritis—A common condition that causes pain and inflammation in a joint. Arthritis can be caused by a form of autoimmune disease.

atherogenic—Something that promotes the development of atherosclerosis (hardening of the arteries).

atherosclerosis—Hardening of the arteries. Also known as arteriosclerosis. It is caused by high blood pressure, smoking, or high blood cholesterol damaging the internal lining of the blood vessels. That damage leads to the formation of plaque.

Atkins diet—A very low-carbohydrate diet which is used for weight loss.

basal metabolic rate—Energy expenditure under basal, overnight fasted conditions representing the energy needed to maintain life under these basal conditions.

bile—Fluid produced by the liver and stored in the gall bladder that contains bile salts, bile pigments, cholesterol, and other molecules. The bile is secreted into the small intestine where it helps to emulsify fats to aid their digestion by enzymes such as pancreatic lipase.

binge eating disorder—An eating disorder in which a person feels compelled to consume a lot of food in a short period of time and is accompanied by feelings of loss of control, and in many cases, guilt and embarrassment.

bioelectrical impedance analysis (BIA)—A method to calculate percentage of body fat by measuring electrical resistance due to the water content of the body.

body fat—Throughout this book the term "body fat" or "body fat tissue" is used to refer to white adipose tissue which comprises, on average, 87% fat (mostly as triglyceride), 10% water, and 3% protein by weight.

body mass—Body weight expressed in kilograms. Often used by scientists instead of body weight.

body mass index (BMI)—Body mass in kilograms divided by height in meters squared (kg/m^2). An index used as a measure of obesity.

bulimia nervosa—An eating disorder characterized by repeated episodes of binge eating (consumption of large amounts of usually energy-dense foods) followed by purging of the stomach contents, allowing insufficient time for most of the nutrients from the heavy meal to be absorbed.

caffeine—A stimulant drug found in many food products such as coffee, tea, and cola drinks. Stimulates the central nervous system and used as an ergogenic aid to improve sport performance. Caffeine also improves concentration and cognitive function when fatigued.

calorie (cal)—Traditional unit of energy. One calorie expresses the quantity of energy (heat) needed to raise the temperature of 1 g (1 mL) of water 1 °C (e.g., from 14.5 °C to 15.5 °C).

carbohydrate—A compound composed of carbon, hydrogen, and oxygen in a ratio of 1:2:1 (e.g., CH_2O). Carbohydrates include sugars, starches, and dietary fibers.

carcinogenic—A cancer-inducing substance.

carotenoid—Plant pigments responsible for bright red, yellow, and orange hues in many fruits and vegetables. Carotenoids are a class of phytonutrients and are found in the cells of a wide variety of plants.

catechin—A type of natural plant phenol and antioxidant that belongs to the flavanol group of compounds, part of the chemical family of flavonoids.

cell—The smallest discrete living unit of the body.

cellulitis—A potentially serious bacterial infection of the deeper layers of skin that can be painful. Cellulitis may first appear as a red, swollen area that feels hot and tender to the touch. The redness and swelling often spread rapidly unless treated by antibiotics.

cerebrovascular disease—Conditions caused by problems that affect the blood supply to the brain. There are several types of cerebrovascular disease. The four most common types are: stroke (a serious medical condition where one part of the brain is damaged by a lack of blood supply or bleeding into the brain from a burst blood vessel), transient ischemic attack (a temporary fall in the blood supply to one part of the brain, resulting in brief symptoms similar to stroke), subarachnoid hemorrhage (a type of stroke where blood leaks out of the brain's blood vessels on to the surface of the brain), and vascular dementia (a persistent impairment in mental ability resulting from stroke or other problems with blood circulation to the brain).

cholesterol—A lipid transported in the blood in high- and low-density lipoproteins (HDL and LDL, respectively). High HDL levels are somewhat protective against coronary heart disease.

chronic disease—Disease that develops over time such as type 2 diabetes, peripheral vascular disease, and coronary heart disease. Often associated with unhealthy lifestyle behaviors.

chronic obstructive pulmonary disease—Disease in which the airways become blocked causing breathing difficulties.

claudication—Narrowing or blockage of one or more main arteries.

coefficient of digestibility—The percentage energy of food ingested that is digested, absorbed, and available for metabolic processes in the body.

coenzyme—Small molecules that are essential in stoichiometric amounts for the activity of some enzymes. Examples include nicotinamide adenine dinucleotide (NAD), flavin adenine dinucleotide (FAD), pyridoxal phosphate (PLP), thiamin pyrophosphate (TPP), and biotin.

coenzyme A—A molecule that acts as a carrier for acyl or acetyl groups (A stands for acetylation).

colon—The large intestine. This part of the intestine is mainly responsible for forming, storing, and expelling feces consisting of bacteria, cells from the intestines, secretions, and a small amount of food residue.

constipation—Hard stools in rectum making defecation difficult.

coronary heart disease (CHD)—Narrowing of the arteries supplying the heart muscle that can cause heart attacks.

cortisol—A steroid hormone secreted from the adrenal glands in response to stress or low blood sugar.

creatinine—A product of creatine breakdown that is found in the urine. It can be measured to assess overall kidney function. An abnormally elevated blood creatinine level is seen in people with kidney insufficiency and kidney failure.

cytokine—Protein released from cells that acts as a chemical messenger by binding to receptors on other cells. Cytokines include interleukins (IL), tumor necrosis factors (TNF), colony-stimulating factors (CSF), and interferons (IFN).

cytoplasm—The fluid found inside a cell.

daily value (DV)—A term used in food labeling that indicates the percentage of the recommended daily intakes for the macronutrients (carbohydrate, fat, and protein) as well as cholesterol, sodium, and potassium. On a food label, the DV is based on a 2,000 kcal (8.4 MJ) diet recommended for healthy people in the US.

dehydration—A lower than normal body water content that is detrimental to both exercise performance and health and should be prevented by provision of fluids to match water loss. Also known as hypohydration.

dental caries—Erosion or decay of tooth caused by the effects of bacteria in the mouth.

dental plaque—A biofilm of bacteria that grows on surfaces within the mouth. Dental plaque may become acidic causing demineralization of the teeth (also known as dental caries) or harden into dental calculus (also known as tartar).

dementia—An overall term that describes a wide range of symptoms associated with a decline in memory or other thinking skills severe enough to reduce a person's ability to perform everyday activities. Alzheimer's disease accounts for 60 to 80 percent of cases.

deoxyribonucleic acid (DNA)—The compound that forms genes (i.e., the genetic material).

diabetes mellitus—A disorder of carbohydrate metabolism caused by disturbances in production or utilization of insulin. Causes high blood glucose levels and loss of sugar in the urine.

diabetic retinopathy—A condition in which the back of the interior of the eyes (the retina) is damaged which leads to impaired vision and often results in total blindness. In diabetics the relative risk of blindness is five times that of the nondiabetic population.

diarrhea—Frequent passage of a watery fecal discharge because of a gastrointestinal disturbance or infection.

diastolic—The filling phase of the cardiac cycle when the ventricles are relaxed.

diet-induced thermogenesis (DIT)—The energy needed for the digestion, assimilation, and metabolism of food that is consumed (also referred to as thermic effect of food, or TEF). This causes a 3-30% increase in resting metabolic rate for a few hours after consuming a meal. DIT is higher for protein than for carbohydrate or fat.

digestion—The process of breaking down food to its smallest components so that it can be absorbed in the intestine.

diglyceride—Glycerol backbone with two fatty acids. It is formed by the removal of one fatty acid from triglyceride.

disaccharide—Sugars that yield two monosaccharides on hydrolysis. Sucrose, the most common, is composed of glucose and fructose.

dopamine—A catecholamine neurotransmitter and hormone formed by decarboxylation of dehydroxyphenylalanine (dopa). A precursor of epinephrine (adrenaline) and norepinephrine (noradrenaline).

downregulation—Decreased expression of genes or hormone (e.g., insulin) receptors in the target tissues.

dual energy X-ray absorptiometry (DEXA)—A special type of X-ray scan that measures bone mineral density. This type of scan may also be called a DXA scan.

dyslipidemia—An abnormal and unhealthy blood lipid profile with high levels of serum total cholesterol, LDL-cholesterol and triglyceride, and low level of HDL-cholesterol.

eating disorder—A psychological disorder centering on the avoidance or purging of food, such as anorexia nervosa and bulimia nervosa.

Eatwell guide—The latest UK government dietary guidelines published in 2016.

eicosanoids—Derivatives of fatty acids in the body that act as cell-to-cell signaling molecules. They include prostaglandins, thromboxanes, and leukotrienes.

electrolyte—A substance that, when dissolved in water, conducts an electric current. Electrolytes, which include acids, bases, and salts, usually dissociate into ions carrying either a positive charge (cation) or a negative charge (anion).

endocrine—Ductless glands that secrete hormones into the blood.

energy—The ability to perform work. Energy exists in various forms, including mechanical, heat, and chemical energy.

energy balance—The balance between energy intake and energy expenditure.

energy density—The amount of energy (or calories) per gram of food. Lower energy density foods provide fewer calories per gram of food – this means that you can have satisfying portions of these foods with relatively low calorie content.

energy expenditure—The amount of energy used.

enzyme—A protein with specific catalytic activity. They are designated by the suffix *-ase* frequently attached to the type of reaction catalyzed (e.g., oxidase, lipase). Virtually all metabolic reactions in the body are dependent on and controlled by enzymes.

epinephrine—A hormone secreted by the adrenal gland in response to acute stress. It is a stimulant, prepares the body for fight or flight, and is an important activator of fat and carbohydrate breakdown during exercise. Also known as adrenaline.

erythrocyte—Red blood cell that contains hemoglobin and transports oxygen.

essential amino acids—Amino acids that must be obtained in the diet and cannot be synthesized in the body. Also known as indispensable amino acids.

essential body fat—Essential body fat is present in all membranes, nerve tissues, bone marrow, and the vital organs, and we cannot lose this fat without compromising physiological function. Essential body fat is approximately 3% of body mass for men and 12% of body mass for women. It is thought that the reason why women have more essential body fat than men is because of childbearing and hormonal functions.

essential fatty acids—Unsaturated fatty acids that cannot be synthesized in the body and must be obtained in the diet (e.g., linoleic acid and α-linolenic acid).

essential nutrient—A food component that provides energy or promotes growth and repair of tissues and must be obtained from the diet as a deficiency of it will result in ill-health.

fasting—Starvation; abstinence from eating that may be partial or complete.

fat—Fat molecules contain the same structural elements as carbohydrates, but they have little oxygen relative to carbon and hydrogen and are poorly soluble in water. Fats are also known as lipids (derived from the Greek word *lipos*), and fat is a general name for oils, fats, waxes, and related compounds. Oils are liquid at room temperature, whereas fats are solid.

Fatmax—The exercise intensity at which the rate of whole-body fat oxidation is highest.

fatty acid (FA)—A type of fat having a carboxylic acid group (COOH) at one end of the molecule and a methyl (CH_3) group at the other end, separated by a hydrocarbon chain that can vary in length. A typical structure of a fatty acid is $CH_3(CH_2)_{14}COOH$ (palmitic acid or palmitate). Also known as free fatty acid or nonesterified fatty acid.

fiber—Indigestible carbohydrates. Some are fermented by bacteria in the colon.

flavonoid—A diverse group of phytonutrients (plant chemicals) found in almost all fruits and vegetables. Along with carotenoids, they are responsible for the vivid colors in fruits and vegetables. Like many other phytonutrients, flavonoids are powerful antioxidants with anti-inflammatory and immune system benefits. They are not classed as essential but are needed for optimal health.

flexitarian diet—A semi-vegetarian diet which is primarily a plant-based diet but includes meat, dairy, eggs, poultry and fish on occasion or in small quantities.

food addiction—A type of compulsive eating behavior in which a person overeats a certain type of food in a similar fashion to a drug or alcohol addict.

food-combining diet—A type of weight loss diet based on a philosophy that certain foods should not be combined in a meal because it causes a "build-up of toxins" with "negative side effects such as weight gain" despite a lack of any scientific evidence for this.

food efficiency—A phenomenon caused by an adaptive decrease in resting metabolic rate when losing body weight due to insufficient dietary energy intake. When dieting it makes weight loss increasingly difficult after a few weeks or months.

food group—A collection of foods that share similar nutritional properties or biological classifications. Nutrition guides typically divide foods into food groups and recommend daily servings of each group for a healthy diet. Common examples of food groups include dairy, meat, fruit, vegetables, grains, and beans.

fructose—A six-carbon sugar found in fruits. It is converted to glucose in the liver.

gangrene—A serious, life-threatening condition where a loss of blood supply causes body tissue to die. It can affect any part of the body but typically starts in the toes, feet, fingers, and hands. Gangrene can occur as a result of an injury, infection, or a chronic condition that impairs blood circulation.

gastrointestinal tract—Gastrointestinal system or alimentary tract. The main sites in the body used for digestion and absorption of nutrients. It consists of the mouth, esophagus, stomach, small intestine, large intestine, rectum, and anus.

gene—A specific sequence in DNA that codes for a particular protein. Genes are located on the chromosomes. Each gene is found in a definite position (locus).

gestational diabetes—A temporary form of type 2 diabetes that can occur during pregnancy, particularly in overweight women. The hormones produced by the placenta during pregnancy (estrogen, cortisol, and human placental lactogen) can block the actions of insulin putting the mother-to-be at an increased risk of insulin resistance and some women are not able to produce enough insulin to overcome this resistance causing hyperglycemia. The condition develops during the second and third trimester and affects 6-8% of pregnant women.

ghrelin—Peptide hormone secreted by the cells of the stomach when it is empty. Ghrelin stimulates parts of the brain that promote hunger and appetite.

gingivitis—Infection and inflammation of the gums.

glaucoma—A common eye condition where the optic nerve, which connects the eye to the brain, becomes damaged. It's usually caused by fluid building up in the front part of the eye, which increases pressure inside the eye. Glaucoma can lead to loss of vision if it isn't diagnosed and treated early.

glucagon—A peptide hormone produced in the pancreas that has the opposite action to insulin. Glucagon secretion increases when the blood sugar level falls below normal and stimulates the liver to break down stored glycogen into glucose which is released into the circulation.

glucose—Blood sugar and an important fuel for many cells in the body. The brain relies on glucose as its main source of energy so we feel tired, faint, and lethargic if our blood glucose levels drop below normal.

GLUT4—The glucose transporter found in muscle cell membranes that carries glucose from the blood into the muscle cell.

glycated hemoglobin—The addition of glucose or metabolites of glucose to the hemogobin molecules in red blood cells. A level above 6.5% or 48 mmol/mol is used as a diagnostic indicator of type 2 diabetes.

glycemic index (GI)—Increase in blood glucose and insulin in response to a meal. The GI of a food represents how much blood glucose rises over a two-hour period after eating a certain food item containing 50 g carbohydrate and is expressed against a reference food, usually glucose.

glycemic load (GL)—Increase in blood glucose and insulin response to a meal (like the GI) but takes into account the amount of that food that is normally consumed. The GL is obtained by multiplying the GI value by the carbohydrate content of the food and then dividing by 100.

glycerol—Three-carbon molecule that is the backbone structure of triglycerides.

glycogen—Polymer of glucose used as a storage form of carbohydrate in the liver and muscles.

gourd—A fleshy, typically large fruit (though commonly referred to as a vegetable) with a hard skin such as aubergine (eggplant), squash, marrow, melon, and zucchini (courgette). All have a low energy density due to their high water and fiber content.

HbA1c—An abbreviation for glycated hemoglobin. Used as a measure of blood glucose control. High levels (6.5% of more) are used to confirm the diagnosis of type 2 diabetes.

heart rate reserve—A person's maximum heart rate minus their resting heart rate.

hemoglobin—The red, iron-containing respiratory pigment found in red blood cells. Hemoglobin is important in the transport of oxygen and in the regulation of blood pH.

high-density lipoprotein (HDL)—A protein-lipid complex in the blood plasma that facilitates the transport of triglycerides, cholesterol, and phospholipids. HDL removes fatty deposits from blood vessel walls.

high-intensity interval exercise (HIIE)—Repeated bouts of heavy dynamic exercise such as sprinting separated by short recovery intervals.

high-intensity interval training (HIIT)—Repeated bouts of heavy dynamic exercise such as sprinting separated by short recovery intervals that are performed regularly (i.e., at least three times per week).

high quality protein—Dietary protein that contain all the essential amino acid in a proportion needed by the human body. Also known as complete protein.

homeostasis—The tendency to maintain uniformity or stability of the internal environment of the cell or of the body.

hormone—An organic chemical produced in cells of one part of the body (usually an endocrine gland) that diffuses or is transported by the blood circulation to cells in other parts of the body, where it regulates and coordinates their activities.

hyperglycemia—Higher than normal blood glucose concentration. A major characteristic of both type 1 and type 2 diabetes.

hyperinsulinemia—High levels of the hormone insulin in the blood.

hyperlipidemia—Higher than normal levels of blood lipids, particularly serum total cholesterol and triglyceride.

hypersecretion—Higher than normal levels of production and release of a substance such as a hormone like insulin.

hypertension—Higher than normal blood pressure, usually above a threshold of 140/90 mmHg.

hypoglycemia—Drop in the blood glucose concentration below 3 mmol/L that causes symptoms of faintness, dizziness, disorientation, and fatigue.

hypothalamus—Region at base of brain responsible for integration of sensory input and effector responses in regulation of body temperature. Also contains centers for control of hunger, appetite, and thirst.

immune system—Cells and soluble molecules involved in tissue repair after injury and in the protection of the body against infection.

incretin—A hormone that is produced by endocrine cells in the small intestine and stimulates a decrease in blood glucose levels. Incretin is released after eating and increases the secretion of insulin from pancreatic β-cells by a blood glucose-dependent mechanism.

inflammation—The body's response to injury, which includes redness (increased blood flow) and swelling (edema) caused by increased capillary permeability.

insomnia—Difficulty with sleeping.

insulin—A hormone secreted by the pancreas, involved in carbohydrate metabolism, particularly in the control of the blood glucose concentration. Insulin stimulates glucose uptake from the blood by muscle, liver, and adipose tissue.

insulin receptor—A protein located in a target cell's membrane that insulin binds to. This initiates a signaling cascade that brings about the actions of the hormone.

insulin receptor substrate 1 (IRS-1)—Mediates the control of various cellular processes by insulin. When phosphorylated by the insulin receptor IRS-1 binds specifically to various cellular proteins to alter their function and bring about the actions of insulin.

insulin resistance—A condition that occurs when target tissues such as muscle, liver, and adipose tissue become less responsive to the actions of insulin. It is strongly associated with being overweight and having signs of chronic low-level inflammation.

insulin sensitivity—How responsive target tissues are to the action of insulin.

interleukin—Type of cytokine produced by leukocytes and some other tissues. Acts as a chemical messenger, rather like a hormone, but usually with localized effects.

intermittent fasting diet (IFD)—A form of dieting that involves fasting or very low calorie intake in between periods of normal eating (e.g., fasting or only eating about 500 kcal on two or three days of the week).

interstitial fluid—The fluid that fills any spaces that lie between cells.

joule (J)—Unit of energy according to the Systeme Internationale. One joule is the amount of energy needed to move a mass of 1 g at a velocity of 1 m/s. One calorie equals 4.184 joules.

ketone bodies (or ketones)—Acidic organic compounds produced during the incomplete oxidation of fatty acids in the liver. Contain a carboxyl group (-COOH) and a ketone group (-C=O). Examples include acetoacetate and β-hydroxybutyrate.

kilocalorie (kcal)—Unit of energy equal to 1,000 calories.

kilojoule (kJ)—Unit of energy equal to 1,000 joules.

lactic acid—Metabolic end product of anaerobic glycolysis.

lactose—Milk sugar, a disaccharide linking a molecule of glucose and a molecule of galactose.

lean body mass (LBM)—All parts of the body, excluding fat.

legume—The high-protein fruit or pod of vegetables, including beans, peas, and lentils.

leptin—Regulatory hormone produced by adipose tissue. When released into the circulation, it influences the hypothalamus to control appetite.

leukocyte—White blood cell. Important in inflammation and immune defense.

linoleic acid—An essential fatty acid.

α-linolenic acid—An essential fatty acid.

lipid—A compound composed of carbon, hydrogen, oxygen, and sometimes other elements. Lipids dissolve in organic solvents but not in water and include triglyceride, fatty acids, cholesterol, and phospholipids. Lipids are commonly called fats.

lipoprotein—A complex of lipid (fat) in the form of triglyceride, cholesterol, and phospholipid with protein that is used for fat transport in the circulation.

low-density lipoprotein (LDL)—A protein-lipid complex in the blood plasma that facilitates the transport of triglycerides, cholesterol, and phospholipids. It deposits fatty material on blood vessel walls. High blood levels of LDL are associated with increased incidence of atherosclerosis and coronary heart disease.

lymphocyte—Type of white blood cell important in the acquired immune response. Includes both T cells and B cells. The latter produce antibodies.

M1 macrophage—Pro-inflammatory type of white blood cell that infiltrates tissues and causes inflammation.

M2 macrophage—Anti-inflammatory type of white blood cell that infiltrates tissues and dampens inflammation.

macronutrients—Nutrients ingested in relatively large amounts (carbohydrate, fat, protein, and water).

macrophage or monocyte—Type of white blood cell that can ingest and destroy foreign material and initiate the acquired immune response.

maltose—A disaccharide that yields two molecules of glucose upon hydrolysis.

melatonin—A hormone produced mainly by the pineal gland, which regulates wakefulness. As a medicine, it is used to treat insomnia and may help you get to sleep more quickly.

meta-analysis—A type of study or report that uses a statistical approach to combine the results from multiple studies in an effort to increase power (over individual studies), improve estimates of the size of the effect, and/or is used to resolve uncertainty when reports disagree.

metabolic syndrome—The co-occurrence of several known cardiovascular disease risk factors, including insulin resistance, obesity, high blood cholesterol, and high blood pressure (hypertension).

metabolizable energy—The net energy remaining of ingested food energy after fecal and urinary energy losses are subtracted from the chemical energy of the food. The metabolizable energy represents the energy available for growth or reproduction and for supporting metabolic processes such as work (locomotion), biosynthesis, thermoregulation, maintenance metabolism, etc.

metformin—Usually the first medication prescribed for type 2 diabetes. It works by improving the sensitivity of your body tissues to insulin so that insulin works more effectively to promote tissue glucose uptake. Metformin also lowers glucose production in the liver.

methylglyoxal—A compound produced by metabolism when blood glucose concentrations are chronically high. Methylglyoxal binds to proteins which is harmful for people with type 2 diabetes.

microbiota—The population of micro-organisms that are found in a particular environment or location such as those that occupy the gut or the skin.

micronutrients—Organic vitamins and inorganic minerals that must be consumed in relatively small amounts in the diet to maintain health.

Mifflin-St. Jeor equation—An equation that can be used to estimate a person's resting metabolic rate based on their sex, age, weight, and height.

millimole (mmol)—One thousandth of a mole which is the amount of a chemical compound whose mass in grams is equivalent to its molecular weight, which is the sum of the atomic weights of its constituent atoms. Usually used to express a concentration of a substance such as blood glucose in millimoles per liter (mmol/L).

mineral—An inorganic element found in nature though the term is usually reserved for those elements that are solid. In nutrition, the term mineral is usually used to classify dietary elements essential to life processes. Examples are calcium and iron.

mitochondria—Oval or spherical organelle containing the enzymes of the tricarboxylic acid cycle and electron-transportchain. Site of oxidative phosphorylation (resynthesis of ATP involving the use of oxygen).

molecular epidemiology studies—The patterns and causes of disease in defined populations.

molecule—An aggregation of at least two atoms of the same or different elements held together by special forces (covalent bonds) and having a precise chemical formula (e.g., O_2, H_2O, $C_6H_{12}O_6$).

monosaccharide—A simple sugar that cannot be hydrolyzed to smaller units (e.g., glucose, fructose, and galactose).

monounsaturated fat—Fats that have one double bond in the fatty acid hydrocarbon chain with all of the remainder carbon atoms being single-bonded. Olive oil is an example of a type of oil that contains monounsaturated fats.

MyPlate—The current nutrition guide published by the USDA Center for Nutrition Policy and Promotion – a food circle (i.e., a pie chart) depicting a place setting with a plate and glass divided into five food groups.

net metabolizable energy—The net energy remaining of ingested food energy after fecal and urinary energy losses are subtracted from the chemical energy of the food and after taking into account the energy lost as heat in its metabolism.

neuroendocrine system—The interaction between the nervous system (including the brain) and the hormone producing endocrine glands or cells in the body that function in an integrated manner to collectively regulate a physiological or behavioral state such as reproduction, metabolism, blood glucose, eating and drinking behavior, energy utilization, fluid balance, and blood pressure.

neurotransmitters—Signaling molecules that transfer information from one nerve ending to the next (e.g., acetyl choline, dopamine, serotonin).

nitrate—A small molecule (NO_3^-) that is naturally abundant in beetroot and rhubarb. It is used by athletes (usually in the form of concentrated beetroot juice) to improve endurance performance as it reduces the oxygen cost of exercise. It can also lower resting blood pressure so can be used as a remedy to treat mild hypertension.

non–insulin-dependent diabetes mellitus (NIDDM)—Also known as type 2 diabetes.

nutrient—Substances found in food that provide energy or promote growth and repair of tissues.

nutrient dense—Term used to describe a food that has a relatively large amount of essential nutrients per unit of energy in the food.

nutrient density—Amount of essential nutrients expressed per unit of energy in the food.

nutrition—The total of the processes of ingestion, digestion, absorption, and metabolism of food and the subsequent assimilation of nutrient materials into the tissues. Also used as a general term meaning the food and beverages that we consume.

obesity—An excessive accumulation of body fat. The term obesity is usually reserved for people who are 20% or more above the average weight for their size or have a BMI of 30 kg/m² or more.

optimal health—Not just the absence of illness or disease but the best your health can be and a state which is associated with reduced risk of developing chronic disease.

oral glucose tolerance test (OGTT)— A clinical diagnostic test for diabetes that is used to assess the blood glucose response for up to two hours after consuming a glucose solution that contains 75 g of glucose. For a normal, healthy person, the peak blood glucose value occurs after one hour and does not exceed 9-10 mmol/L or 160-180 mg/dL and blood glucose should return to its pre-test fasting value within two hours. Someone with a reading of 11 mmol/L (200 mg/dL) or higher after two hours may indicate diabetes, whereas a reading of 7.8-10.9 mmol/L (140-199 mg/dL) indicates prediabetes.

osteoarthritis—The most common form of arthritis. It occurs when the protective cartilage on the ends of your bones wears down over time. Although osteoarthritis can damage any joint in your body, the disorder most commonly affects joints in your hands, knees, hips, and spine.

osteoporosis—A weakening of the bone structure that occurs when the rate of demineralization exceeds the rate of bone formation.

palatability—Pleasure provided by foods or fluids that are agreeable to the palate (sensed by taste buds on the tongue), which often varies relative to the homeostatic satisfaction of nutritional, water, or energy needs.

Paleo diet—A dietary plan based on foods similar to what might have been eaten during the Paleolithic era, which dates from approximately 2.5 million to 10,000 years ago. A Paleo diet typically includes lean meats, fish, fruits, vegetables, nuts, and seeds – foods that in the past could be obtained by hunting and gathering. A Paleo diet avoids or limits foods that became common when farming emerged about 10,000 years ago such as dairy products, legumes, and grains.

pancreas—An organ located below and behind the stomach. It secretes insulin and glucagon (involved in plasma glucose regulation) and pancreatic enzymes involved in the digestion of carbohydrate, fat, and protein in the small intestine.

pancreatitis—Inflammation of the pancreas, the accessory digestive organ that secretes insulin and glucagon. Inflammation can be caused by infection or physical damage sometimes caused by gall stones becoming trapped. The condition can cause symptoms similar to type 1 diabetes due to impaired insulin secretion.

pathogen—Microorganism that can cause symptoms of disease. A pathogen can be a bacterium or a virus.

peptide—Small compound formed by the bonding of two or more amino acids. Larger chains of linked amino acids are called polypeptides or proteins.

peripheral vascular disease—A disease of blood vessels outside the heart. Peripheral vascular disease affects the arteries or veins of the peripheral circulation, as opposed to the cardiac circulation.

pescatarian diet—A diet which typically includes vegetables, grains, and pulses along with fish and other seafood, but generally excludes meat, poultry, and sometimes dairy products.

phospholipid—A phosphorus containing lipid (fat) that is a major component of cell membranes.

phytonutrients—Certain organic components of plants that are thought to promote human health but are non-nutrients. They differ from vitamins because they are not considered an essential nutrient, meaning that without them people will not develop a nutritional deficiency. Examples include the carotenoids, flavonoids, and coumarins.

plant sterol—A plant-based lipid (fat) compound that is similar in structure to cholesterol and can compete with dietary cholesterol to be absorbed by the intestines, resulting in lower blood cholesterol levels. Plant sterols may also have some effect in cancer prevention.

plaque—A deposit on blood vessel walls that is made up of fat, cholesterol, calcium, and other substances found in the blood. Atherosclerosis is a disease in which plaque builds up inside your arteries. Another form of plaque is dental plaque which is a biofilm of bacteria that grows on surfaces within the mouth. Dental plaque may become acidic causing demineralization of the teeth (also known as dental caries) or harden into dental calculus (also known as tartar).

plasma—The liquid portion of the blood in which the blood cells are suspended. Typically accounts for 55% to 60% of the total blood volume. Differs from serum in that it contains fibrinogen, the clot-forming protein.

pneumonia—A severe respiratory illness caused by bacterial or viral infection, in which the lungs become inflamed and the air sacs fill with pus making breathing difficult. A potentially fatal condition if not treated quickly.

polycystic ovarian syndrome—A set of symptoms that are usually caused by elevated androgens (male hormones) in females. Signs and symptoms include irregular or no menstrual periods, heavy periods, excess body and facial hair, acne, pelvic pain, difficulty getting pregnant, and patches of thick, darker, velvety skin.

polyphenols—A large class of naturally occurring compounds that includes the flavonoids, flavonols, flavonones, and anthocyanidins. These compounds contain a number of phenolic hydroxyl (-OH) groups attached to ring structures, which confers them with powerful antioxidant activity.

polysaccharide—Polymers of (arbitrarily) more than about 10 monosaccharide residues linked together by glycosidic bonds in branched or unbranched chains. Examples include starch and glycogen.

polyunsaturated fat—Fats that contain a high proportion of fatty acids more than one carbon–carbon double bond in the hydrocarbon chain. Polyunsaturated fats are considered to be healthier in the diet than saturated fats.

power—The ability to exert a maximal force in as short a time as possible, as in accelerating, jumping, and throwing implements. While strength is the maximal force you can apply against a load, power is proportional to the speed at which you can apply this maximal force. So power is the amount of work performed per unit of time.

prediabetes—A "pre-diagnosis" of diabetes—you can think of it as a warning sign. It's when your blood glucose level (blood sugar level) is higher than normal, but it's not high enough to be considered diabetes. Appropriate changes to diet and exercise habits at this stage can prevent prediabetes from developing into type 2 diabetes.

probiotic—A supplement usually derived from dairy foods or a dietary supplement containing live bacteria that replace or add to the beneficial bacteria normally present in the gut.

protein—Biological macromolecules composed of a chain of covalently linked amino acids. Proteins may have structural or functional roles (e.g., as enzymes, receptors, and membrane transporters).

recommended dietary allowance (RDA)—Recommended intake of a particular nutrient that meets the needs of nearly all (97%) healthy individuals of similar age and gender.

reference daily intake—Nutrient intake standards set by the FDA based on the 1968 recommended dietary allowance (RDA) for various vitamins and minerals. Reference daily intakes have been set for infants, toddlers, people over four years of age, and pregnant and lactating women.

renal threshold—The concentration level up to which a substance (such as glucose) in the blood is completely reabsorbed in the kidney tubules and so is prevented from passing through the kidneys into the urine. For glucose this level is normally 8.8-10.0 mmol/L.

resistance exercise—Exercise in which a muscle contraction is opposed by force. The resistance is often applied by using weights. Regular resistance exercise results in increased muscle size, strength and power.

resting energy expenditure—Energy expenditure under resting conditions. The resting energy expenditure includes the resting metabolic rate plus the small (10-30%) transient increases in energy expenditure that occur following feeding.

resting metabolic rate (RMR)—The energy required for the maintenance of normal body functions and homeostasis in resting conditions. The RMR is the largest component of daily energy expenditure in a relatively inactive person.

retina—Cells at the back of the eye responsible for vision. Damage to the retina can cause loss of sight.

saccharide—Generic name for sugars including monosaccharides such as glucose and disaccharides such as sucrose.

salt—Sodium chloride: a white crystalline substance which gives seawater its characteristic taste and is used for seasoning or preserving food. In chemistry a salt is any chemical compound formed from the reaction of an acid with a base, with all or part of the hydrogen of the acid replaced by a metal or other cation.

sarcopenia—Loss of muscle mass that occurs with aging.

satiety—Sensation of fullness and satisfaction following eating that inhibits further desire to consume food.

saturated fat—A type of fat containing a high proportion of fatty acid molecules with only single bonds and no double bonds in the hydrocarbon chain. Saturated fat is considered to be less healthy in the diet than unsaturated fat.

serotonin—A brain neurotransmitter. Also known as 5-hydroxytryptamine (5-HT).

sleep quality—How well we sleep and feel refreshed in the morning. Poor sleep quality may be due to lack of sleep time or frequent awakenings.

sodium—A silvery-white chemical element (symbol Na) which combines with other chemicals. Salt is a sodium compound in which the sodium is combined with chlorine (Cl) to form sodium chloride (NaCl).

sodium-glucose-cotransporter 2—One of a family of glucose transporters found in the proximal tubule of the kidney nephrons that assist with renal glucose reabsorption. Also known as sodium-glucose linked transporter 2 (SGLT2).

starch—A carbohydrate made of multiple units of glucose attached together by bonds that can be broken down by human digestion processes. Starch is also known as a complex carbohydrate.

steroid—A complex molecule derived from the lipid cholesterol containing four interlocking carbon rings.

stroke—A stroke is a serious life-threatening medical condition that occurs when the blood supply to part of the brain is cut off. Strokes are a medical emergency and urgent treatment is essential. Strokes may be caused by a brain blood vessel blockage or rupture.

sucrose—A disaccharide consisting of a combination of glucose and fructose; table sugar from cane or beet.

sugar—Any of the class of soluble, crystalline, typically sweet-tasting carbohydrates found in plant and animal tissues and exemplified by glucose and sucrose.

sugar-sweetened beverage (SSB)—A drink that contains added sugars for sweetness and energy.

sulfonylureas—Sulfonylureas are a group of medicines used to treat type 2 diabetes. These drugs work by increasing the release of insulin from the pancreas.

sympathetic nervous system—One of the two main divisions of the autonomic nervous system. Its general action is to mobilize the body's fight-or-flight response. It increases heart rate, reduces blood flow to the skin, gut, and kidneys, causes the pupils to dilate, increases alertness, and opens up the airways.

Systeme Internationale (SI)—International Unit System, a worldwide uniform system of metric units.

systolic—Indicating the maximum arterial pressure during contraction of the left ventricle of the heart.

T-regulatory lymphocyte—A specialized subpopulation of T cells (a type of white blood cell) that act to suppress inflammation and the immune response, thereby maintaining homeostasis and self-tolerance. T regulatory cells (Tregs) are able to inhibit T lymphocyte proliferation and cytokine production and play a critical role in limiting inflammation and preventing autoimmunity.

thermic effect of exercise (TEE)—The energy required for exercise. Increased muscle contraction increases energy expenditure and heat production due to the inefficiency of energy transformations.

thermic effect of food (TEF)— The increased energy expenditure following feeding that is due to the energy needed for the digestion, assimilation, and metabolism of food after it is consumed (also referred to as diet-induced thermogenesis).

thermogenesis—The production of heat. Metabolic processes in the body generate heat constantly.

time-restricted feeding—A daily eating pattern in which all your food is eaten within an 8- to 12-hour timeframe every day, with no deliberate attempt to alter nutrient quality or quantity.

tissue—An organized association of similar cells that perform a common function (e.g., muscle tissue).

toll-like receptor—Family of evolutionary conserved cell membrane receptors present on macrophages that detect the presence of bacteria and viruses and initiate the acquired immune response to pathogens.

toxemia—The presence of toxins in the blood.

trans—A prefix indicating that geometrical isomer in which like groups are on opposite sides of a double bond with restricted rotation.

trans fatty acids—Unsaturated fatty acids that contain at least one double bond in the trans configuration. Found in hydrogenated fats. They are harmful to health.

triglyceride—The storage form of fat composed of three fatty acid molecules linked to a three-carbon glycerol molecule. Also known as triacylglycerol.

tumor necrosis factor—A cytokine that promotes inflammation.

type 1 diabetes mellitus—Insulin-dependent diabetes mellitus. A chronic condition in which the pancreas produces little or no insulin. Usually a consequence of an autoimmune destruction of the β-cells in the pancreas at an early age.

type 2 diabetes mellitus—Non-insulin-dependent diabetes mellitus. Usually a consequence of being overweight or obese and not doing enough regular exercise. Prevalence increases with age.

unit of alcohol—One unit equals 10 milliliters or 8 grams of pure alcohol, which is the amount of alcohol the average adult can process in an hour. The number of units in a drink is based on the size of the drink, as well as its alcohol strength. For example, a pint of strong lager contains three units of alcohol, whereas the same volume of low-strength lager has just over two units. One glass of wine contains about 1.5 units.

unsaturated fat—A type of fat containing a high proportion of fatty acid molecules with at least one double bond in the hydrocarbon chain. Unsaturated fats are, considered to be healthier in the diet than saturated fat.

upper respiratory tract infection—Viral or bacterial infections of the throat and upper airways like colds and flu.

urea—End product of protein metabolism. Chemical formula: $CO(NH_2)_2$

urinary tract infection—A bacterial infection of the urinary tract (i.e., the urethra and/or bladder).

urine—Fluid produced in the kidney and excreted from the body. Contains urea, ammonia, and other metabolic wastes.

vegan—Vegetarian who eats no animal products.

vegetarian—One whose food is of vegetable or plant origin. Some versions of the diet allow the consumption of dairy products (e.g., milk, cheese, yogurt) and/or eggs.

very low energy diet—Restriction of the dietary energy intake to less than 1,000 kcal per day in order to lose weight.

visceral fat—Body fat that is stored within the abdominal cavity and is therefore stored around a number of internal organs such as the intestines, liver, and pancreas. It is commonly known as belly fat and is associated with increased risks of a number of health problems including type 2 diabetes.

vitamin—An organic substance necessary in small amounts for the normal metabolic functioning of the body. Must be present in the diet because the body cannot synthesize it (or an adequate amount of it).

Warrior diet—An unconventional intermittent fast type of diet in which you fast during the day, are encouraged to do some hard exercise, and eat only at night, avoiding all processed foods.

water retention—An increase in the body water content. Water is the universal solvent of life (H_2O). The average adult human body is composed of 60% water.

white blood cell—Important cells of the immune system that defend the body against invading microorganisms. Also known as a leukocyte.

weight cycling—A cycle in which the considerable effort applied to achieve weight loss is exceeded by the effort required to maintain the new lower body weight. After the weight is lost, it is regained in a relatively short period. Also referred to as the yo-yo effect.

waist-to-hip ratio (WHR)—The circumference around the waist in centimeters divided by the circumference around the hips in centimeters.

yo-yo effect—See weight cycling.

Zone diet— The Zone Diet is about eating a certain balance of macronutrients to get in a "zone" for specific health benefits and to facilitate weight loss. To get into the zone you have to eat a specific ratio of 40% carbohydrate, 30% protein, and 30% fat. As part of the diet, carbohydrates should have a low glycemic index, protein should be lean, and fat should be mostly monounsaturated.

References

This is a list of reference sources I have used in putting together this book. You can find the journal articles on the PubMed website (https://www.ncbi.nlm.nih.gov/pubmed). PubMed is a search engine that comprises more than 27 million papers and review articles from the biomedical literature, life science journals, and online books. Just type in the title of the article or a few author surnames to bring up a 250-word abstract of the article; for many articles you can click on a link to get the full article for free. The other reference sources in the list are books and websites where you will find helpful information on particular topics.

Firstly, here are my top 10 recommended websites (in alphabetical order) for information relevant to type 2 diabetes and its serious health consequences:

American Heart Association: https://www.heart.org/

Centers for Disease Control and Prevention National Diabetes Education Program (NDEP): https://www.cdc.gov/diabetes/ndep/index.html

Cleveland Clinic: https://www.my.clevelandclinic.org/health/diseases/

Diabetes UK: https://www.diabetes.co.uk/

International Diabetes Federation: https://www.idf.org

Mayo Clinic: https://www.mayoclinic.org/

National Health Service (NHS) UK 111: https://www.111.nhs.uk/

National Institute of Diabetes and Digestive and Kidney Diseases (NIDDK): https://www.niddk.nih.gov/health-information/diabetes

National Institutes of Health (NIH) USA: https://www.nih.gov/

Royal National Institute of Blind People (RNIB): https://www.rnib.org.uk/

LIST OF REFERENCE SOURCES

Abbott, Howard, Christin, et al. (1988). Short-term energy balance: Relationship with protein, carbohydrate and fat balances. *Am J Physiol* 255(3 Pt 1):E332-E337.

Achten, Gleeson, and Jeukendrup. (2002). Determination of the exercise intensity that elicits maximal fat oxidation. *Med Sci Sports Exerc* 34(1).92-97.

Achten, Venables, and Jeukendrup. (2003). Fat oxidation rates are higher during running compared to cycling over a wide range of intensities. *Metabolism* 52(6):747-752.

Afshar, Richards, Mann, et al. (2015). Acute immunomodulatory effects of binge alcohol consumption. *Alcohol* 49(1):57-64.

Age UK website. https://www.ageuk.org.uk/

Ajala, English, and Pinkney. (2013). Systematic review and meta-analysis of different dietary approaches to the management of type 2 diabetes. *Am J Clin Nutr* 97(3):505-516.

Alzheimer's Society website. https://www.alzheimers.org.uk/

American Alliance for Health, Physical Education, Recreation and Dance (AAHPERD) website. https://www.aahperd.org

American College of Sports Medicine (ACSM) website. https://www.acsm.org

American College of Sports Medicine. (2015). Protein intake for optimal muscle maintenance. https://www.acsm.org/docs/default-source/files-for-resource-library/protein-intake-for-optimal-muscle-maintenance.pdf

American Dietetic Association. (1997). Health implications of dietary fiber. *Am Diet Assoc* 97:1157-1160.

American Heart Association website. https://www.heart.org/

American Physiological Society website. https://www.the-aps.org

American Psychiatric Association. (2013). *Diagnostic and Statistical Manual of Mental Disorders.* 5th ed. Washington, DC: American Psychiatric Association.

Andersen. (1990). Diagnosis and treatment of males with eating disorders. In Andersen (Ed.), *Males With Eating Disorders,* pp. 133-162. New York: Brunner/Mazel.

Andersen. (1995). Eating disorders in males. In Brownell and Fairburn *(Eds.), Eating Disorders and Obesity: A Comprehensive Handbook*, pp. 177-192. London: Guildford Press.

Andrews, Balart, and Bethea. (1998). *Sugar Busters.* London: Vermillion.

Angellotti and Pittas. (2017). The role of vitamin D in the prevention of type 2 diabetes: To D or not to D? *Endocrinology* 158(7):2013-2021.

Anton, Hida, Heekin, et al. (2017). Effects of popular diets without specific calorie targets on weight loss outcomes: Systematic review of findings from clinical trials. *Nutrients* 9(8):E822.

Aranow. (2011). Vitamin D and the immune system. *J Invest Med* 59:881-886.

Archundia Herrera, Subhan, and Chan. (2017). Dietary patterns and cardiovascular disease risk in people with type 2 diabetes. *Curr Obes Rep* 6(4):405-413.

Areosa Sastre, Vernooij, González-Colaço Harmand, and Martínez. (2017). Effect of the treatment of type 2 diabetes mellitus on the development of cognitive impairment and dementia. *Cochrane Database Syst Rev* 6:CD003804.

Armbruster, Evans, and Sherwood-Laughlin. (2018). *Fitness and Wellness*. Champaign, IL: Human Kinetics.

Atkins: Low Carb Diet Program and Weight Loss Plan website. https://www.atkins.com/

Atkins. (1992). *Doctor Atkins' New Diet Revolution.* New York: Avon Books.

Atkinson, Foster-Powell, and Brand-Miller. (2008). International table of glycemic index and glycemic load values: 2008. *Diab Care* 31(12):2281-2283.

Aune, Giovannucci, Boffetta, et al. (2017). Fruit and vegetable intake and the risk of cardiovascular disease, total cancer and all-cause mortality: A systematic review and dose-response meta-analysis of prospective studies. *Int J Epidemiol* 46(3):1029-1056.

Australian Dietary Guidelines. (2015). https://www.eatforhealth.gov.au/guidelines/about-australian-dietary-guidelines.

Australian Food, Supplement and Nutrient (AUSNUT) Database. https://www.foodstandards.gov.au/science/monitoringnutrients/ausnut/foodnutrient/

Australian National Nutrient Database. https://www.foodstandards.gov.au/science/monitoringnutrients/ausnut/ausnutdatafiles/Pages/foodnutrient.aspx

Bachman, Deitrick, and Hillman. (2016). Exercising in the fasted state reduced 24-hour energy intake in active male adults. *J Nutr Metab* 2016:1984198, Epub.

Ballor and Keesey. (1991). A meta-analysis of the factors affecting exercise-induced changes in body mass, fat mass and fat-free mass in males and females. *Int J Obes* 15(11):717-726.

Barnosky, Hoddy, Unterman, and Varady. (2014). Intermittent fasting vs daily calorie restriction for type 2 diabetes prevention: A review of human findings. *Transl Res* 164(4):302-311.

Baumgartner, Chumlea, and Roche. (1990). Bioelectric impedance for body composition. *Exerc Sport Sci Rev* 18:193-224.

BBC Good Food website. https://www.bbcgoodfood.com/recipes

Bell, McHugh, Stenenson, and Howatson. (2014). The role of cherries in exercise and health. *Scand J Med Sci Sports* 24(3):477-490.

Bender and Bender. (1997). *Nutrition. A Reference Handbook*. Oxford: Oxford University Press.

Bendik, Friedel, Roos, et al. (2014). Vitamin D: A critical and essential micronutrient for human health. *Front Physiol* 5:248.

Beisswenger. (2014). Methylglyoxal in diabetes: link to treatment, glycaemic control and biomarkers of complications. *Biochem Soc Trans* 42(2):450-456.

Bennell, Matheson, and Heevwisse. (1999). Risk factors for stress fractures. *Sports Med* 28:91-122.

Bermon, Castell, Calder, et al. (2017). Consensus statement: Immunonutrition and exercise. *Exerc Immunol Rev* 23:8-50.

Beumont (1995). The clinical presentation of anorexia and bulimia nervosa. In Brownell and Fairburn *(Eds.), Eating Disorders and Obesity: A Comprehensive Handbook*, pp. 151-158. London: Guildford Press.

Bischoff-Ferrari, Orav, Willett, and Dawson-Hughes. (2014). The effect of vitamin D supplementation on skeletal, vascular, or cancer outcomes. *Lancet Diabetes Endocrinol* 2(5):363-364.

Blaak. (2001). Gender differences in fat metabolism. *Curr Opin Clin Nutr Metab Care* 4(6):499-502.

Blair, Kohl, Paffenbarger, et al. (1989). Physical fitness and all-cause mortality: a prospective study of healthy men and women. *J Am Med Assoc* 262:2395-2401.

Blüher. (2016). Adipose tissue inflammation: a cause or consequence of obesity-related insulin resistance? *Clin Sci* 130(18):1603-1614.

Blüher. (2019). Obesity: global epidemiology and pathogenesis. *Nat Rev Endocrinol* 15(5):288-298.

Blundell, Gibbons, Caudwell, et al. (2015). Appetite control and energy balance: impact of exercise. *Obes Rev Suppl* 1:67-76.

Blundell, Stubbs, Hughes, et al. (2003). Cross talk between physical activity and appetite control: Does physical activity stimulate appetite? *Proc Nutr Soc* 62(3):651-661.

Bonaventura and Montecucco. (2019). The STOP DIABETES study: when prevention works. *Acta Diabetol* 56(5):501-504.

Bouchard. (1994). Genetics of obesity: Overview and research directions. In Bouchard (Ed.), *The Genetics of Obesity*, pp. 223-233. Boca Raton, FL: CRC Press.

Bouchard, Tremblay, Despres, et al. (1990). The response to long-term overfeeding in identical twins. *N Engl J Med* 322(21):1477-1482.

Bouchard, Tremblay, Després, et al. (1994). The response to exercise with constant energy intake in identical twins. *Obes Res* 2(5):400-410.

Boutcher. (2011). High-intensity intermittent exercise and fat loss. *J Obesity* 2011:868305, Epub.

Bradbury, Appleby, and Key. (2014). Fruit, vegetable and fiber intake in relation to cancer risk: Findings from the European Prospective Investigation into Cancer and Nutrition (EPIC). *Am J Clin Nutr* 100 (Suppl 1):394S-398

British Association of Sport and Exercise Sciences (BASES) website. https://www.bases.org.uk

British Heart Foundation website. https://www.bhf.org.uk/

British Society for Immunology (BSI) website. https://www.immunology.org

Brouwer, Wanders, and Katan. (2010). Effect of animal and industrial trans fatty acids on HDL and LDL cholesterol levels in humans: A quantitative review. *PLoS One* 5(3):e9434.

Brown and Walker. (2016). Genetics of insulin resistance and the metabolic syndrome. *Curr Cardiol Rep* 18(8):75

Burgomaster, Howarth, Phillips, et al. (2008). Similar metabolic adaptations during exercise after low volume sprint interval and traditional endurance training in humans. *J Physiol* 586(1):151-160.

Buttriss, Welch, Kearney, and Lanham-New (Eds.). (2017). *Public Health Nutrition*, 2nd Edition. London: Wiley-Blackwell.

Byrne and Byrne. (1993). The effect of exercise on depression, anxiety and other mood states: A review. *J Psychosomatic Res* 37:565-574.

Calder. (2006). N-3 polyunsaturated fatty acids, inflammation and inflammatory diseases. *Am J Clin Nutr* 83:1505S-1519S.

Calder. (2017). Omega-3 fatty acids and inflammatory processes: from molecules to man. *Biochem Soc Trans* 45(5):1105-1115.

Calle, Thun, Petrelli, et al. (1999). Body-mass index and mortality in a prospective cohort of US adults. *N Engl J Med* 341(15):1097-1105.

Cancer Research UK website. https://www.cancerresearchuk.org/

Cavan. (2014). *Reverse Your Diabetes: The Step-by-Step Plan to Take Control of Type 2 Diabetes*. London: Vermilion.

Centers for Disease Control and Prevention. (2013). Alcohol and Public Health: Alcohol-Related Disease Impact (ARDI) application, 2013 Available at https://www.cdc.gov/ARDI

Centers for Disease Control and Prevention. (2017). National Diabetes Statistics Report, 2017. Available at https://www.cdc.gov/diabetes/pdfs/data/statistics/national-diabetes-statistics-report.pdf

Centers for Disease Control and Prevention Division of Diabetes Translation website. http://www.cdc.gov/diabetes/data

Centers for Disease Control and Prevention National Diabetes Education Program (NDEP). https://www.cdc.gov/diabetes/ndep/index.html

Chaker, Ligthart, Korevaar, et al. (2016). Thyroid function and risk of type 2 diabetes: a population-based prospective cohort study. *BMC Med* 14(1):150.

Chatterjee, Khunti, and Davies. (2017). Type 2 diabetes. *Lancet* 389(10085):2239-2251.

Cho, Shaw, Karuranga, et al. (2018). IDF Diabetes Atlas: Global estimates of diabetes prevalence for 2017 and projections for 2045. *Diabetes Res Clin Pract* 138:271-281.

Cities Changing Diabetes website. http://www.citieschangingdiabetes.com/.

Cleveland Clinic website. https://www.my.clevelandclinic.org/health/diseases/

Cohen, Doyle, Alper, et al. (2009). Sleep habits and susceptibility to the common cold. *Arch Intern Med* 169(1):62-67.

Crowe, Appleby, Travis, and Key. (2013). Risk of hospitalization or death from ischemic heart disease among British vegetarians and nonvegetarians: results from the EPIC-Oxford cohort study. *Am J Clin Nutr* 97(3):597-603.

Davis and Runyan. (2017). *Conquer Type 2 Diabetes With A Ketogenic Diet.* Gutsy Badger Publishing.

de Castro. (1987). Macronutrient relationships with meal patterns and mood in the spontaneous feeding behavior of humans. *Physiol Behav* 39(5):561-569.

de Castro and Elmore. (1988). Subjective hunger relationships with meal patterns in the spontaneous feeding behavior of humans: Evidence for a causal connection. *Physiol Behav* 43(2):159-165.

DeFronzo, Ferrannini, Groop, et al. (2015). Type 2 diabetes mellitus. *Nat Rev Dis Primers* 1:15019.

de Koning, Malik, Kellogg, et al. (2012). Sweetened beverage consumption, incident coronary heart disease and biomarkers of risk in men. *Circulation* 125:1735-1741.

Devries, Sithamparapillai, Brimble, et al. (2018). Changes in kidney function do not differ between healthy adults consuming higher- compared with lower- or normal-protein diets: a systematic review and meta-analysis. *J Nutrition* 148(11):1760–1775.

Diabetes UK website. https://www.diabetes.co.uk/

Diaz, Krupka, Chang, et al. (2015). Fitbit®: An accurate and reliable device for wireless physical activity tracking. *Int J Cardiol* 185:138-140.

DiNicolantonio, O'Keefe, and Lucan. (2015). Added fructose: a principal driver of type 2 diabetes mellitus and its consequences. *Mayo Clin Proc* 90(3):372-381.

Djoussé, Gaziano, Buring, and Lee. (2009). Egg consumption and risk of type 2 diabetes in men and women. *Diabetes Care* 32(2):295–300.

Doherty and Smith. (2005). Effects of caffeine ingestion on rating of perceived exertion during and after exercise: A meta-analysis. *Scand J Med Sci Sports* 15(2):69-78.

Dohm, Beeker, Israel, and Tapscott. (1986). Metabolic responses after fasting. *J Appl Physiol* 61(4):1363-1368.

Douglas, Hemila, Chalker, and Treacy. (2007). Vitamin C for preventing and treating the common cold. *Cochrane Database Syst Rev 18(3)*:CD000980.

Dulloo and Jacquet. (1998). Adaptive reduction in basal metabolic rate in response to food deprivation in humans: A role for feedback signals from fat stores. *Am J Clin Nutr* 68(3):599-606.

Durnin and Womersley. (1974). Body fat assessed from total body density and its estimation from skin fold thickness: Measurements on 481 men and women aged from 16 to 72 years. *Br J Nutr* 32(1):77-97.

Edwards, Margaria, and Dill. (1934). Metabolic rate, blood sugar and the utilization of carbohydrate. *Am J Physiol* 108:203-209.

Eshak, Iso, Kokubo, et al. (2012). Soft drink intake in relation to incident ischemic heart disease, stroke and stroke subtypes in Japanese men and women: The Japan Public Health Centre-based study cohort *Am J Clin Nutr* 96:1390-1397.

Esposito and Giugliano. (2014). Mediterranean diet and type 2 diabetes. *Diabetes Metab Res Rev* 30 Suppl 1:34-40.

European College of Sports Science (ECSS) website. https://www.sport-science.org

Evenson, Goto, and Furberg. (2015). Systematic review of the validity and reliability of consumer-wearable activity trackers. *Int J Behav Nutr Phys Act* 12:159.

Everyday Health website. https://www.everydayhealth.com/

Færch, Borch-Johnsen, Vaag, et al. (2010). Sex differences in glucose levels: a consequence of physiology or methodological convenience? The Inter99 study. *Diabetologia* 53: 858-865.

Fast Diet website. https://thefastdiet.co.uk/

Ferguson, Rowlands, Olds, and Maher. (2015). The validity of consumer-level, activity monitors in healthy adults worn in free-living conditions: A cross-sectional study. *Int J Behav Nutr Phys Act* 12:42.

Ferreira and Behnke. (2011). A toast to health and performance! Beetroot juice lowers blood pressure and the O_2 cost of exercise. *J Appl Physiol* 110(3):585-586.

Field, Byers, Hunter, et al. (1999). Weight cycling, weight gain and risk of hypertension in women. *Am J Epidemiol* 150(6):573-579.

Flatt. (1995). Use and storage of carbohydrate and fat. *Am J Clin Nutr* 61:952S-959

Fogelholm, Koskinen, and Laasko. (1993). Gradual and rapid weight loss: Effects on nutrition and performance in male athletes. *Med Sci Sports Exerc* 25:371-377.

Fontani, Corradeschi, Felici, et al. (2005). Cognitive and physiological effects of Omega-3 polyunsaturated fatty acid supplementation in healthy subjects. *Eur J Clin Invest* 35:691-699.

Food and Nutrition Board. (2005). *Dietary Reference Intakes for Energy, Carbohydrate, Fiber, Fat, Fatty Acids, Cholesterol, Protein and Amino Acids (Macronutrients).* Washington, DC: National Academies Press.

Forbes and Cooper. (2013). Mechanisms of diabetic complications. *Physiol Rev* 93(1):137-188.

Fung, Malik, Rexrode, et al. (2009). Sweetened beverage consumption and risk of coronary heart disease in women. *Am J Clin Nutr* 89(4):1037-1042.

Galbo. (1983). *Hormonal and Metabolic Adaptation to Exercise.* New York: Verlag.

GBD 2016 Alcohol Collaborators. (2018). Alcohol use and burden for 195 countries and territories, 1990–2016: a systematic analysis for the Global Burden of Disease Study 2016. *Lancet* 392(10152):1015-1035.

Gearhardt, Corbin, and Brownell. (2009). Preliminary validation of the Yale Food Addiction Scale. *Appetite* 52:430-436.

Gearhardt, White, Masheb, et al. (2012). An examination of the food addiction construct in obese patients with binge eating disorder. *Int J Eating Disorders* 45:657-663.

Geer EB and Shen W. (2009). Gender differences in insulin resistance, body composition, and energy balance. *Gend Med* 6 Suppl 1: 60-75.

Geleijnse, Launer, Van der Kuip, et al. (2002). Inverse association of tea and flavonoid intakes with incident myocardial infarction: The Rotterdam Study. *Am J Clin Nutr* 75(5):880-886.

Gibala and McGee. (2008). Metabolic adaptations to short-term high-intensity interval training: A little pain for a lot of gain? *Exerc Sport Sci Rev* 36(2):58-63.

Gibney, Macdonald, and Roche (Eds.). (2008). *Nutrition and Metabolism* (the Nutrition Society textbook). Oxford: Blackwell Science.

Gibson. (1996). Are high-fat, high-sugar foods and diets conducive to obesity? *Int J Food Sci Nutr* 47(5):405-415.

Gill and Panda. (2015). A smartphone app reveals erratic diurnal eating patterns in humans that can be modulated for health benefits. *Cell Metab* 22:789–798.

Girgis, Clifton-Bligh, Turner, et al. (2014). Effects of vitamin D in skeletal muscle: Falls, strength, athletic performance and insulin sensitivity. *Clin Endocrinol* 80:169-181.

Gleeson. (2013). Exercise, nutrition and immunity. In Calder and Yaqoob (Eds.), *Diet, Immunity and Inflammation*, pp. 652-685. Cambridge: Woodhead Publishing.

Gleeson. (2015). Effects of exercise on immune function. *Sports Sci Exch* 28(151):1-6.

Gleeson. (2016). Immunological aspects of sport nutrition. *Immunol Cell Biol* 94:117-123.

Gleeson. (2020). *Eat, Move, Sleep, Repeat.* Meyer and Meyer.

Gleeson, Bishop, Stensel, et al. (2011). The anti-inflammatory effects of exercise: Mechanisms and implications for the prevention and treatment of disease. *Nat Rev Immunol* 11:607-615.

Gleeson, Bishop, and Walsh. (Eds.). (2013). *Exercise Immunology.* Abingdon: Routledge.

Going, Massett, Hall, et al. (1993). Detection of small changes in body composition by dual-energy x-ray absorptiometry. *Am J Clin Nutr* 57(6):845-850.

GoodtoKnow website. https://www.goodtoknow.co.uk

Graudal, Galloe, and Garred. (1998). Effects of sodium restriction on blood pressure, renin, aldosterone, catecholamines, cholesterols and triglyceride: A meta-analysis. *JAMA* 279(17):1383-1391.

Hall, Moore, Harper, and Lynch. (2009). Global variability in fruit and vegetable consumption. *Am J Prev Med* 36(5):402-409.

Hall, Bemis, Brychta, et al. (2015). Calorie for calorie, dietary fat restriction results in more body fat loss than carbohydrate restriction in people with obesity. *Cell Metab* 22 (3):427-436.

Hall, Chen, Guo, et al. (2016). Energy expenditure and body composition changes after an isocaloric ketogenic diet in overweight and obese men. *Am J Clin Nutr* 104(2):324-333.

Hall and Guo. (2017). Obesity energetics: Body weight regulation and the effects of diet composition. *Gastroenterology* 152(7):1718-1727.

Halson. (2013). Nutritional interventions to enhance sleep. *Sports Sci Exch* 26(116):1-5.

Hamasaki. (2018). Interval exercise therapy for type 2 diabetes. *Curr Diabetes Rev*14(2):129-137.

Hamilton, Hamilton, and Zderic. (2014). Sedentary behavior as a mediator of type 2 diabetes. *Med Sport Sci* 60:11-26.

Hao, Lu, Dong, et al. (2011). Probiotics for preventing acute upper respiratory tract infections. *Cochrane Database Syst Rev* (September 7): CD006895.

Hargreaves. (1995). *Exercise Metabolism*. Champaign, IL: Human Kinetics.

Harper. (1999). Nutritional essentiality: Evolution of the concept. *Nutr Today* 36:216-222.

Harvard Health website. https://www.health.harvard.edu/topics/staying-healthy

Haskell, Lee, Pate, et al. (2007). Physical activity and public health: Updated recommendation for adults from the American College of Sports Medicine and the American Heart Association. *Med Sci Sports Exerc* 39:1423-1434.

Hawley, Burke, Phillips, and Spriet (2011). Nutritional modulation of training-induced skeletal muscle adaptations. *J Appl Physiol* 110:834-845.

Health website. https://www.health.com/

Healthline website. https://www.healthline.com/

HelpGuide website. https://www. helpguide.org/category-pages/healthy-living.htm

Hemmingsen, Gimenez-Perez, Mauricio, et al. (2017). Diet, physical activity or both for prevention or delay of type 2 diabetes mellitus and its associated complications in people at increased risk of developing type 2 diabetes mellitus. *Cochrane Database Syst Rev* 12:CD003054.

Henry, Lightowler, Stirk, et al. (2005). Glycaemic index and glycaemic load values of commercially available products in the UK. *Br J Nutr* 94:922-930.

Henson, Dunstan, Davies, and Yates. (2016). Sedentary behaviour as a new behavioural target in the prevention and treatment of type 2 diabetes. *Diabetes Metab Res Rev* 32 Suppl 1:213-220.

Hertog, Feskens, Hollman, and Katan. (1993). Dietary antioxidant flavonoids and risk of coronary heart disease: The Zutphen elderly study. *Lancet* 342:1007-1011.

Hickson. (2015). Nutritional interventions in sarcopenia: A critical review. *Proc Nutr Soc* 74(4):378-386.

Holloszy and Coyle. (1984). Adaptations of skeletal muscle to endurance exercise and their metabolic consequences. *J Appl Physiol* 56(4):831-838.

Hooper, Martin, Abdelhamid, and Davey Smith. (2015). Reduction in saturated fat intake for cardiovascular disease. *Cochrane Database Syst Rev* (June 10): CD011737.

Howatson, Bell, Tallent, et al. (2012). Effect of tart cherry juice (Prunus cerasus) on melatonin levels and enhanced sleep quality. *Eur J Nutr* 51(8):909-916.

Howell and Kones. (2017). "Calories in, calories out" and macronutrient intake: The hope, hype and science of calories. *Am J Physiol Endocrinol Metab* 313(5):E608-E612.

Hoy, Goldman, and Sebastian (2016). Fruit and vegetable intake of US adults estimated by two methods: What We Eat in America, National Health and Nutrition Examination Survey 2009-2012. *Public Health Nutr* 19(14):2508-2512.

Hoy and Goldman. (2014). Fiber Intake of the US Population: What We Eat in America, National Health and Nutrition Examination Survey 2009-2010. Food Surveys Research Group Dietary Data Brief No. 12. Available at https://www.ars.usda.gov/ARSUserFiles/80400530/pdf/DBrief/12_fiber_intake_0910.pdf

Hruby, Manson, Qi, et al. (2016). Determinants and consequences of obesity. *Am J Public Health* 106(9):1656-1662.

Hsu, Chen, and Sheu. (2015). Glycemic variability and diabetes retinopathy: a missing link. *J Diabetes Complications* 29(2):302-306.

Hu, Huang, Wang, et al. (2014). Fruits and vegetables consumption and risk of stroke: A meta-analysis of prospective cohort studies. *Stroke* 45(6):1613-1619.

Hubert, King, and Blundell. (1998). Uncoupling the effects of energy expenditure and energy intake: Appetite response to short-term energy deficit induced by meal omission and physical activity. *Appetite* 31:9-19.

Huxley, Barzi, and Woodward. (2006). Excess risk of fatal coronary heart disease associated with diabetes in men and women: meta-analysis of 37 prospective cohort studies. *Br Med J* 332:73-78.

International Diabetes Federation website: https://www.idf.org

International Federation of Sports Medicine (FIMS) website. https://www.fims.org

International Glycemic Index (GI) Database (Sydney University, Australia). https://researchdata. ands.org.au/international-glycemic-index-gi-database/11115 and https://www. glycemicindex.com/foodSearch.php

International Society of Exercise and Immunology (ISEI) website. https://www.isei.dk

Jackson and Pollock. (1978). Generalized equations for predicting body density of men. *Br J Nutr* 40(3):497-504.

Jeffery, Hellerstedt, French, and Baxter. (1995). A randomized trial of counseling for fat restriction versus calorie restriction in the treatment of obesity. *Int J Obes Relat Metab Disord* 19(2):132-137.

Jeppesen and Kiens. (2012). Regulation and limitations to fatty acid oxidation during exercise. *J Physiol* 590(5):1059-1068.

Jeukendrup. (2002). Regulation of skeletal muscle fat metabolism. *Ann N Y Acad Sci* 967:217-35.

Jeukendrup and Gleeson. (2018). *Sport Nutrition*. 3rd ed. Champaign, IL: Human Kinetics.

Johnstone. (2007). Fasting—The ultimate diet? *Obesity Rev* 8:211-222.

Kadowaki, Yamauchi, Kubota, et al. (2006). Adiponectin and adiponectin receptors in insulin resistance, diabetes, and the metabolic syndrome. *J Clin Invest* 116(7):1784-1792.

Kagan, Harris, Winkelstein, et al. (1974). Epidemiologic studies of coronary heart disease and stroke in Japanese men living in Japan, Hawaii and California: Demographic, physical, dietary and biochemical characteristics. *J Chronic Dis* 27(7-8):345-364.

Kaiser, Shikany, Keating, and Allison. (2013). Will reducing sugar sweetened beverage consumption reduce obesity? Evidence supporting conjecture is strong, but evidence when testing effect is weak. *Obes Rev* 14:620-633.

Keesey and Hirvonen. (1997). Body weight set-points: Determination and adjustment. *J Nutr* 127(9):1875S-1883S

Key, Appleby, Crowe et al. (2014). Cancer in British vegetarians: updated analyses of 4998 incident cancers in a cohort of 32,491 meat eaters, 8612 fish eaters, 18,298 vegetarians, and 2246 vegans. *Am J Clin Nutr* 100(Suppl 1):378S-385S.

Keys, Menotti, Karvonen, et al. (1986). The diet and 15-year death rate in the seven countries study. *Am J Epidemiol* 124(6):903-915.

King, Burley, and Blundell. (1994). Exercise-induced suppression of appetite: Effects on food intake and implications for energy balance. *Eur J Clin Nutr* 48(10):715-724.

King, Caudwell, Hopkins, et al. (2007). Metabolic and behavioral compensatory responses to exercise interventions: Barriers to weight loss. *Obesity* (Silver Spring) 15(6):1373–1383.

Kirwan, Sacks, and Nieuwoudt. (2017). The essential role of exercise in the management of type 2 diabetes. *Cleve Clin J Med* 84(7 Suppl 1):S15-S21.

Kit, Fakhouri, Park, et al. (2013). Trends in sugar-sweetened beverage consumption among youth and adults in the United States: 1999-2010. *Am J Clin Nutr* 98(1):180-188.

Kim, Lim, Choi, and Park HY. (2015). Hypertension is an independent risk factor for type 2 diabetes: the Korean genome and epidemiology study. *Hypertens Res* 38(11):783-789.

Kivimaki, Luukkonen, Batty, et al. (2017). Body mass index and risk of dementia: Analysis of individual-level data from 1.3 million individuals. *Alzheimer's and Dementia* 1-9.

Knapik, Meredith, Jones, et al. (1988). Influence of fasting on carbohydrate and fat metabolism during rest and exercise in men. *J Appl Physiol* 64(5):1923-1929.

Kodama, Saito, Tanaka, et al. (2012). Fasting and post-challenge glucose as quantitative cardiovascular risk factors: a meta-analysis. *J Atheroscler Thromb* 19(4):385-396.

Kodama, Tanaka, Heianza, et al. (2013). Association between physical activity and risk of all-cause mortality and cardiovascular disease in patients with diabetes: a meta-analysis. *Diabetes Care* 36(2):471-479.

Kohrt. (1995). Body composition by DXA: Tried and true? *Med Sci Sports Exerc* 27(10):1349-1353.

Kolbs. and Martin. (2017). Environmental/lifestyle factors in the pathogenesis and prevention of type 2 diabetes. *BMC Med* 15(1):131.

Laakso and Kuusisto. (2014). Insulin resistance and hyperglycaemia in cardiovascular disease development. *Nat Rev Endocrinol* 10(5):293-302.

Lanou and Barnard. (2008). Dairy and weight loss hypothesis: An evaluation of the clinical trials. *Nutr Rev* 66(5):272-279.

Lansley, Winyard, Fulford, et al. (2011). Dietary nitrate supplementation reduces the O_2 cost of walking and running: A placebo-controlled study. *J Appl Physiol* 110(3):591-600.

Larsen, Schiffer, Borniquel, et al. (2011). Dietary inorganic nitrate improves mitochondrial efficiency in humans. *Cell Metab* 13(2):149-159.

Layman and Walker. (2006). Potential importance of leucine in treatment of obesity and the metabolic syndrome. *J Nutr* 136(1 Suppl):319S-323S.

Lean, Leslie, Barnes, et al. (2018). Primary care-led weight management for remission of type 2 diabetes (DiRECT): an open-label, cluster-randomised trial. *Lancet* 391(10120):541-551.

Ledikwe, Blanck, Kettel Khan, et al. (2006). Dietary energy density is associated with energy intake and weight status in US adults. *Am J Clin Nutr* 83(6):1362-1368.

Leibel, Rosenbaum, and Hirsch. (1995). Changes in energy expenditure resulting from altered body weight. *N Engl J Med* 332(10):621-628.

Libianto and Ekinci. (2019). New agents for the treatment of type 2 diabetes. *Crit Care Clin* 35(2):315-328.

Lichtenstein. (2014). Dietary trans fatty acids and cardiovascular disease risk: Past and present. *Curr Atheroscler Rep* 16(8):433.

Lichtenstein, Ausman, Jalbert, and Schaefer. (1999). Effects of different forms of dietary hydrogenated fats on serum lipoprotein cholesterol levels. *N Engl J Med* 340(25):1933-1940.

Lim, Hollingsworth, Aribisala, et al. (2011). Reversal of type 2 diabetes: normalisation of beta cell function in association with decreased pancreas and liver triacylglycerol. *Diabetologia* 54(10):2506-2514.

Lin, Rexrode, Hu, et al. (2007). Dietary intakes of flavonols and flavones and coronary heart disease in US women. *Am J Epidemiol* 165(11):1305-1313.

Linde, Barrett, Wolkart, et al. (2006). Echinacea for preventing and treating the common cold. *Cochrane Database Syst Rev* CD000530.

Liu, Liu, Huang, et al. (2017). Dietary total flavonoids intake and risk of mortality from all causes and cardiovascular disease in the general population: A systematic review and meta-analysis of cohort studies. *Mol Nutr Food Res* 61(6).

Logue, Walker, Colhoun, et al. (2011). Do men develop type 2 diabetes at lower body mass indices than women? Diabetologia 54: 3003-3006.

Longo and Panda. (2016). Fasting, circadian rhythms, and time restricted feeding in healthy lifespan. Cell Metab 23:1048–1059.

Ma, Wang, and Li. (2015). Insulin resistance and cognitive dysfunction. *Clin Chim Acta* 444:18-23.

Malik, Pan, Willett, and Hu. (2013). Sugar-sweetened beverages and weight gain in children and adults: a systematic review and meta-analysis. *Am J Clin Nutr* 98:1084-1102.

Malik, Schulze, and Hu. (2006). Intake of sugar-sweetened beverages and weight gain: A systematic review. *Am J Clin Nutr* 84:274-288.

Mann and Truswell. (2002). *Essentials of Human Nutrition*. Oxford: Oxford University Press.

Martin, Heilbronn, de Jonge, et al. (2007). Effect of calorie restriction on resting metabolic rate and spontaneous physical activity. *Obesity (Silver Spring)* 15(12):2964-2973.

Matthews, Ockene, Freedson, et al. (2002). Moderate to vigorous physical activity and the risk of upper-respiratory tract infection. *Med Sci Sports Exerc* 34:1242-1248.

Maughan and Gleeson. (2010). *The Biochemical Basis of Sports Performance.* 2nd ed. Oxford: Oxford University Press.

Maughan, Gleeson, and Greenhaff. (1997). *Biochemistry of Exercise and Training.* Oxford: Oxford University Press.

Mayo Clinic website. https://www.mayoclinic.org/

McMurray, Ben-Ezra, Forsythe, and Smith. (1985). Responses of endurance-trained subjects to caloric deficits induced by diet or exercise. *Med Sci Sports Exerc* 17(5):574-579.

Medical News Today website. https://www.medicalnewstoday.com/

MedicineNet website. https://www.medicinenet.com/

MedlinePlus website. https://medlineplus.gov/

Melkani and Panda. (2017). Time-restricted feeding for prevention and treatment of cardiometabolic disorders. *J Physiol* 595(12):3691-3700.

Meneton, Jeunemaitre, de Wardener, and MacGregor. (2005). Links between dietary salt intake, renal salt handling, blood pressure, and cardiovascular diseases. *Physiol Rev* 85:679-715.

Mengheri. (2008). Health, probiotics and inflammation. *J Clin Gastroenterol* 42(2):S177-S178.

Mental Health Foundation website. https://www.mentalhealth.org.uk/

Mikkelsen, Toubro, and Astrup. (2000). Effect of fat-reduced diets on 24-h energy expenditure: Comparisons between animal protein, vegetable protein and carbohydrate. *Am J Clin Nutr* 72(5):1135-1141.

Moore, Churchward-Venne, Witard, et al. (2015). Protein ingestion to stimulate myofibrillar protein synthesis requires greater relative protein intakes in healthy older versus younger men. *J Gerontol Ser A Biol Sci Med Sci* 70:57-62.

Moseley. (2012). Type 2 diabetes and bone fractures. *Curr Opin Endocrinol Diabetes Obes* 19(2):128-135.

Mosley. (2015). *The 8-week Blood Sugar Diet*. London, UK: Short Books.

Mosley. (2019). *The Fast 800. How To Combine Rapid Weight Loss And Intermittent Fasting For Long-Term Health*. London, UK: Short Books.

Mosley and Spencer. (2014). *The Fast Diet: Lose Weight, Stay Healthy, Live Longer*. New York: Atria Books.

Muoio and Newgard. (2008). Mechanisms of disease: Molecular and metabolic mechanisms of insulin resistance and beta-cell failure in type 2 diabetes. *Nat Rev Mol Cell Biol* 9(3):193-205.

Mursu, Voutilainen, Nurmi, et al. (2008). Flavonoid intake and the risk of ischaemic stroke and CVD mortality in middle-aged Finnish men: The Kuopio Ischaemic Heart Disease Risk Factor Study. *Br J Nutr* 100(4):890-895.

My Fitness Pal website. https://www.myfitnesspal.com/

National Cancer Institute website. https://www.cancer.gov/

National Health Service (NHS) UK 111 Online website. https://111.nhs.uk/

National Health Service (NHS) UK Conditions website. https://www.nhs.uk/conditions/

National Health Service (NHS) UK Weight loss plan. https://www.nhs.uk/live-well/healthy-weight/start-the-nhs-weight loss-plan/

National Institute for Health Care and Excellence UK website. https://www.nice.org.uk/

National Institutes of Diabetes and Digestive and Kidney Diseases (NIDDK) website. https://www.niddk.nih.gov/

National Institutes of Health (NIH) USA website. https://www.nih.gov/

National Kidney Foundation website. https://www.kidney.org/

National Osteoporosis Foundation website. https://www.nof.org/

National Sleep Foundation website. https://sleepfoundation.org/

Nieman. (1994). Exercise, infection and immunity. *Int J Sports Med* 15(Suppl 3):S131-S141.

Nieman, Henson, Austin, and Sha. (2011). Upper respiratory tract infection is reduced in physically fit and active adults. *Br J Sports Med* 45:987-992.

Nitzke, Freeland-Graves, and American Dietetic Association. (2007). Position of the American Dietetic Association: Total diet approach to communicating food and nutrition information. *J Am Dietetic Assoc* 107(7):1224-32.

Noakes and Windt. (2017). Evidence that supports the prescription of low-carbohydrate high-fat diets: A narrative review. *Br J Sports Med* 51(2):133-139.

Noerman, Kärkkäinen, Mattsson, et al. (2019). Metabolic profiling of high egg consumption and the associated lower risk of type 2 diabetes in middle-aged Finnish men. *Mol Nutr Food Res* 63(5):e1800605.

Nolan, Damm, and Prentki. (2011). Type 2 diabetes across generations: from pathophysiology to prevention and management. *Lancet* 378(9786):169-181.

Nutrition Society website. https://www.nutritionsociety.org

Office On Women's Health website. https://www.womenshealth.gov/

Olefsky and Glass. (2010). Macrophages, inflammation, and insulin resistance. *Annu Rev Physiol* 72:219-246.

Olsen and Heitmann. (2009). Intake of calorically sweetened beverages and obesity. *Obes Rev* 10:68-75.

Oral Health Foundation website. https://www.dentalhealth.org/

Paffenbarger, Hyde, Wing, and Hsieh. (1986). Physical activity, all-cause mortality, and longevity of college alumni. *N Engl J Med* 314:605–613.

Pandey, Chawla, and Guchhait. (2015). Type-2 diabetes: Current understanding and future perspectives. *IUBMB Life* 67(7):506-513.

Pedersen and Febbraio. (2008). Muscle as an endocrine organ: Focus on muscle-derived interleukin-6. *Physiol Rev* 88:1379-1406.

Pendergast, Horvath, Leddy, and Venkatraman. (1996). The role of dietary fat on performance, metabolism and health. *Am J Sports Med* 24(6):S53-S58.

Perry and Wang. (2012). Appetite regulation and weight control: The role of gut hormones. *Nutr Diabetes* 2(1):e26.

Perry, Heigenhauser, Bonen, and Spriet. (2008). High-intensity aerobic interval training increases fat and carbohydrate metabolic capacities in human skeletal muscle. *Appl Physiol Nutr Metab* 33(6):1112-1123.

Perusse and Bouchard. (2000). Gene-diet interactions in obesity. *Am J Clin Nutr* 72(5 Suppl):1285S-1290.

Petersen and Shulman. (2017). Roles of diacylglycerols and ceramides in hepatic insulin resistance. *Trends Pharmacol Sci* 38(7):649-665.

Phillips. (2011). The science of muscle hypertrophy: Making dietary protein count. *Proc Nutr Soc* 70:100-103.

Phillips. (2015). Nutritional supplements in support of resistance exercise to counter age-related sarcopenia. *Adv Nutr* 6(4):452-460.

Phillips. (2016). Optimising the person-centred management of type 2 diabetes. *Br J Nurs* 25(10):535-538.

Phinney, Horton, Sims, et al. (1980). Capacity for moderate exercise in obese subjects after adaptation to a hypocaloric, ketogenic diet. *J Clin Invest* 66:1152-1161.

Physiological Society website. https://www.physoc.org

Polivy and Herman. (1995). Dieting and its relation to eating disorders. In Brownell and Fairburn (Eds.), *Eating Disorders and Obesity: A Comprehensive Handbook*, pp. 83-86. London: Guildford Press.

Poppitt and Prentice. (1996). Energy density and its role in the control of food intake: Evidence from metabolic and community studies. *Appetite* 26(2):153-174.

Pories, Swanson, MacDonald, et al. (1995). Who would have thought it? An operation proves to be the most effective therapy for adult-onset diabetes mellitus. *Ann Surg* 222(3):339-350.

Prietl, Treiber, Pieber, and Amrein. (2013). Vitamin D and immune function. *Nutrients* 5(7):2502-2521.

Public Health England. Composition of foods integrated dataset (CoFID). https://www.gov.uk/government/publications/composition-of-foods-integrated-dataset-cofid

PubMed website. https://www.ncbi.nlm.nih.gov/pubmed/

QuickStats. (2017). Percentage of total daily kilocalories consumed from sugar-sweetened beverages among children and adults, by sex and income level: National Health and Nutrition Examination Survey, United States, 2011-2014. *MMWR Morb Mortal Wkly Rep* 66(6):181.

Rachek. (2014). Free fatty acids and skeletal muscle insulin resistance. *Prog Mol Biol Transl Sci* 121:267-292.

Rankinen, Perusse, Weisnagel, et al. (2002). The human obesity gene map: The 2001 update. *Obes Res* 10(3):196-243.

Ren, Semenkovich, Gulve, et al. (1994). Exercise induces rapid increases in GLUT4 expression, glucose transport capacity and insulin-stimulated glycogen storage in muscle. *J Biol Chem* 269(20):14396-14401.

Rennie. (2005). Body maintenance and repair: How food and exercise keep the musculoskeletal system in good shape. *Exp Physiol* 90:427-436.

Rimm, Katan, Ascherio, et al. (1996). Relation between intake of flavonoids and risk for coronary heart disease in male health professionals. *Ann Intern Med* 125(5):384-389.

Rippe and Angelopoulos. (2016). Sugars, obesity and cardiovascular disease: Results from recent randomized control trials. *Eur J Nutr* 55(Suppl 2):45-53.

Robertson, Kato, Rhoads, et al. (1977). Epidemiologic studies of coronary heart disease and stroke in Japanese men living in Japan, Hawaii and California: Incidence of myocardial infarction and death from coronary heart disease. *Am J Cardiol* 39(2):239-243.

Romeo, Warnberg, Nova, et al. (2007). Moderate alcohol consumption and the immune system. A review. *Br J Nut* 98(1):S111-S116.

Royal National Institute of Blind People (RNIB) website. https://www.rnib.org.uk/

Royal Society of Biology website. https://www.rsb.org.uk/

Rugg-Gunn. (2013). Dental caries: Strategies to control this preventable disease. *Acta Med Acad* 42(2):117-130.

Sami, Ansari, Butt, and Hamid. (2017). Effect of diet on type 2 diabetes mellitus: A review. *Int J Health Sci (Qassim)* 11(2):65-71.

Schlundt, Hill, Pope-Cordle, et al. (1993). Randomized evaluation of a low-fat ad libitum carbohydrate diet for weight reduction. *Int J Obes Relat Metab Disord* 17(11):623-629.

Schoenfeld, Aragon, and Krieger. (2013). The effect of protein timing on muscle strength and hypertrophy: A meta-analysis. *J Int Soc Sports Nutr* 10:53.

Schofield and Sutherland. (2012). Disordered insulin secretion in the development of insulin resistance and Type 2 diabetes. *Diabet Med* 29(8):972-979.

Schulte, Avena, and Gearhardt. (2015). Which foods may be addictive? The roles of processing, fat content, and glycemic load. *PLoS One* 10(2):e0117959.

Schwingshackl, Hoffmann, Lampousi, et al. (2017). Food groups and risk of type 2 diabetes mellitus: a systematic review and meta-analysis of prospective studies. *Eur J Epidemiol* 32(5):363-375.

Scott, de Courten, and Ebeling. (2016). Sarcopenia: a potential cause and consequence of type 2 diabetes in Australia's ageing population? *Med J Aust* 205(7):329-333.

Sears. (1995). *The Zone: A Dietary Road Map*. New York: Harper Collins.

Seidelmann, Claggett, Cheng, et al. (2018). Dietary carbohydrate intake and mortality: a prospective cohort study and meta-analysis. *Lancet Public Health* 3(9):e419-e428.

SELF Nutrition Data website. https://nutritiondata.self.com/

Senate Select Committee on Nutrition and Human Needs. (1977). *Dietary Goals for the United States*. Washington, DC: US Government Printing Office.

Shan, Ma, Xie, et al. (2015). Sleep duration and risk of type 2 diabetes: a meta-analysis of prospective studies. *Diabetes Care* 38(3):529-537.

Shaw (2019). *Conquer Type 2 Diabetes: How A Fat, Middle-Aged Man Lost 31 Kilos And Reversed His Type 2 Diabetes*. London: Hammersmith.

Sheppard, Kristal, and Kushi. (1991). Weight loss in women participating in a randomized trial of low-fat diets. *Am J Clin Nutr* 54(5):821-828.

Shils, Olson, Shike, et al. (Eds.). (2005). *Modern Nutrition in Health and Disease*. Baltimore: Williams and Wilkins.

Skeaff and Miller. (2009). Dietary fat and coronary heart disease: Summary of evidence from prospective cohort and randomised controlled trials. *Ann Nutr Metab* 55(1-3):173-201.

Slyper. (2013). The influence of carbohydrate quality on cardiovascular disease, the metabolic syndrome, type 2 diabetes and obesity: An overview. *J Pediatr Endocrinol Metab* 26(7-8):617-629.

Sport2Health website. https://www.sport2health.com

Stackpool, Porcari, Mikat, et al. (2014). The accuracy of various activity trackers in estimating steps taken and energy expenditure. *J Fitness Res* 3:32-48.

Steven and Taylor. (2015). Restoring normoglycaemia by use of a very low calorie diet in long- and short-duration Type 2 diabetes. *Diabet Med* 32(9):1149-1155.

Stubbs, Harbron, and Prentice. (1996). Covert manipulation of the dietary fat to carbohydrate ratio of isoenergetically dense diets: Effect on food intake in feeding men ad libitum. *Int J Obes Relat Metab Disord* 20(7):651-660.

Stubbs, Ritz, Coward, and Prentice. (1995). Covert manipulation of the ratio of dietary fat to carbohydrate and energy density: Effect on food intake and energy balance in free-living men eating ad libitum. *Am J Clin Nutr* 62(2):330-337.

Symons, Sheffield-Moore, Wolfe, and Paddon-Jones. (2009). A moderate serving of high-quality protein maximally stimulates skeletal muscle protein synthesis in young and elderly subjects. *J Am Diet Assoc* 109:1582-1586.

Tamez, Virtanen, and Lajous. (2016). Egg consumption and risk of incident type 2 diabetes: a dose-response meta-analysis of prospective cohort studies. *Br J Nutr* 115(12):2212-2218.

Tappy. (1996). Thermic effect of food and sympathetic nervous system activity in humans. *Reprod Nutr Dev* 36(4):391-397.

Tappy and Lê. (2010). Metabolic effects of fructose and the worldwide increase in obesity. *Physiol Rev* 90(1):23-46.

Tappy and Lê. (2015). Health effects of fructose and fructose-containing caloric sweeteners: Where do we stand 10 years after the initial whistle blowings? *Curr Diab Rep* 15(8):54.

Taylor (2013). Type 2 diabetes: etiology and reversibility. *Diabetes Care* 36(4):1047-1055.

Te Morenga, Mallard, and Mann. (2013). Dietary sugars and body weight: Systematic review and meta-analysis of randomized controlled trials and cohort studies. *BMJ* 346:e7492.

Thorning, Raben, Tholstrup, et al. (2016). Milk and dairy products: Good or bad for human health? An assessment of the totality of scientific evidence. *Food Nutr Res* 60:32527.

Thrasher (2017). Pharmacologic management of type 2 diabetes mellitus: available therapies. *Am J Med* 130(6S):S4-S17.

Threapleton, Greenwood, Evans, et al. (2013). Dietary fibre intake and risk of cardiovascular disease: Systematic review and meta-analysis. *BMJ* 347:f6879.

Tippett and Cleveland (Eds.). (1999). How current diets stack up: Comparison with dietary guidelines. *Agriculture Information Bulletin* 750:51-70.

Trapp, Chisholm, Freund, and Boutcher. (2008). The effects of high-intensity intermittent exercise training on fat loss and fasting insulin levels of young women. *Int J Obesity* 32(4):684-691.

Tudor-Locke, Han, Aguiar, et al. (2018). How fast is fast enough? Walking cadence (steps/min) as a practical estimate of intensity in adults: a narrative review. *Br J Sports Med* 52:776–788.

UK Food Standards Agency. (2013). *Food Hygiene: A Guide For Businesses*. © Crown Copyright 2013. Available at https://www.food.gov.uk/business-guidance/food-hygiene-for-your-business

UK Food Standards Agency website. https://www.food.gov.uk/

UK Government Dietary Recommendations. (2016). Government dietary recommendations: The Eatwell Guide. https://www.gov.uk/government/publications/the-eatwell-guide

UK Food Standards Agency website. https://www.food.gov.uk/business-industry/food-hygiene

UK National Diet and Nutrition Survey Rolling Programme for 2008/2009 to 2011/2012. (2014). https://www.gov.uk/government/collections/national-diet-and-nutrition-survey

UK National Diet and Nutrition Survey Rolling Programme for 2012/2013 to 2013/2014. (2016). https://www.gov.uk/government/uploads/system/uploads/attachment_data/file/551352/NDNS_Y5_6_UK_Main_Text.pdf

UK National Nutrient Database. Composition of foods integrated dataset (CoFID). https://www. gov.uk/government/publications/composition-of-foods-integrated-dataset-cofid

US Centers for Disease Control and Prevention website. http://www.cdc.gov/

US Department of Agriculture. (2000). *Dietary Guidelines for Americans, 2000.* https://www. health.gov/dietaryguidelines/dga2000/document

US Department of Agriculture. Agricultural Research Service. USDA Food Composition Databases website. https://ndb.nal.usda.gov/ndb/search/list

US Department of Agriculture. (2005). *Dietary Guidelines for Americans, 2005.* https://www. health.gov/dietaryguidelines

US Department of Agriculture. (2015). *2015-2020 Dietary Guidelines for Americans.* https:// health.gov/dietaryguidelines/2015/guidelines

US Department of Agriculture Food Composition and Branded Food Products Databases. https:// ndb.nal.usda.gov/ndb/search/list

US Food and Drug Administration Food website. https://www.fda.gov/food

US Food and Drug Administration website. https://www.fda.gov/Food/default.htm

US National Diabetes Education Program (NDEP) website. https://www.cdc.gov/diabetes/ ndep/index.html

US National Institute of Diabetes and Digestive and Kidney Diseases (NIDDK) website. https:// www.niddk.nih.gov/health-information/diabetes

Valenti, Bugianesi, Pajvani, and Targher. (2016). Nonalcoholic fatty liver disease: cause or consequence of type 2 diabetes? *Liver Int* 36(11):1563-1579.

van Greevenbroek, Schalkwijk, and Stehouwer. (2013). Obesity-associated low-grade inflammation in type 2 diabetes mellitus: causes and consequences. *Neth J Med* 71(4):174-187.

Virtanen, Mursu, Tuomainen, et al. (2015). Egg consumption and risk of incident type 2 diabetes in men: the Kuopio ischaemic heart disease risk factor study. *Am J Clin Nutr* 101(5):1088-1096.

Walsh, Gleeson, Pyne, et al. (2011). Position statement part two: Maintaining immune health. *Exerc Immunol Rev* 17:64-103.

Walsh, Gleeson, Shephard, et al. (2011). Position statement part one: Immune function and exercise. *Exerc Immunol Rev* 17:6-63.

Wang, Han, and Hu. (2017). Fasting insulin, insulin resistance and risk of hypertension in the general population: A meta-analysis. *Clin Chim Acta* 464:57-63.

Wannamethee, Papacosta, Lawlor, et al. (2012). Do women exhibit greater differences in established and novel risk factors between diabetes and non-diabetes than men? The British Regional Heart Study and British Women's Heart Health Study. *Diabetologia* 55: 80-87.

Web MD website. https://www.webmd.com/

Weck, Bornstein, and Blüher. (2012). Strategies for successful weight reduction: Focus on energy balance. *Dtsch Med Wochenschr* 137:2223-2228.

Weigle, Breen, Matthys, et al. (2005). A high-protein diet induces sustained reductions in appetite, ad libitum caloric intake and body weight despite compensatory changes in diurnal plasma leptin and ghrelin concentrations. *Am J Clin Nutr* 82(1):41-48.

Westerterp. (2013). Metabolic adaptations to over-and-underfeeding: Still a matter of debate? *Eur J Clin Nutr* 67:443-445.

Westerterp, Donkers, Fredrix, and Boekhoudt. (1995). Energy intake, physical activity and body weight: A simulation model. *Br J Nutr* 73:337-347.

Weyers, Mazzetti, Love, et al. (2002). Comparison of methods for assessing body composition changes during weight loss. *Med Sci Sports Exerc* 34(3):497-502.

WHO. (2015). *Guideline: Sugars Intake for Adults and Children*. Geneva: WHO Press.

WHO. (2015). Healthy Diet Factsheet. https://www.who.int/mediacentre/factsheets/fs394/en

Wicks. (2015). *Lean in 15*. London: Bluebird.

Willems, van den Heuvel, Schoemaker, et al. (2017). Diet and exercise: a match made in bone. *Curr Osteoporos Rep* 15:555–563.

Willett. (2000). Diet and cancer. *Oncologist* 5:393-404.

Women's Health website. https://www.womenshealthmag.com/

Wu, Ding, Tanaka, and Zhang. (2014). Risk factors contributing to type 2 diabetes and recent advances in the treatment and prevention. *Int J Med Sci* 11(11):1185-1200.

Wynne, Stanley, McGowann, and Bloom. (2005). Appetite control. *J Endocrinol* 184:291-318.

Yin, Jin, Shan, et al. (2017). Relationship of sleep duration with all-cause mortality and cardiovascular events: a systematic review and dose-response meta-analysis of prospective cohort studies. *J Am Heart Assoc* 6(9): e005947.

Zemel, Richards, Mathis, et al. (2005). Dairy augmentation of total and central fat loss in obese subjects. *Int J Obes (Lond)* 29(4):391-397.

Zheng, Ley, and Hu. (2018). Global aetiology and epidemiology of type 2 diabetes mellitus and its complications. *Nat Rev Endocrinol* 14(2):88-98.

Zone Diet website. https://www.zonediet.com/the-zone-diet/

About the Author

Michael Gleeson is Emeritus Professor at Loughborough University, UK. He retired in 2016. He was previously Professor of Exercise Biochemistry in the School of Sport, Exercise and Health Sciences of Loughborough University. His first degree was in Biochemistry at the University of Birmingham, graduating in 1976. His PhD research was carried out at the University of Central Lancashire in collaboration with Queen's College, London and concerned the effects of diet and exercise training on energy metabolism. He carried out postdoctoral research in exercise physiology and metabolism at Salford University for three years, and this was followed by three years as a temporary lecturer at the University of Edinburgh. He conducted further research on diet–exercise interactions as a senior research fellow at the University of Aberdeen for three years, and then joined Coventry University as a senior lecturer in 1987.

He moved to the University of Birmingham in 1996 where he progressed from senior lecturer to professor in the School of Sport and Exercise Sciences, being awarded a personal chair in exercise biochemistry in 1999. He joined Loughborough University's School of Sport, Exercise and Health Sciences in 2002. Loughborough is renowned for its excellence in sport and sport science. His main research interests have been in the metabolic responses to exercise, sports nutrition, and the effects of acute and chronic exercise on the function of the immune system. He was the physiology section editor for the *Journal of Sports Sciences* and an associate editor of *Exercise Immunology Review*.

He has published over 200 research papers in scientific and medical journals, contributed chapters to over 30 books, and has co-authored textbooks entitled *Biochemistry of Exercise and Training* (Oxford University Press 1997), *The Biochemical Basis of Sports Performance* (Oxford University Press 2004 and 2010), *Sport Nutrition* (Human Kinetics 2004, 2010, and 2019), *Immune Function in Sport and Exercise* (Elsevier 2006), and *Exercise Immunology* (Routledge 2013). He is a Fellow of the British Association of Sport and Exercise Sciences (BASES) and the European College of Sport Science (ECSS), as well as a past president of The International Society of Exercise and Immunology (ISEI). He has taught thousands of BSc sport science students, hundreds of MSc exercise physiology and sport nutrition students, and supervised 17 PhD students.

He has featured in several national radio and TV programs in the UK, and his research has attracted interest from local, national, and international media. He is still an active science writer, and in the past few years has contributed to international expert consensus reviews sponsored by the IOC (training load and illness, 2016), ISEI (immuno-nutrition, 2017), and UEFA (nutrition in football, 2019), as well as completing the third edition of his popular book *Sport Nutrition* (Human Kinetics 2019) which he coauthors with Professor Asker Jeukendrup, and his first solo book *Eat, Move, Sleep, Repeat* (Meyer and Meyer 2020).

Credits

Cover design: Falcon Oast Graphic Art Ltd.

Interior design: Katerina Georgieva

Layout: Zerosoft

Figures: © Mike Gleeson, unless otherwise noted

Photos: © AdobeStock, unless otherwise noted

Managing editor: Elizabeth Evans

Copyeditor: sarahcomms@btinternet.com